The Woman Who Walked into the Sea

The Woman Who Walked into the Sea

Huntington's and the Making of a Genetic Disease

Alice Wexler

Yale University Press
New Haven & London

Set in Electra and Trajan type by Tseng Information Systems, Inc.

Printed in the United States of America by Sheridan Books, Ann Arbor, Michigan

Library of Congress Cataloging-in-Publication Data
Wexler, Alice, 1942–
The woman who walked into the sea : Huntington's and the making of a genetic disease / Alice Wexler.
p. cm.
Includes bibliographical references and index.
ISBN 978-0-300-10502-5 (cloth : alk. paper) 1. Hedges, Phebe, 1764–1806. 2. Huntington, George, 1850–1916. 3. Muncey, E. B. 4. Huntington's chorea—New York (State)—History—19th century. 5. Huntington's chorea—New York (State)—History—20th century. I. Title. II. Title: Huntington's and the making of a genetic disease.
[DNLM: 1. Hedges, Phebe, 1764–1806. 2. Huntington, George, 1850–1916. 3. Muncey, E. B. 4. Eugenics—history—New York. 5. Huntington Disease—history—New York. 6. History, 19th Century—New York. 7. History, 20th Century—New York. WL 11 AN6 W545W 2008]
RC394.H85W52 2008
616.8′510097471—dc22
2008006389

A catalogue record for this book is available from the British Library.

The paper in this book meets the guidelines for permanence and durability of the Committee on Production Guidelines for Book Longevity of the Council on Library Resources.

10 9 8 7 6 5 4 3 2 1

For the memory of my father, Milton Wexler, 1908–2007

Why resurrect it all now. From the Past. History, the old wound. The past emotions all over again. To confess to relive the same folly. To name it now so as not to repeat history in oblivion. To extract each fragment by each fragment from the word from the image another word another image the reply that will not repeat history in oblivion.

—Theresa Hak Kyung Cha, *Dictee*

Contents

Foreword

Nancy S. Wexler

Alice Wexler brings a unique perspective to understanding the nineteenth-century families affected with what we today know as Huntington's disease (HD) and they called St. Vitus's dance or the magrums. Alice and I are their sisters. We watched our own mother be undone by Huntington's, which causes uncontrollable movements in all parts of the body, cognitive decline, and emotional distress. It is irrevocably fatal over ten to twenty years. It is also hereditary. Alice and I each have a 50–50 chance of inheriting it ourselves.

Alice's empathy with the families affected by St. Vitus's dance gives a novel slant to this tale. With new lenses, she reads the old newspaper articles, journals, wills, ledgers, photographs, and medical daybooks of the Huntington doctors from East Hampton as if translating the Rosetta stone. She understands the language of Huntington's disease and interprets it in her own DNA.

I was part of the team that in 1983 identified a genetic marker for Huntington's disease and in 1993 discovered the Huntington's gene. The gene is very near the top of chromosome 4. The Huntington's disease gene makes a protein called huntingtin. Everyone has this gene that makes the huntingtin protein. This gene always contains a sequence of repeated CAGs—base pairs of DNA that spell out the amino acid glutamine. What matters is the length of this sequence, or how many CAGs your gene contains. We found that an expanded sequence of CAGs is the essential molecular mistake in the gene. Too much glutamine in your huntingtin protein means you will eventually get the disease.

HD is called a dominant genetic disease. This means that each child of a parent with HD has a 50 percent chance of inheriting it. It also means that if you inherit the expanded gene and you live a normal life span, the disease will certainly appear. Usually the disease appears in your thirties or forties but it can manifest as early as two and occasionally, if you are lucky, as late as eighty-two.

From 1976 to 1978 I had the honor of serving as the executive director of the congressional Commission for the Control of Huntington's Disease and Its Consequences. This was a commission mandated by Congress to investigate the needs of families with Huntington's nationwide and to draw up policy and research proposals. It was a particular privilege to serve with two co-chairs who had intimate personal knowledge of this illness: Marjorie Guthrie, widow of the songwriter and singer Woody Guthrie, who died of HD in 1967, and my father, Milton Wexler, who started the Hereditary Disease Foundation after my mother was diagnosed with HD in 1968.

We held hearings in all parts of the country, where hundreds of people testified, mainly family members, who had never before been given a public voice. The urgency of their need and the power of their strength were overwhelming. What those hearings also made clear was the secrecy and shame that surrounded this disease, and the prejudice and hostility many families reported encountering, even from some health professionals. What the hearings did not reveal as clearly was the history behind these attitudes, especially the role of the eugenics movement, which Alice traces so succinctly in this book.

The story of Huntington's in East Hampton, Long Island, especially fascinates me because of my own experience doing research in very different communities where the disease has also existed for at least two hundred years. For more than twenty years I spent six weeks each year in two small Venezuelan communities along the shores of Lake Maracaibo. When we were working with the families in San Luis and Barranquitas, I would sometimes find myself thinking of George Huntington, who had grown up in East Hampton among the families he described in his classic paper, and who knew not only the individuals with St. Vitus's dance but also their siblings without it—a key factor, as Alice shows, in his analysis of its pattern of inheritance. It still amazes me that George Huntington and Gregor Mendel, the founding figure of modern genetics, were almost contemporaries, albeit on opposite sides of the globe, and that George Huntington delivered his classic paper "On Chorea" just six years after Mendel published his famous study of pea plants (in 1866), although Huntington knew nothing about it.

In San Luis and in Barranquitas we observed that the families affected by *San Vito,* as they call it, were treated by their neighbors within the community with a combination of acceptance and rejection. Outsiders, however, tended to stigmatize the entire community, in a kind of democracy of fear. The histories of East Hampton, on the one hand, and Barranquitas and San Luis, on the other, form a fascinating study in contrasts, and in the differential impact of an identical disease gene in distinct social and cultural circumstances.

It is tempting to think that the hero of this book is the town of East Hampton, because the families with St. Vitus's dance in the nineteenth century do not appear to have been ostracized or isolated, and some of them were leaders in the town. And yet, as Alice shows, the story is more complicated, because the same criteria that led to the acceptance of these specific families—descendants of the seventeenth-century English town founders—also to led the exclusion of others; indeed the insider/outsider status of the Huntington doctors themselves may have helped enable their special insights into the malady they observed in their neighbors.

But one conclusion seems unambiguous: our fate is not in our genes, irrevocable and inexorable as the illness may be. Whatever the size of our Huntington's disease gene—since we all have this gene—we are not defined by it. We and our genes are not identical. In our current era of romantic fascination with DNA, this fact alone is a source of hope. Alice's book gives us a mirror backward and a path forward to change our future.

Acknowledgments

First, I wish to thank my sister, Nancy Wexler, who brought her keen intelligence and deep knowledge of Huntington's and of science to multiple readings of this manuscript. Her encouragement and comradeship were a great gift throughout the research and writing of this book. I am also immensely grateful to the descendants of George Huntington, whom I had the pleasure of meeting at an early stage of this project. They graciously gave me access to the medical daybooks, school notebooks, family memoirs, diaries, and photographs in their possession, sharing my enthusiasm for their famous forebear. I am indebted to Jean K. Lominska, Elizabeth Lominska Johnson, Charles Gardiner Huntington 3rd, the late Doris Huntington, Susan Lominska Mills, and Bob Lominska for their generosity and interest throughout this project, and for wonderful conversations over tea in Pasadena, at the Huntington Library (no relation).

The many people who smiled when I said I was traveling to East Hampton for "research," did not know about the wonderful Pennypacker Long Island Collection at the East Hampton Library, a treasure trove of archival materials. When I first visited in 1997, the library was undergoing renovation, and most of the archives were "under plastic." Nonetheless, the former archivist and town historian, Dorothy King, at great inconvenience to herself, immediately brought out the materials I was looking for, and she continued to do so for all the years of this project. It was Dorothy who introduced me to the riches of the Long Island Collection and generously shared her deep knowledge of the town. I am also grateful to Averill Dayton Geus, whose intimate understanding of East Hampton history helped inform my own. The "town crier" Hugh King educated me about many dimensions of local history, as did the late Carleton Kelsey over cups of tea. Diana Dayton, who succeeded Dorothy King as head of the Long Island Collection, cheerfully tolerated endless requests for manuscripts, while Marci Vail, who followed next, located photographs with an expert eye. Many other East Hampton and Amagansett residents also shared their memories and facilitated access to East Hampton's past. I especially wish to thank the Reverend John Ames and Barbara Borschart of the First Presbyterian Church for making available the Sessions Records; Ethan Bassford and Clarence Bennett; Anne Collins for access to the whaling log of Joseph Redfield, who sailed with Hiram B. Hedges aboard the *Monmouth;* Elizabeth Davis, Kathy and David McHugh, Shirley Payne and Tony Prohaska, and Martha Kalser of the East Hampton Oral History Project; Helen Rattray, Ann Roberts, Peggy Sherrill, the Reverend Robert Stuart of the Amagansett Presbyterian Church; the late Edward Welles; and Irene Silverman and Fred Yardley. Sheila and Jim Dunlop always made me feel at home in their home.

Over the years of researching and writing this book, I have had the pleasure and privilege of learning from colleagues and friends in several communities whose distinct perspectives on science, medicine, disability, and illness pushed me to think about Huntington's disease in multiple conceptual frames. Moshe Sluhovsky and Emily Abel brought their historical acumen and sharp insights to the whole manuscript at a crucial stage and offered invaluable criticisms and suggestions throughout. I am also immensely grateful to Cornelia Dayton for sharing her understanding of early American culture, for her critical readings of several chapters, and for her hospitality. Diane Paul's deep knowledge of eugenics, in all its manifestations, and her many trenchant readings helped me grasp that "normal people thought like" that when I resisted this essential insight. I have also learned much from conversations with Ellen Dwyer, Elizabeth Lord, Sandra Harding, Deborah Heath, Howard Kushner, Maria Lepowsky, Philippa Levine, Kaori Muto, Yoshio Nukaga, Jenny Price, Rickie Solinger, and Sharon Traweek, whose work as philosophers, anthropologists, sociologists, and biologists as well as historians challenged me to think more deeply about the social and cultural contexts of bodies, in sickness and in health. Robert Rosenstone's experimental approach to historical narrative has been a continuing stimulus, while Ellen DuBois, Alice Echols, Marla Stone, and Lois Banner have inspired me as committed scholars as well as generous colleagues and friends. Victoria Lewis, Mary Felstiner, Felicity Nussbaum, and the late Miriam Silverberg pushed me to think about Huntington's in terms of disability as well as disease. Wendy Belcher, Janet Brodie, Mary Bush, Sharla Fett, Ellen Krout-Hasegawa, Kathleen McHugh, Harryette Mullen, Lynn Sacco, and Devra Weber—distinguished writers and cherished members of my reading and writing groups—read and reread chapters and parts of chapters, gave supportive criticism, made suggestions, and reminded me of the pleasures of writing when I could no longer remember. And I doubt I could have finished without Ellen Krout-Hasegawa's critical enthusiasm and affection, Doris Baizley's playwright's eyes and ears, and Devra Weber's historian's acumen.

While researching Huntington's in the past, I have learned much from members of the HD community about how present-day social contexts shape the meanings of living as part of a family affected by this disease. In this regard I am especially grateful to Christiane Lohkamp, for her wisdom, her courage, and her generosity. Thanks also to the many scientists and clinicians with whom I discussed Huntington's disease in the present. In particular I thank Gillian Bates, Marie-Françoise Chesselet, Arthur Golding, David Housman, Carl Johnson, Edward Kravitz, Bernhard Landwehrmeyer, Richard Mulligan, Michael Rawlins, Leslie Thompson, and Anne B. Young, who patiently answered questions and helped me appreciate the thinking of contemporary scientists and doctors, and the challenges of biomedicine today. Michael Rawlins also generously read the entire manuscript at a late date, asked pertinent questions, and saved me from some medical mistakes. I am deeply grateful to all, not only for their intellectual inspiration, but also for their healing actions at a difficult personal time.

Many librarians and archivists have helped locate materials over the years. I wish to thank Beth Horrocks, formerly of the American Philosophical Society Library; Clare Clark at the Archives of the Cold Spring Harbor Laboratory; Suzan Habib at the John Jermain Memorial Library at Sag Harbor; Ann M. Gill and Samuel Scott of the Whaling Museum at Cold Spring Harbor; Michael Dyer of the Kendall Whaling Museum; James D. Folts of the New York State Archives; Susan Richardson at the Greenwich (Conn.) Historical Society; Toby A. Appel of the Cushing/Whitney Medical Library at Yale University; Katherine E. S. Donahue, Russell A. Johnson, and Teresa G. Johnson at the History and Special Collections of the Louise M. Darling Medical Library of UCLA; Caroline Duroselle-Melish of the New York Academy of Medicine; Nava Hall at College of Physicians of Philadelphia; and Linda Krell of the Connecticut Valley Hospital. Thanks also to archivists at the Huntington Library, the Manuscript Division of the Library of Congress, the New York Hospital Cornell Medical Center Archives, the Countway Medical Library at Harvard University, the New York Public Library, the New York Genealogical Society, the Wood Library of the College of Physicians of Philadelphia, the New England Biographical and Genealogical Society Library, the Connecticut State Library, the Connecticut Historical Society, the New Bedford Whaling Museum, and the Rhode Island Historical Society. At an early stage, Wayne Tillinghast helped unravel Long Island–Rhode Island connections. Jacqueline Jackson of the Hereditary Genomics Division of the Department of Medical and Molecular Genetics, Indiana University School of Medicine, provided support for a reanalysis of Elizabeth Muncey's pedigrees.

The UCLA Center for the Study of Women has been an important academic home and feminist community over the years of this project. I wish especially to thank Sandra Harding, the late Miriam Silverberg, Kathleen McHugh, and Van Nguyn for their support. I was fortunate to receive fellowships from the American Council of Learned Societies and the John Simon Guggenheim Memorial Foundation, as well as a Publication Grant from the National Library of Medicine. I also benefited greatly from the opportunity to present part of this research at a meeting in London on Diversity, Difference, and Deviance: Ethics in Human Biology, sponsored by the Society for the Study of Human Biology; in Tokyo, thanks to Yoshio Nukaga, at a conference on Empirical Bioethics in Cultural Context: Genetic Confidentiality, Ownership, and Public Participation in the United States and Japan; and at meetings of the American Association for the History of Medicine and as part of the Medical Classics series at UCLA. Part of this book appeared, in a different form, in the *Bulletin of the History of Medicine*, vol. 76 (Fall 2002).

It has been a joy and privilege, for more than twenty years, to work with Frances Goldin, mentor, friend, and risk-taker. Sydelle Kramer has also guided this book through the pitfalls of publication, untying knots of all sorts with consummate skill. I am grateful also to everyone at Yale University Press for making this book happen, especially to Chris Rogers and Laura Davulis for their patience and commitment, to James J. Johnson for his keen eye, and to Dan Heaton for his expertise, elegance, and good humor in a process that for me remains mind-boggling and arcane. My deep appreciation also to Vija Celmins, for allowing me to use her luminous ocean drawing of 1970 for the cover.

My father, Milton Wexler, followed the progress of this book with unflagging enthusiasm, but he did not live to see it completed. Without his love, strength, insight, and sense of humor, I doubt whether I could have faced the challenge of Huntington's in our family, nor would research on this illness have made such significant advances. His grace and determination as he approached his ninety-ninth year provided a model to me of how to live a rich full life in the face of disability. He once said that he would like a few of his ashes scattered in the Palisades park rose garden near his home, a place he loved, so that when my sister or I faced a difficult problem we might go there to think and get comfort from his presence. I write these lines among the roses, and dedicate this book to him.

INTRODUCTION

In the seaside town of East Hampton, New York, at the far eastern end of Long Island, in a cemetery shadowed by an old windmill, a simple slate gravestone marks the life and death of Stafford Hedges, son of a woman named Phebe Hedges, who walked into the sea and drowned on a summer night in 1806. A few blocks away on East Hampton's Main Street stands an old house facing south, where a family of physicians called the Huntingtons lived and practiced medicine for almost the entire course of the nineteenth century, counting among their patients some like Stafford Hedges, and his mother and grandmother and daughter as well, all of whom died with the illness they called St. Vitus's dance, later known as Huntington's chorea, and after that Huntington's disease. It was named after George Huntington, youngest of three generations of Huntington doctors, who in 1872, at the age of twenty-one, described the dominant inheritance pattern of this illness in a classic paper based on families in this town. Though East Hampton today is known more for its celebrities than for its contributions to medical science, these traces of the past speak to a historical moment when families and physicians in this town invented new knowledge of heredity and illness, lived out in the contours of a devastating family disease.

What, then, is Huntington's disease? Clinicians today define Huntington's as both a neurological and a psychiatric disease, one that involves disturbances of movement, mind, and mood. It is one of the more common genetic disorders worldwide, reported in all racial and ethnic groups. In the United States some thirty thousand persons are affected, with another seventy-five thousand gene carriers who will someday develop the disease if they live long enough. The most dramatic symptom is the movement disorder: awkward, intrusive, involuntary movements of the body that make eating, walking, and talking increasingly difficult. Those affected develop an unsteady staggering gait that often gives the appearance of drunkenness; eventually they lose the ability to walk altogether. Speech grows mushy, with communication increasingly difficult. Eating becomes a major challenge, swallowing perilous. Personality changes and emotional disturbances may also develop, with apathy, irritability, and sometimes depression leading to suicide. Although most people remain aware of their surroundings, they develop cognitive changes, with impairment of judgment and memory leading sometimes in the end stages to dementia. Typically starting in the thirties or forties—although it can also begin much earlier or later—the disease progresses slowly but inexorably over a period of ten to twenty years. Especially devastating for affected families is the knowledge that this illness is hereditary (following a dominant pattern of inheritance), and that each child of an affected parent faces a 50 percent risk of developing the disease.[1]

In *Making Sense of Illness: Science, Society, and Disease,* the physician Robert Aronowitz argues that disease identity "is neither a necessary nor an inevitable consequence of biological processes, but rather is contingent on social factors. Knowing the details of a disease's particular social construction matters," he writes, "because it is only with such knowledge that we can make sense of disease, especially chronic disease."[2]

Aronowitz's point seems especially relevant to Huntington's as a disease that has long been known to be hereditary, and one that involves both physical and mental disability. Yet for all its heightened visibility over the past two decades, only a few authors have attempted to survey its history, almost all of them either geneticists or clinicians. To speak about Huntington's disease in the past, of course, immediately poses problems of definition. Even the terms are confusing. Chorea—meaning involuntary "dancelike" movements (from the Greek word for dance)—has been known to doctors at least since the sixteenth century. Physicians, using Latin, spoke of *Chorea Sancti Viti* while lay people adopted the literal translation. The name derived from the frenzied mass dancing in the aftermath of European plague epidemics in the fourteenth, fifteenth, and sixteenth centuries. Apart from these epidemics, sufferers from anxiety and malaise made annual June pilgrimages—June 15 being the saint's day—to the chapels of St. Vitus in towns such as Ulm, in present-day southern Germany, and Echternacht, in Luxembourg, where they danced and danced until their symptoms disappeared: the dance, in short, was both disease and cure.[3]

By the nineteenth century the popular term *St. Vitus's dance* circulated widely in the United States, Europe, and Latin America to describe a broad range of conditions, from temporary fidgets and nervous agitation to chronic states of involuntary and disabling movement. The most common sort of St. Vitus's dance was a childhood disease (technically known as Sydenham's chorea) that usually went away on its own. People also spoke of St. Vitus's dance in certain families where it did not go away, however, and where it primarily affected the adults. In parts of New England and New York people referred also to "the migrims" or "the magrums"—a term similar to an old dialect word used in the northern English county of Lancashire, meaning "in a state of temper or rage."[4]

Physicians, as we shall see, did not define "hereditary chorea" as a single disease entity until the mid-nineteenth century. And yet their testimony, along with accounts from letters, newspapers, and other sources, makes clear that ordinary folks in certain communities had long recognized St. Vitus's dance and the magrums as a distinct illness, affecting the same families as those in whom the doctors later diagnosed hereditary or Huntington's chorea. In this book I will use *St. Vitus's dance* or *magrums* when speaking of popular usage, *hereditary* or *Huntington's chorea* when referring to medical discourse from 1872 to about 1972, and *Huntington's disease* for the period following, when clinicians and family members decided that since chorea was only one of the many symptoms of this malady, it should not be privileged in the name.

This book had its origins in a sociological quest. While writing an earlier autobiographical book about Huntington's disease, *Mapping Fate: A Memoir of Family, Risk, and Genetic Research*, I became eager to learn more about the earliest North American families to be associated with this disorder—my biosocial if not my biological ancestors—and how they lived in their communities. My mother, grandfather, and maternal uncles had all died with this disease, and I was well acquainted with the stigma and silences surrounding it in the late twentieth century. But I wanted to know whether it had always been this way, or whether in the past this illness—and those affected by it—may have been viewed differently. As a historian, I had learned to see disability and disease as socially as well as biologically constructed, and as conditions whose meaning could change over time and across place. I had also learned the importance of the "patient perspective," as many new social histories of medicine termed it, and of viewing medicine from the point of view of the sufferer. Indeed, as a feminist, but also as a member of a family affected by Huntington's, I wanted to begin my story from the perspective of the sufferers rather than with a portrait of George Huntington, as so many of the texts on Huntington's disease began. I was impressed by Nora Groce's landmark 1985 study, *Everyone Here Spoke Sign Language*, showing that hereditary deafness on Martha's Vineyard, an island off the coast of Massachusetts, was not a handicap and that the deaf were wholly integrated into the local society at a time, in the eighteenth and nineteenth centuries, when deaf people on the mainland were severely stigmatized. If deafness was regarded so differently on Martha's Vineyard in the eighteenth and nineteenth centuries, could individuals and families affected by St. Vitus's dance/Huntington's chorea also have been viewed distinctly?[5]

What especially piqued my curiosity were the claims of a psychiatrist named Percy R. Vessie in Stamford, Connecticut, who had published a pair of influential papers in the 1930s that are cited even today. In tracing the ancestry of one of his own patients with Huntington's, Vessie identified a group of colonial settlers in the New Haven colony (in present-day Connecticut) whom he described as scoundrels, outcasts, and suspected witches—individuals whose allegedly antisocial behavior revealed them to be possible progenitors of the disease. He portrayed their descendants as mean and greedy people who were ostracized and shunned by their neighbors, down to the present, as "living examples of sin." What especially disturbed me was that Vessie wrote almost as if these men and women deserved the hostility they provoked. He seemed to blame them for bringing the disease to America. Moreover, when I consulted local histories and archives in the towns where these families lived, I found the same men and women portrayed as relatively typical English settlers and even, in some cases, prominent as leaders, wealthy landowners, and literate respected women and wives.[6]

Why were these portrayals so different, I wondered. Did local historians omit disturbing truths, or did Vessie project twentieth-century assumptions onto a seventeenth-century past? I had hoped to trace some of the men and women in Vessie's narrative using a historical ethnographic approach to explore their social experience in early Stamford and Greenwich, Connecticut. Lack of evidence precluded this project, however, and I decided to look elsewhere. George Huntington's hometown, East Hampton, Long Island, proved much more fruitful in terms of archival and other sorts of records. Here doctors and patients lived together in a small community, and here George Huntington made his observations on a few affected families. Here his father and grandfather practiced medicine, and their patients were the ones whom he described. Here other physicians too, such as Edward Osborn and Elizabeth B. Muncey, made observations and recorded their views.

Famous as a glamorous vacation spot, the town of East Hampton has a rich history going back to the mid-seventeenth century, when English Puritans settled there and, along with men and women of African and Indian origins, created a farming and fishing community with strong ties to New England. Most important, the East Hampton Library has the superb Pennypacker Long

Island Collection, with a wealth of local materials such as diaries, letters, wills, tax lists, censuses, whaling logs, ledgers, account books, and local newspapers, testifying to the lives of ordinary people in this town. The East Hampton families with St. Vitus's dance in the nineteenth century included prominent and not-so-prominent individuals, whose lives I could trace through several generations. Judging by the local offices they held, the people they married, the roles they played in church, the places they lived, they appeared to be full members of the community, or, as one local historian called herself, "one of ours."[7]

Investigating this history was not straightforward. The written evidence alluding to the disease was fragmentary, elusive. There were no extant diaries or letters written by a sufferer or close relative of one. Moreover, an inherited illness that is stigmatized today, especially in relation to employment and insurance, presents obstacles to an interviewer in small-town settings where the privacy and confidentiality of the families must be the highest priority. I did not want to stir up talk about who did or did not have this disease, especially since I was studying not only those actually affected in the nineteenth century—a relatively small number of people—but also certain of their siblings, ancestors, and descendants. Indeed, when I visited East Hampton in the late 1990s, some descendants of those who were patients of the Huntington doctors did not know about St. Vitus's dance among their ancestors: the disease had disappeared in their families, and the memory of it as well.

Fortunately, local historians sensitive to the situation provided me with valuable contacts. I was able to talk to members of affected families, who generously shared their memories and histories with me. They wanted to have the story told. Initially I had planned to change the names of the families, although no one in this history is still living and most have been deceased for more than a century. Yet after talking to many members of these families as well as professional colleagues, I decided against changing the names of people who had lived in the eighteenth and nineteenth centuries, especially since part of my aim was to honor the historical presence of these individual lives. Most of these names had already appeared in print in early medical papers on Huntington's chorea or in a newspaper; others appeared in letters readily available in libraries and archives, or could be inferred (through the diagnosis of a son or daughter). Moreover there is no relation between the names of persons from the affected families in this book and the names of persons and families affected today. Although medical confidentiality is a critical value, I believe there is a fine line between protecting confidentiality and perpetuating secrecy and shame. One local historian put it this way: "My suggestions to you (for what they are worth) are to keep the names, keep the town intact, and don't change anything. This disease should not be a shameful thing . . . and it may help future historians to understand our people and happenings in greater depth." The descendants and relatives with whom I spoke all supported the decision to use real names.[8]

Overcoming shame was, in fact, another incentive for writing this book. My mother had always been very secretive about Huntington's disease in her father's family. Although he had died of this illness in 1929, when she was fifteen, she never mentioned it to my sister and me until after her own diagnosis in 1968, when we were both in our twenties. This sudden revelation of the family secret came as a shock, and I felt angry at her failure to inform us earlier. Yet as I worked on this book, I came to understand that the decades when my mother had come of age, the 1920s and 1930s, were also some of the most influential years of that scientific and social movement called eugenics—the crusade that, in the United States, sought to "improve" the human race by preventing the births of those deemed "unfit" and encouraging the "fittest" to reproduce. I wanted, then, to place the experience of families like mine into the social context of eugenics, while also viewing eugenics through the lens of Huntington's disease.[9]

Starting from the premise that disease cannot be understood apart from its social and historical contexts, this book differs from other historical accounts of Huntington's disease in several respects. First, it begins from the perspective of the patient and family rather than from that of the physicians, emphasizing the social experience of families prior to the definition of "Huntington's chorea" as a distinct clinical entity. It also looks at the social experience of the early doctors who helped define this disease, since they came from the same communities as the people whose lives they described—as observers they occupied the same space as the observed. Third, this book places Huntington's chorea within the context of the cultural history of heredity, including the eugenics movement of the late nineteenth and early twentieth centuries, a context that is often missing in medical histories of this disease.

Within this frame, I make several arguments here. First, I argue that the social experience of families with the magrums, St. Vitus's dance, and Huntington's chorea differed considerably across communities, shaped by distinct local cultures and histories as well as by variations in the expression of the disease. While families in some towns may have been marginalized and ostracized, in others they were accepted and respected, their members prominent figures in town and church affairs; the disease was not central to their identity.

I also suggest that hereditary chorea emerged as a discrete clinical entity in the early nineteenth century not because of increases in life expectancy, as some have argued, but because of social, cultural, and medical changes that led physicians to reconfigure the symptoms around the concept of heredity. Most important, the earliest accounts of magrums and hereditary chorea, in the 1830s and 1840s, coincided with the emergence of what the historians Hans-Jörg Rheinberger and Staffan Müller-Wille have called a new "epistemic" or conceptual space of biological heredity.[10] In the context of new botanical gardens, natural history museums, hospitals, breeders' societies, genealogical practices, zoos, and chemical and physical laboratories, biological heredity moved to the forefront of an array of social and scientific concerns. Still, it was not until the 1880s, with the consolidation of neurology as a medical specialty and increasingly pessimistic notions of degeneration and decline in society, that "Huntington's chorea" became an "interesting" and significant disease.

Finally, I argue that to understand the lived experience of Huntington's chorea after 1900, it is essential that we situate it within the context of eugenics. Although eugenics, as we shall see, did not create the stigma that surrounded this disease in the twentieth century, eugenics helped to intensify the secrecy and silences associated with this malady throughout the modern era. Moreover, viewing North American eugenics through the lens of Huntington's extends the interpretation of a number of scholars that hereditarian ideology and practices persisted long after the end of World War II. I argue here that, in the United States at least, the most hostile representations of people with Huntington's chorea in the medical literature surfaced in the 1930s, 1940s, and 1950s rather than in the decades before.

Several caveats are in order here. Because of the fragmentary nature of the historical sources relevant to the everyday practices surrounding St. Vitus's dance/Huntington's chorea, many aspects of this study must remain speculative. Mentions of this illness are few and far between, in private as well as public papers. But while I cannot make claims based on the abundance of evidence I would have liked, I have tried to wrest meanings from the available traces with the conviction that even limited historical evidence can illuminate important dimensions of this disease. Indeed, I hope that placing St. Vitus's dance/Huntington's chorea in its social and historical contexts will illuminate the stakes involved, for different stakeholders, in the making and living of this disease.

Some may wonder why I draw on the testimony of a eugenics worker, Dr. Elizabeth Muncey—the fieldworker employed at the Eugenics Record Office by Charles Davenport, the leading North American eugenicist—when we know that most of the eugenic studies of the early twentieth century were scientifically worthless. Part of my project in this book is to read Muncey's testimony against the grain, and to listen to her subjects' voices and emotions within the text of her field notes. While her diagnoses of Huntington's may have been medically unreliable, even by the standards of her time, Muncey was nonetheless a trained clinician, and her clinical skills at times transcended the eugenic framework of her assignment; her notes include narrative testimony that occasionally allows the voices of her subjects to emerge.

I also wish to note that while I have organized this book into separate sections in order to highlight three different types of discourse—the popular discourse of people in several communities, the formal medical discourse of doctors, and both the scientific and popular discourse of the supporters of eugenics—this separation is artificial, as all these domains interconnect. Illuminating these interconnections is another of my aims in this book.

Finally, I apologize for the primarily North American orientation of this history. Although one of the myths about Huntington's disease is that nothing was known about it before 1993, or before 1977, depending upon whom you read, in fact the medical literature on this malady was considerable by the early twentieth century. Focusing primarily on English-language sources and on the United States side of the story, this book represents a partial history, an intervention into a global subject that I hope others will want to continue.[11]

Family/Community

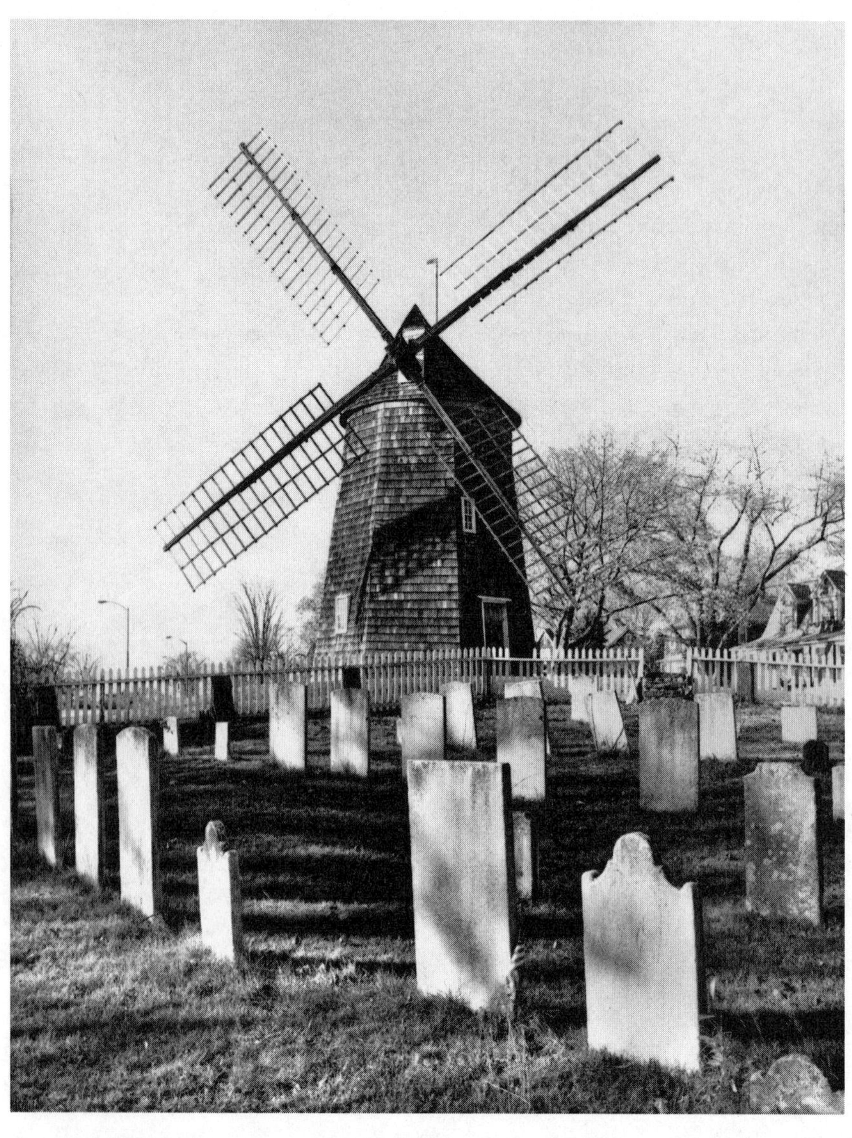

Hook Mill in East Hampton, viewed from the North End Burying Ground.
Library of Congress, Prints and Photographs Division, Historic
American Engineering Record, HAER no. NY 105

1

THE DEATH OF PHEBE HEDGES

> It has become our duty to publish the following melancholy circumstance, which took place at Easthampton a few weeks since:—Capt. David Hedges returned to his home in the evening, and found Mrs. Hedges ironing clothes, and apparently in health—he retired to bed and left her at that employment, but on awaking in the morning she was not to be found. After considerable search and enquiry, her footsteps were traced from the house thro' fields of grain to the shore; and there is every reason to believe she has precipitated herself into the surf which washes the south shore. Mrs. Hedges was about 40 years of age, and was much esteemed by her neighbors. This extraordinary step is attributed to her extreme dread of the disorder called St. Vitus' dance, with which she began to be affected, and which her mother now has to a great degree. From some arrangements of her clothing it appears she had for some time contemplated her melancholy end.
>
> —The *Suffolk Gazette* (East Hampton, New York), June 30, 1806

In the year of her birth, 1764, a revival swept the town, the people—mainly the young people—gathering day after day in the house of the minister, the Reverend Samuel Buell, and "making the most mournful declarations of their exceeding sinfulness before God." The great English preacher George Whitefield had traveled all through New England and New York that year, stirring up revivals everywhere he went, including East Hampton, this triracial farming and fishing town founded by Puritans at the eastern tip of Long Island, a region that had been home to the native Montauks for thousands of years. As news of the Lord's work flew around the town, the spirit of prayer seemed to pour forth in a celestial torrent, according to Buell, and throngs of new converts joined the church, though it appears her parents were not among them.[1]

And so Phebe Tillinghast began her life, with the cries of the sinners in her infant ears, the resistance of the patriot rebels at her back, and the protests of the much-diminished Montauk people rising against the danger "of being crowded out of all their ancient Inheritance, and of being rendered Vagabonds upon the Face of the earth."[2] She was the third child of seven born to the former Phebe Mulford, who traced her ancestry to several prominent East Hampton families. Phebe Mulford's mother, Anna Chatfield Mulford (who had died five years earlier at the age of fifty), was the daughter of a justice of the peace who later became a judge of the Court of Common Pleas for Suffolk County, a position of considerable prestige. Phebe's father, John Mulford, one of the few called "Esquire" in this vicinity, descended from a long line of respected figures, including one of the town founders and several judges and "gentlemen." He had suffered a great tragedy in his youth, when his father, mother, and four siblings had died within two months' time, probably of the "sweating sickness" that desolated several families in the winter of 1726–27, leaving fifteen-year-old John and two sisters orphaned. Nonetheless, the resilient John grew up to become, at the age of twenty-nine, a town trustee—one of twelve or so leaders who oversaw all town affairs—a post to which he was reelected almost yearly for the next twenty-three years.[3]

Showing her independent nature, the twenty-two-year-old Phebe Mulford had married, in 1761, a man "from away," a young mariner named Joseph Tillinghast from a prominent family of distillers in the town of Newport, Rhode Island. Later, Rhode Island came to figure in several legends about how St. Vitus's dance came to East Hampton. Some said the malady began as a curse on those who had persecuted Roger Williams, the founder of the Rhode Island colony. Others traced it to an unnamed Rhode Island family with five daughters who supposedly married into five East Hampton families. On the other hand, Judge Henry P. Hedges (a distant relation of Phebe Hedges), who was born in East Hampton in 1817 and wrote a history of the town, was told as a young man that the disease was introduced by "the intermarriage of an Easthampton Mulford with a Howell woman from Southampton"—a description that fit Phebe Mulford's paternal grandparents—although whether this story was true no one really knew.[4]

East Hampton in the late eighteenth century was less a compact settlement than a collection of scattered villages and hamlets—Amagansett, Springs, and Freetown among others—counting about 1,250 white people and some 67 "Negroe" slaves who lived in the homes of the white people. There were about 34 Montauk Indian families, too. Some of these were also servants, and others lived on the outskirts of the villages, their numbers much reduced by disease and depression of the spirit since the English had begun encroaching on their lands one hundred years earlier. In the village of East Hampton—the "capital" of East Hampton town—several hundred people lived within hearing of the old church bell, the plain unpainted houses of the gentry lined up along a wide, muddy Main Street, their home lots stretching out behind the houses, for they all planted crops to feed their families, no matter what else they did as well. They had all been whalers for a few decades back in the seventeenth century, some forming small companies—a practice known as "the whale design"—to catch the whales that swam off the Atlantic coast, until the whales no longer appeared close to shore and their pursuers had to go farther afield, and whaling became a global industry. But the whale design produced a more stratified town in which some families, like that of Phebe Mulford, were distinctly wealthier than others.[5]

Besides whaling, farming, and fishing, they raised cattle and other livestock. "The people are more properly Graziers than farmers," wrote the local historian David Gardiner, author of a series of newspaper essays in the 1840s that were later published as the *Chronicles of Easthampton*; "they raise large droves of cattle and sheep for sale; but very little [else] except flaxseed and cord wood." During the late eighteenth and early nineteenth centuries residents of East Hampton lived lives closely attuned to the rhythms of an animate nature and the uncertainties of divine Providence. They still valued "trade and commerce" as "in general a benefit to mankind," though the far-reaching relations with Boston, London, and the West Indies that had begun soon after the town's settlement appear to have diminished by this time. Some among them had begun to question the old Calvinist religious orthodoxies about the inherent sinfulness of men and women and the importance of deference to God's inscrutable will. These "farmers and mechanics of a bolder tone of mind" were exploring the new secular Enlightenment thought—the ideas of Thomas Paine, Voltaire, and Thomas Jefferson—what the orthodox young preacher Lyman Beecher would later call "French infidelity" and try to stamp out with his Morals Society. Like many white inhabitants of New York—the northern colony with highest percentage and greatest number of African slaves—some here remained slaveholders. At the start of the Revolution in 1776, thirty-five East Hampton households had at least one slave, including the elder Phebe's father and the local minister, who each owned three.[6]

Young Phebe Tillinghast was twelve on that harrowing September day in 1776, just after British forces defeated Washington's armies at the Battle of Long Island and the patriot government urged white women and children and their slaves to flee. She boarded a sloop, most likely in Sag Harbor, along with her mother, father, four siblings (nine-month-old Henry had died the previous May), several

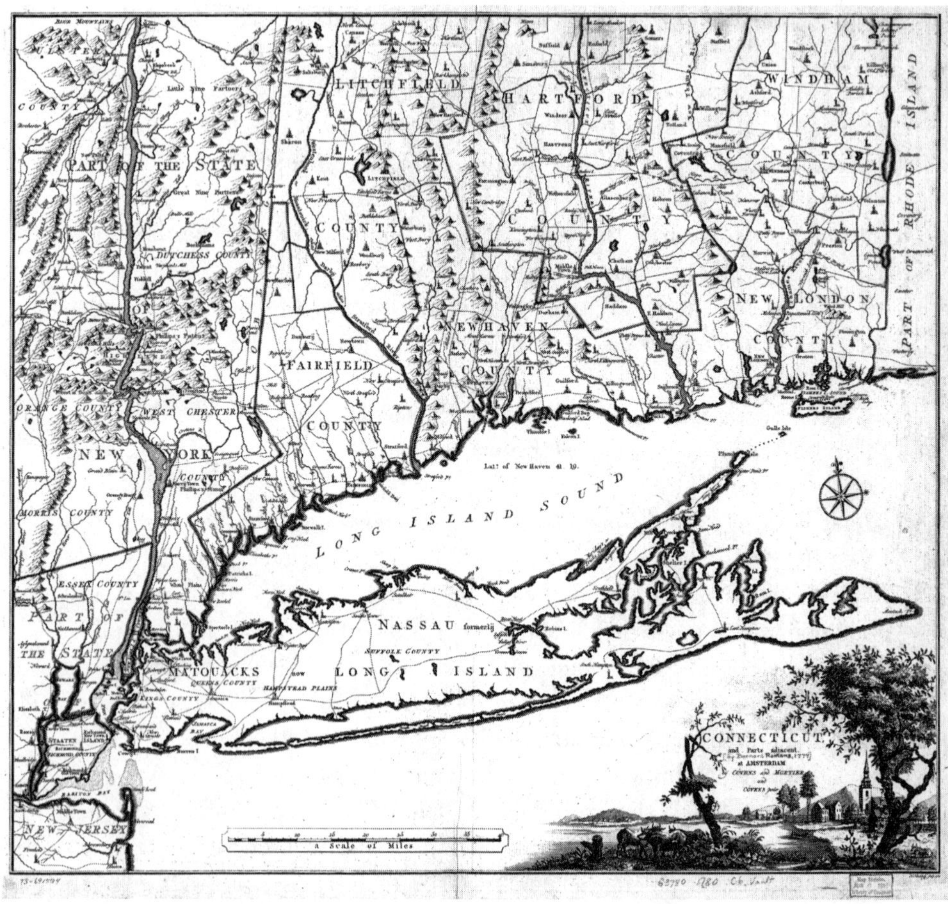

H. Klockhoff and B. Romans, "Connecticut and Parts Adjacent" (Amsterdam: Covens and Mortier and Covens Jr., 1780) Library of Congress, Geography and Map Division

loads of corn, three cows, and a horse. They traveled across Long Island Sound and up the Connecticut River to Haddam, where the family joined a community of refugees. As the British occupied all of Long Island, a third of the people of East Hampton left (apart from the young men who had already joined the patriot army)—those most unwilling to submit to British rule, those with fewer resources to protect, or simply those who had the means and mobility to leave. According to the elder Phebe, those who left valued "the peaceable Injoyment of our Liberties" over "our pleasant and Profitable Dwelling places." But dysentery, smallpox, and diphtheria raged in Connecticut in the early years of the Revolution. Joseph Tillinghast died in September 1777, leaving the younger Phebe and her siblings fatherless, and his thirty-eight-year-old widow pregnant and far from home, with five children and, soon, a new infant to feed.[7]

They held out in Haddam for nearly three more years. But by the spring of 1780 the elder Phebe was growing desperate. She and her friend Hannah Cooper, another war widow and Long Island refugee, petitioned the patriot government for permission to go home, including in their request the obligatory self-deprecation and expressions of humility. Finding themselves now "with the Care of a number of small Children to bring up in Each of our Families," and having "exhosted al that Treasure we brought over with us for our Supporte," the two women were "Redused to the Disagreeable Nessessety of Supplicating your Honours for Relief." They urged "your Honours to take our Pitiful Cases into your Wise Consideration and give Each of us The Liberty to Transport our Selves and Small Children" back home. They wished to carry in addition "two cows three swine our household stuff and Furniture with Sum provision for the present Support of our Families."[8]

Their petition granted within the month, the two Phebes, mother and daughter, traveled by sloop back across the Sound to Long Island, along with the other Tillinghast children, Hannah Cooper and her family, the cows, pigs, two barrels of fish, and six bushels of flour. They returned to a village with fields stripped bare and livestock much reduced by raids from both sides. Though the patriots were in the ascendant, the British fleet remained anchored in Gardiner's Bay, off the coast of East Hampton, the officers fraternizing with some of the residents at the widow Huntting's "publick house" (saloon) on Main Street. Under duress, those who had remained in East Hampton had all taken oaths of loyalty to the king, including the wily pastor, Samuel Buell, who maneuvered energetically between loyalists and patriots, so much so that some later accused him of Tory sympathies. The people here were more pragmatic than passionate. Henry Hedges defended his neighbors. "What should they do?" he asked in 1907. "Take the oath and live? Refuse, and die?"[9]

By the time the fighting ended, in 1783, East Hampton was impoverished and devastated, with a heavy burden of taxation to boot. As Henry Hedges described it, "Agriculture had declined; commerce had been ruined; estates swept away; and when the first thrilling, triumphant transports of a free, victorious people were over, they wept at the surrounding desolation." But in truth, not everyone here was free. The state of New York did not begin gradual emancipation of slaves until 1799, and slavery was not entirely outlawed until 1827. The institution persisted in Suffolk County, and in East Hampton, long after the Revolutionary war had ended.[10]

In 1785, in the midst of yet another of East Hampton's periodic revivals—this "outpouring of the divine spirit" as the Reverend Buell phrased it—the young Phebe Tillinghast, now twenty-one, married David Hedges, twenty-four, who also traced his ancestors to the town's English founders. David's mother, Mary Miller, was the daughter of a longtime member of the New York State Assembly who, like Phebe's grandfather, was called "Esquire." David's father, Stephen Hedges, was typical of the wealthy men in the town, the owner of extensive lands and several slaves. The Hedges family had played, and continued to play, a prominent role in the town, from the silversmith Colonel David Hedges Jr., to the shoemaking Hedges brothers, to the future judge Henry P. Hedges. Hedgeses were deacons, captains, and colonels. The men were town supervisors and whaling masters, and some of the women taught school. The Hedges men had a well-earned reputation for longevity. A number of them lived into their eighties and even nineties, a trait relevant to George Huntington's later characterization of "hereditary chorea," as we shall see.[11]

Phebe and David Hedges set up housekeeping in a section called "the Hook" at the north end of town, where their grandchildren later lived. In 1786 their first child was born, named Stafford after Joseph's Rhode Island Tillinghast relatives. Four years later Phebe gave birth to another son, christened Stephen after his paternal grandfather. In five years' time, a daughter, Betsy, joined the family, her name more evocative of the revolutionary generation than of family genealogy. But there were no more children that we know of, and the family remained atypically small, just three surviving children born over a period of eleven years, one approximately every four or five years, as opposed to the usual two or three.[12]

By the mid-1790s Phebe's husband had begun to hold local office, becoming part of the inner circle of men elected at the annual town meeting. Captain David Hedges, as he was called, served first as sheep and swine pounder (responsible for ensuring that sheep and swine stayed within the enclosure called a pound at night rather than roaming about town, destroying crops and fences), then as overseer of highways and tax assessor, and, most often, as a town trustee, elected at least every other year for the next decade. He may have been among those progressive local farmers drawn to Enlightenment thought—those whom Lyman Beecher called "infidels"—for his name appears often in the account books of the Clinton Academy, the center of liberal thought in East Hampton and one of the first public coeducational schools in New York. He owned no slaves.[13]

White women too may have joined the infidels, as old patterns of deference weakened and the wartime struggles of women without men led some of them to adopt a more independent and secular stance. But in rural East Hampton the lives of most women remained more constrained than those of the men, so much so that one female visitor considered East Hampton "a frog pond, without the music of it." As she wrote a friend in 1803, "Here we are so still, so quiet, so dull, so inactive, that we have forgotten . . . that there are wars, murders, and violence abroad in the earth; that there are society, and friendship, and intercourse, and social affection, and science, and pleasure, and life, and spirit, and gayety, and good-humor, alive still among the sons of earth."[14]

When the twenty-one-year-old physician Abel Huntington—grandfather of the future George Huntington—came from his hometown of Norwich, Connecticut, to East Hampton in 1797 to take over the medical practice of the aging Dr. Ebenezer Sage, he noticed a peculiar malady that, as his grandson reported many years later, seemed "well established" in this town. Dr. Huntington had apprenticed with a noted physician, the Yale University graduate Dr. Philomen Tracy, scion of a prominent Norwich medical family, who was noted for his "patient and thorough investigation of chronic diseases" at a time when most people died of acute conditions. So it was perhaps his training with Dr. Tracy that led Abel Huntington to pay particular attention to this malady, St. Vitus's dance, which was nothing if not long and lingering.[15]

It is worth recalling that for lay people and the learned alike in late-eighteenth-century Anglo-America, diseases were not, for the most part, distinct, well-demarcated conditions. They tended to slide into one another, protean and dynamic, "a changed state of being affecting the whole" body rather than a specific response to a defined pathogen. With the exception of a few culturally resonant disorders such as small pox, physicians thought in terms not of specific diseases but of the individual suffering body and its special characteristics—for instance, whether it was overexcited or enfeebled, and whether the humours were out of balance. They relied on a handful of therapies such as bleeding and purging, and on a variety of powerful drugs. The eighteenth-century medicine in which Abel Huntington was trained treated symptoms rather than diseases, regarding "fever" or "convulsions" or "agitation of the nerves" as disorders in themselves rather than as signs of an underlying pathology.[16]

Still, by 1797, St. Vitus's dance, or "chorea Sancti Viti," had existed in the literature of medicine and in popular discourse at least since the mid-sixteenth century, when the famous Basel physician known as Paracelsus used the Latin term to describe disorders of involuntary movement (including the so-called dancing manias of the fourteenth, fifteenth, and sixteenth centuries), which were almost always accompanied by mental distress. Robert Burton, author of *The Anatomy of Melancholy*, published in 1621, referred to "Chorus sancti Viti, or Saint Vitus dance," as one of the "Diseases of the Minde." Burton explained that the name—which referred, confusingly, to both the disease and the cure—arose because "the parties so troubled were wont to goe to Saint Vitus for helpe, & after they had danced there a while, they were certainly freed." By the late seventeenth century, the name was so much a part of popular discourse that the English physician Thomas Sydenham could write of "a certain kind of convulsion, which is called by the common people Chorea Sancti Viti." Sydenham referred to the frightening but self-limiting childhood disease that often followed rheumatic fever (or "rheumatism," as it was called), but the symptoms he described in 1696 were those of chorea more generally:

> He that is affected with this Disease, can by no means keep his hand in the same Posture for one Moment, if it be brought to the Breast or any other part, but it will be distorted to another position or Place by a certain Convulsion, let the Patient do what he can. If a Cup of Drink be put into his Hand, he represents a thousand Gestures, like Juglers, before he brings it to his Mouth; for whereas he cannot carry it to his Mouth in a Rightline, his hand being drawn hither and thither by the Convulsion, he turns it often about for some time, till at length happily reaching his Lips, he flings it suddenly into his Mouth, and drinks it greedily, as if the poor Wretch designed only to make sport.[17]

Thereafter the childhood disease became known to physicians as Sydenham's chorea or chorea minor, while laypeople still commonly referred to St. Vitus's dance. This name shows up in the daybooks and diaries of early New England healers, such as the Maine midwife Martha Ballard, who in 1785 listed "St. Vitas daunce" among the maladies she knew how to treat. People in the late eighteenth and early nineteenth centuries used the term *St. Vitus's dance* broadly (as physicians used the term *chorea*) to describe a wide range of disordered movement, from ordinary fidgetiness and nervousness to tics, seizures, and other disturbances of motion, in adults as well as in children. Popular medical manuals such as the Edinburgh physician William Buchan's best-selling *Domestic Medicine,* first published in Edinburgh in 1769 and thereafter in many editions on both sides of the Atlantic, explained that St. Vitus's dance was not due to "the effects of witchcraft," as "the common people" were wont to believe. Rather, it was a nervous disorder closely allied with epilepsy and commonly ascribed to similar causes, including fright of the pregnant mother, blows to the head, worms or other intestinal disturbances, and "violent passions or affections of the mind." Nervous disorders generally, in Buchan's view, were characterized by "low spirits, timorousness, melancholy, and fickleness of temper," leading many people to believe wrongly that such disorders were "entirely diseases of the mind." In fact, according to Buchan, such maladies had physiological as well as psychological causes. Buchan considered that St. Vitus's dance was usually curable through "repeated bleedings and purges," along with appropriate drugs such as Peruvian bark, snakeroot, and chalybeate waters, a popular mineral tonic.[18]

No notes of Abel Huntington on chorea have survived, so we do not know precisely how he conceived of St. Vitus's dance in East Hampton, or whether residents had used that name before his arrival in 1797. But Edward Osborn, a local physician from an old East Hampton family, writing in the late nineteenth century, affirmed that it had been present in the community for two hundred years, handed down in families from the early settlers. Evidence also indicates that a "deep-seated popular belief in the hereditary nature of the disease" was circulating in other New York towns by the 1860s, suggesting that such beliefs had arisen long before. Certainly Abel Huntington's generation, lay and learned alike, believed that hereditary influences played a role in many disorders, such as consumption, gout, epilepsy, syphilis, and especially "insanity," which since antiquity had been thought to run in families.[19]

In the seventeenth and eighteenth centuries, nervous disorders deemed hereditary were likely to be considered especially resistant to cure, although this theory was subject to debate. Nicolas Culpepper's popular *Complete Family Physician*, which first appeared in 1652 and was often reprinted, advised that "all species and degrees of madness which are hereditary . . . are very likely to be incurable." Similarly, the influential New England preacher and physician Cotton Mather warned in his 1723 text *The Angel of Bethesda*, "If an Epilepsy, be Hereditary; or if it comes after Thirty years of Age; tis very hardly curable." Maladies that were inherited and incurable had serious consequences for marriage, for once a disease was "contracted and rivetted in the habit, it is entailed upon posterity." Even William Buchan considered "the gout, scurvy, or the king's evil" a "dreadful inheritance" to pass on to the next generation. How much better, he advised, for "the heir of many a great estate, had he been born a beggar, rather than to inherit his father's fortunes at the expence of inheriting his diseases!"[20]

Historians such as John Waller have claimed that fears of marrying into "hereditarily tainted families" were already well entrenched by the late eighteenth century, at least in England among the upper classes, and that "parents often sedulously examined the relatives of their children's suitors for evidence of chronic disease." On the other hand Buchan, perhaps referring to those outside the elite, found it "amazing" how little regard his late-eighteenth-century contemporaries paid to the health of prospective spouses and their parents, despite the wealth of warnings about the dangers of hereditary ills. What is certain is that members of families with a history of illness, especially mental illness, sometimes felt great anxiety on this account. In his 1812 classic *Medical Inquiries and Observations upon Diseases of the Mind*, the great Philadelphia physician Benjamin Rush told the story of an anguished American Revolutionary War officer who confided to a friend that he hoped "'he might not live to be old, that he might die suddenly, and that if he married, he might have no issue.'" According to Rush, the officer explained to his friend that "he was descended from a family in which madness had sometimes appeared about the fiftieth year of life." For this reason, "he did not wish to incur the chance of inheriting, and propagating it to a family of children." Here was a man who had reached a high position as a military officer, yet he was so haunted by the knowledge that he was heir to a family legacy of mental illness that he wished for—and received—an early death.[21]

It is important to note, however, that prevailing ideas about the meanings of heredity in the late eighteenth and early nineteenth centuries differed from conceptions that arose later on. For one thing, hereditary influences were more metaphoric than material. They were "soft" rather than "hard." They were anything you got from your parents, whether biological or social or psychological. Most naturalists considered hereditary influences to include not only elements directly transmitted from the parents but also those of embryonic and early infant development. Heredity did not end at birth. In addition, almost everyone believed that acquired influences could be transmitted from one generation to the next. This so-called Lamarckian view of inheritance was almost universally accepted, by lay and learned people alike. Not until the late nineteenth century would this theory be directly challenged.[22]

Notions of hereditary disease also differed from later conceptualizations. Only very rarely was a disease itself thought to be directly inherited. For the most part, Abel Huntington's contemporaries believed that parents transmitted to their offspring not a disease but a predisposition, a constitutional "endowment," or what doctors later called a "diathesis," that rendered a person vulnerable to certain maladies. Hereditary influences were an important contributing element (or remote cause) in the etiology of many ills, but a proximate or immediate cause was usually required for symptoms to appear.[23]

Heredity, then, was never seen as the sole factor that underlay disease. Although an inherited disease might be resistant to cure once the symptoms actually appeared, healthy habits could often overcome a hereditary predisposition, forestalling their appearance. "Those who inherit any family disease ought to be very circumspect in their manner of living," advised the optimistic Dr. Buchan. "They should consider well the nature of such diseases, and guard against it by a proper regimen." Since a predisposition required exciting or triggering factors to initiate the development of symptoms, vulnerable individuals could try to avoid them through a proper diet and healthy living. Until the latter part of the nineteenth century, learned writers and uneducated people alike considered most "hereditary" influences malleable and open to change: while the effects of bad habits could be passed down to the next generation, so too could the beneficial influences of proper diet and healthy living. Buchan believed that family diseases could even be "wholely eradicated" by appropriate care. "Family constitutions are as capable of improvement as family estates," he stated firmly. Medically speaking, "heredity" was by no means destiny.[24]

Bringing with him to East Hampton "the imposing name of Huntington" (Samuel Huntington, a distant cousin, had been president of the Continental Congress and governor of the state of Connecticut), Abel Huntington soon won the respect of his Main Street neighbors, who regarded him as a brilliant physician and an exceptionally able surgeon, with a reputation for blunt speech and occasional humorous profanity. He became skilled at a wide range of procedures, from venesection (bleeding), pulling teeth, delivering babies, giving enemas, and setting broken legs to lancing abscesses, prescribing drugs, and simply giving "advice." He was also the first physician on Long Island to perform the operation of lithotomy, a dangerous procedure involving the surgical removal of stones from the bladder. An enthusiastic partisan of the Enlightenment, he introduced into East Hampton what he called "the Varicola Vaccina or Kine Pox" based on Edward Jenner's discovery that inoculation with relatively mild cowpox (vaccination, after the Latin *vacca,* cow) pustules produced immunity to smallpox. At a time when vaccination remained highly controversial, Abel Huntington vaccinated his own sister, the first to undergo the procedure in the town.[25]

Within a short time, the young Abel Huntington had become the Hedgeses' family physician. He vaccinated Phebe Hedges, her daughter Betsy, and another member of the household for smallpox on May 20, 1802. On other occasions he prescribed laudanum and "dressings" for Phebe, camphor for the children, opium pills number four, and "sundries." He extracted one of ten-year-old Betsy's teeth on November 1, 1805. Each year on November 21 he collected his one-year "subscription"—three dollars—a sort of early health insurance policy common in this community. The Hedgeses, like many families, paid a small additional fee for each visit, with "cash to balance" or more often, with "horse-keeping," "a sorrel mare," "tallow," "4 Dunghill Fowl," "2 bushels corn, old cord wood/very good." Abel Huntington recorded all these transactions in his account book, marking them also in a separate ledger at the end of the year. In the Long Island

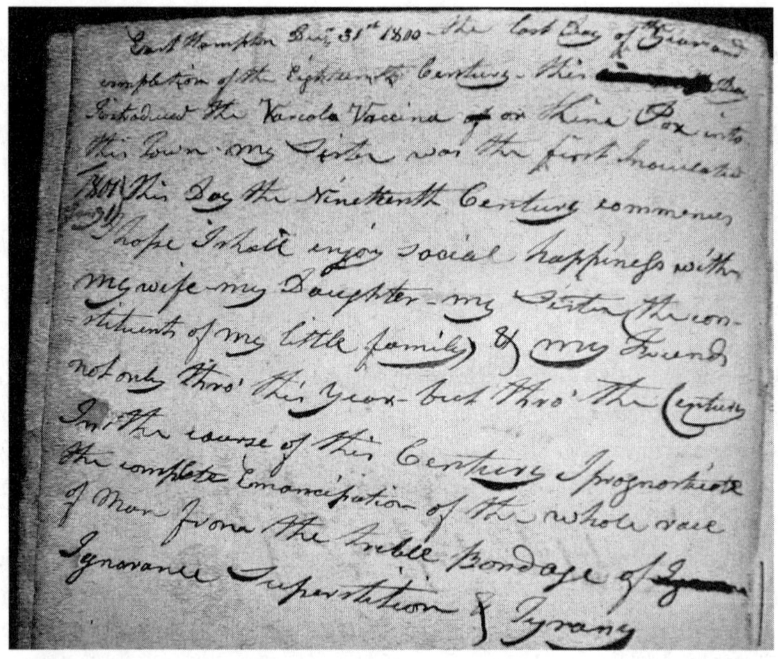
East Hampton Dec. 31st 1800 - the last Day of the Year and
completion of the Eighteenth Century - this Day
Introduced the Variola Vaccina or Kine Pox into
this Town - my Sister was the first Inoculated
1801 This Day the Nineteenth Century commences
Jany 1 I hope I shall enjoy social happiness with
my wife - my Daughter - my Sister (the con-
-stituents of my little family) & my Friends
not only thro' this year - but thro' the Century
In the course of this Century I prognosticate
the complete Emancipation of the whole race
of Man from the treble Bondage of Ig
Ignorance Superstition & Tyranny

Abel Huntington (1777–1858) account book, January 1, 1800: "In the course of this Century I prognosticate the complete Emancipation of the whole race of Man from the treble Bondage of Ignorance, Superstition, & Tyranny." Courtesy Pennypacker Long Island Collection, East Hampton Library

Room of the East Hampton Library, you can still see the notations in his long, narrow, suede-covered volumes, an entire universe of lives, hopes, and deaths.[26]

Spring 1805. Phebe's mother, the widow Tillinghast, was in her mid-sixties, old by the standards of the time, though not yet "ancient," as some here were called. Like many widows of her time, she had not remarried after her husband died, back in 1777. She owned her own long-roofed house, a ten-acre home lot at the north end of town on the low rise called "the Hook," and two pieces of woodland, property worth $250. She paid taxes. But by 1805 she was no longer able to manage on her own.[27]

In March of that year, Phebe Tillinghast's adult children made an arrangement with their mother to guarantee her support for the rest of her life. Such arrangements were common, a means of ensuring support for aging parents while passing on family property to the next generation. The timing, however, suggests that Phebe's son and daughters were concerned about their mother's growing incapacity, and that she herself may have shared this concern. On March 4, 1805, Phebe Tillinghast willed her house, home lot, woodlands, furniture, and household goods to her youngest daughter, Lydia Bennett, then twenty-eight years old, and her son-in-law William Bennett, in exchange for their agreement to care for her for the rest of her life. Suggesting their strong familial bonds, all of the widow Tillinghast's children and their spouses, including Phebe and Captain David Hedges, signed the document establishing the Bennetts as her heirs.[28]

Phebe Hedges was now forty-one years old, a woman "much esteemed by her neighbors," the mother of two sons, nineteen-year-old Stafford and fifteen-year-old Stephen, and a daughter, Betsy, who was just ten. Captain David Hedges was one of the wealthier men in the community, active in local affairs, and currently a town trustee. But toward the end of December 1805, as he was driving a wagon loaded with flour, "his horses took fright by which he was thrown from his seat and the waggon wheels passed over his breath." Many others had died from just such falls, and the *Suffolk Gazette* reported that Captain Hedges's recovery was "as yet doubtful."[29]

In cases of accident or illness, East Hampton folk commonly went to church to ask for prayers from the congregation. Even if they were not members—as many were not—most people attended church on the Sabbath, on holidays and other special occasions, or in times of illness or hardship. So it is likely that Phebe Hedges was present four days after her husband's fall, on New Year's Day, 1806, at the old Presbyterian church, where she would have heard the minister, Lyman Beecher, deliver a sermon on the "General History of the Town of East Hampton." The historical sermon was a popular convention, so, too, the jeremiad focusing on the sins and guilt of the community: the familiar story of the Fall, well-known to all East Hampton Christians. But Beecher framed this sermon with a pointed family metaphor, warning that "the iniquity of the fathers is imitated by and is visited upon the children." Unlike his predecessor, the Reverend Buell, who tended to speak in more general terms, the young Lyman Beecher aimed straight for the heart, "every sermon with my eye on the gun to hit somebody," as he later boasted.[30]

Comparing East Hampton to a beautiful garden once filled with "the choicest vine," Beecher asked, "Is not the hand of God conspicuous in planting the town with such men as your fathers?" He insisted that "the first inhabitants of a town determine the complexion of their descendants to distant generations." The current generation, however, fell "short of their excellent standard." Indeed, it tottered on the edge of a moral precipice, endangering future generations as well. For Beecher, the solution lay not in the future but the past. "Imitate your fathers," he urged; return to the example of "the first settlers of this town." Since they had transmitted "a glorious inheritance," the question now was, "Shall this inheritance perish in your hands, or shall it continue?" Each one bore a responsibility for the rest, "for your sins added together constitute an awful weight of guilt; and your combined influence continued will ruin the town. From day to day the degeneracy may not be perceived," he allowed, "but its progress is certain and its influence fatal."[31]

Let us imagine that Phebe Hedges, worried about her injured husband, melancholy over the advancing illness of her mother, and anxious about changes she noticed in herself, might have read personal meanings into his warnings, brooding over the "awful weight of guilt" and internalizing his allusions to "degeneracy" and ruin. What, after all, was her inheritance, and what inheritance would she leave her children? Few Christians in a town like East Hampton could have entirely escaped the suspicion that illness and accidents represented some form of divine punishment, or at least a test from God. Even among those most drawn to secular, Enlightenment thought—the skeptics, Deists, and "infidels"—these emotional associations with "the judgment of God" would have been hard to resist. The best men and women still reeked of sin. As one woman from nearby Shelter Island had reminded her daughter a few years earlier, "we are in a state of trial in this life, tho God's ways are ways of pleasantness & all his paths are peace, yet we have so much remaining Corruption & Sin left in us[,] that makes all our trouble—how can creatures that have so much of Hell & so much of Heaven in them expect to be happy with two such opposite principles[?]" Throughout the nineteenth century, most people accepted both naturalistic and supernatural explanations of illness, particularly mental illness, and did not see these two domains as being mutually exclusive or contradictory. A sense that "there is little unhappiness in this life for which sin in some shape is not accountable" probably lingered in the minds of even the most irreverent, long after any literal belief in the material reality of sin had disappeared.[32]

Spring 1806. On May 23 Mrs. Phebe Hedges sends for Dr. Huntington, who dispenses no drugs but offers "advice." He charges the usual twenty-five cents. Four days later, she sends for him again, apparently in more distress. This time he gives her spirits of turpentine, a stimulant. He also prescribes tonics—chamomile flowers, commonly used for their antispasmodic effects, and chalybeate powder number twelve, an iron supplement. In his account book Abel Huntington notes the charges, eighty-eight cents. He probably observes her carefully, noting the early signs of the malady that he will later describe to his son.[33]

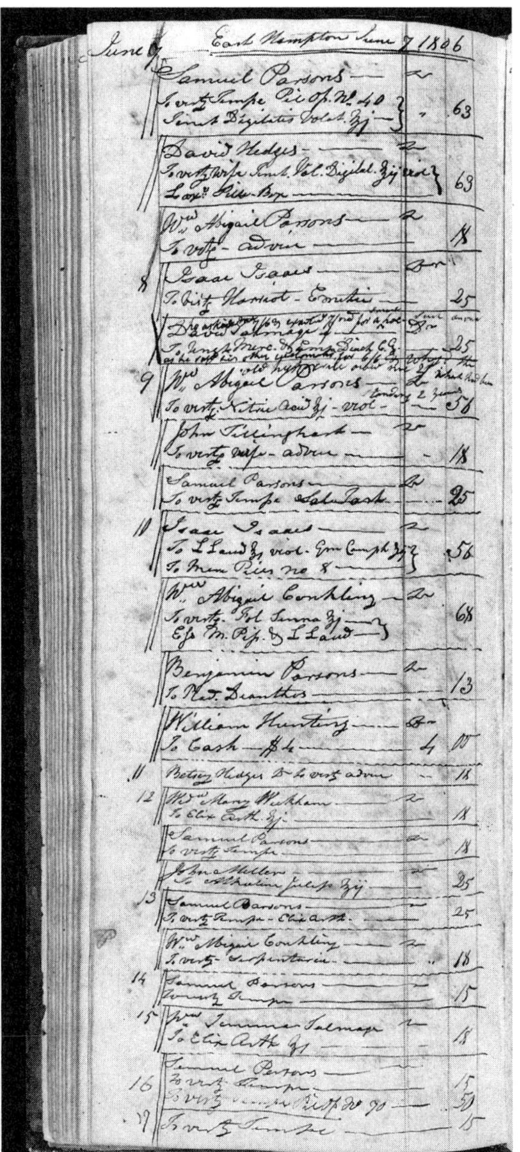

Abel Huntington account book, June 7–14, 1806.
Courtesy Pennypacker Long Island Collection,
East Hampton Library

But Phebe Hedges calls for Dr. Huntington yet again eleven days later, on June 7, evidently with continuing malaise and melancholy. This time he gives her a box of laxative pills along with digitalis, used to lower the pulse and diminish the body's irritability, and tincture of valerian, which doctors prescribed for many nervous disorders as an antispasmodic drug. If Phebe Hedges confides her fears to the physician, he does not make a note in his daybook, except to record charges of sixty-three cents that her husband will pay later with "cash and tallow to balance."[34]

On June 10 Captain David Hedges returns in the evening to find his wife ironing clothes. Possibly he has been out late overseeing construction of the new windmill in the Hook, of which he is a part owner. He has been working on this project since April, although construction itself began just eight days earlier and is now in its most intensive phase. At home he sees nothing out of the ordinary and goes to bed. But the next morning the villagers awaken to the news that Mrs. Phebe Hedges is missing. They mobilize a search, inquiring in every house for her whereabouts. Finally they trace her footsteps from her home through the fields of grain to the shore. Dr. Huntington, who usually sees three or four patients a day, suspends his regular practice today and sees only one person, eleven-year-old Betsy Hedges. We may imagine that he gives her chamomile tea to calm her sobbing, tries to comfort her in her grief. But Phebe Hedges does not return, not that day, or the next, or any day after. Timothy Miller, a resident of East Hampton who notes in his journal the passing of his neighbors, records that "the wife of Captain David Hedges walked into the surf and walked in and drowned."[35]

A week later, June 18, Dr. Huntington records no patients in his ledger, a highly unusual omission. Possibly on this day the body is found, washed up on the beach at Montauk, twenty miles to the east. East Hampton physicians often had to preside over inquests on the bodies of drowning victims on the beach, so Abel Huntington may have traveled out to Montauk for this purpose. The newspaper at nearby Sag Harbor considers the Hedges family of sufficient importance to note the death of Phebe Hedges in a full paragraph, along with its usual anti-Federalist diatribes, Republican entreaties, and advertising for "A Negro Girl" to be "purchased for any term of time over three years." As we have seen, the *Suffolk Gazette* speculated that Mrs. Hedges may have taken her drastic step because of "her extreme dread of the disorder known as St. Vitus dance," which her mother now suffered "to a great degree" and which had begun to affect her as well. The newspaper does not mention that June 15, five days after her death, vances, and are not behind many of their elder sisters in these respects. As it is generally acknowledged that examples of excellence tend greatly to facilitate improvement in whatever is honorable and praise-worthy, by exciting a laudable emulation, I hope it will not be considered partiality in me to mention *Durham* as a village, whose inhabitants of all classes, if we may trust to the assertions of strangers, have attained to improvements which are excelled but by few towns in the state. Liberal encouragement is given to *Newspaper* circulation, *Schools* and *Music*. In vocal, we are not excelled in this state, and we have an elegant band of instrumental music. There is an excellent *Library* in extensive circulation, and a *Society* has lately been established for moral and literary purposes, founded upon liberal and permanent principles, and aided by a number of gentlemen of science and information, which will undoubtedly be of great utility to its members. *Durham, June*, 1806.

Reader, have you not observed that the Federalists, in speaking of the British depredations and outrages upon our commerce, say very little against their British friends; but are vehement against our own government and lay the blame upon them? If you have read their newspapers, or listened to their conversation, you know this to be a fact.—Let every man draw his own inference from it. [*Pittsfield Sun.*

It appears that a distinguished *Federalist*, at the head of one of the *Federal* insurance offices in New-York, invited the British frigates to take their station on our coast. Yet the *Federalists*, for electioneering purposes, have united in a general party clamour, on account of British depredations, not, however, against the British perpetrators of those outrages, but against our government for not building a navy to match the British fleets. [*ib.*

Died, in Fairfield, Mr. John Bradshaw, who was born on Long-Island, June 7, 1701, O. S. aged 104 years, 10 months and 20 days. One week before his death he walked near a mile to his neighbors and home again. He was remarkable for his piety to the last, and retained his reason, sight and hearing as well as men in common at the age of 80.

From several parts of this state we have accounts of the ravages committed by a worm, generally called the *Army worm*. We have heard of many fields of wheat, rye and corn, which have been almost totally cut down by this destructive worm. [*Kentucky pap.*

SAG-HARBOR:
MONDAY, JUNE 30, 1806.

[COMMUNICATION.]

A hint to the civil authority of Sag-Harbor.

There is now in this port an itinerant person exhibiting *sleight-of-hand tricks*, and imposing upon the credulous part of community by the lowest species of deceptions. He has exhibited once, and appointed Monday evening the 30th inst. for another. He is picking the pockets of those who are least able to be robbed. Such despicable impostors are an offence to every citizen who has any regard for PUBLIC MORALITY.

A barn and corn-house belonging to Mr. Israel Rose, in Southampton, was struck with lightning, the last week, and consumed.

It has become our duty to publish the following melancholy circumstance, which took place at Easthampton a few weeks since:—Capt. David Hedges returned to his home in the evening, and found Mrs. Hedges ironing clothes, and apparently in health—he retired to bed and left her at that employment, but on awaking in the morning she was not to be found. After considerable search and enquiry, her footsteps were traced from the house thro' fields of grain to the shore; and there is every reason to believe she has precipitated herself into the surf which washes the south shore. Mrs. Hedges was about 40 years of age, and was much esteemed by her neighbors. This extraordinary step is attributed to her extreme dread of the disorder called *St. Vitus' dance*, with which she began to be affected, and which her mother now has to a great degree. From some arrangements of her clothing it appears she had for some time contemplated her melancholy end.

☞ *The Republicans in the vicinity of Sag-Harbor, are invited to join in the celebration of American Independence, on Friday next. A discourse, suited to the occasion, will be delivered by the Rev. Mr. Boge, and an entertainment provided by Capt. Daniel Fordham.*

BY THE COMMITTEE.

WANTED,

A Negro Girl from eighteen to thirty years of age.—She will be purchased for any term of time over three years. She is wanted to live in a small family, and must come well recommended for honesty. For further particulars enquire of the Printer, Sag-Harbor.

WHEREAS Abel Basset and John Whittesey, of Sag-Harbor, in the County of Suffolk, and state of New-

Suffolk Gazette, June 30, 1806

is the feast day of St. Vitus, who is supposed to protect those with epilepsy and chorea.[36]

There is no record of a funeral for Phebe Hedges, or any report that, like her neighbors, she was "buried from the church." I have been unable to locate a gravestone, though the stones of her husband, her children, and many grandchildren still stand in the cemeteries of East Hampton. One would like to think that the preacher Lyman Beecher comforted the Hedgeses with the advice he gave other local families grieving over painful losses, as when he advised a distraught father who had just lost his son, "Do not set in judgment on your son, but give up him and all into the hands of God." Alluding to the possibility of suicide, Beecher urged this father not to "weary your soul by saying, if such and such a thing had not been, for it is done, the providential will of God has come to pass." For the orthodox Beecher, the Calvinist emphasis on the "uncertainty of mere worldly good" and the importance of placing "our affections on things above" did not preclude experiences of profound grief and mourning. If some East Hampton folk were stoic and resigned in the face of sudden death, others were "crushed" with sorrow and "inexpressibly shocked." Even Samuel Buell, the preceding East Hampton minister, had struggled against what he perceived as the excessive sorrow and grief of his parishioners facing the death of loved ones, especially of young people, while evoking in his sermons the tremendous pain of losing those "we justly value and esteem, greatly love and delight in," and the grief of knowing that "we must see their faces no more in this world."[37]

Suicide raised especially painful issues for the family of the deceased. Historically, suicide in England had been both a sin and a crime, self-murder or felo-de-se, with severe penalties for the suicide's survivors, sometimes extending to forfeiture of all property to the state. By the mid-seventeenth century, however, English coroners' juries increasingly interpreted acts of suicide as evidence of mental illness, turning in verdicts of non compos mentis. In the United States, too, according to the historian Howard Kushner, "by the end of the eighteenth century, melancholy behavior followed by suicide was almost uniformly connected with mental illness," though as late as 1810 an occasional coroners' jury in Suffolk County still ruled suicide as felo-de-se. As portrayed by the newspaper report, the suicide of Phebe Hedges was not an act of insanity or a crime or an instance of giving in to temptation, but rather the result of "melancholy" linked to fears of St. Vitus's dance. Her death was "unfortunate," but it was neither criminal nor crazy.[38]

Had Phebe Hedges not suffered from St. Vitus's dance and "walked into the sea and walked in and drowned," we might never have known about her life, nor that of her mother, two white women in the late eighteenth and early nineteenth centuries in this town at the eastern tip of Long Island. As it is, we have the barest outline from scraps of evidence in old town and church records. Phebe Hedges's death, more than her life, stands out in all its poignancy. Yet her name echoes in the archives of chorea, reminding us that real people in the past suffered with this disease, people who bought fancy calimanco shoes from the town cordwainer (shoemaker), who got chalybeate powder and "advice" from the local physician, who gave birth to children and sometimes buried them before the year was out; men and women who had neighbors and friends and joys and sorrows, but whose only traces are brief entries in a doctor's daybook or a shopkeeper's account, the hurried scrawl of the pastor noting who got married and who died.

More important, her action opens a window onto the social experience of families with St. Vitus's dance. Reported in the newspaper and inscribed in the historical record of the town, her death allows us to inquire how it was for the children and grandchildren of the sufferers from St. Vitus's dance in the years before and also after the doctors invented "hereditary chorea" as a clinical category. What stories do their lives tell, about St. Vitus's dance and about illness, disability, and heredity in a nineteenth-century Long Island town?

Seven months after the death of Phebe Hedges, Captain David Hedges remarried, as most widowers did at this time, especially those with small children. When Dr. Abel Huntington paid a medical visit to the family again in 1808, he did not record the fact that this "Mrs. Hedges" was a different woman altogether.[39]

2

THE SOCIAL COURSE OF ST. VITUS'S DANCE

Family trees here are hard to untangle; their branches are intertwined like the lop-fences still discernible along our woodland roads.
—Jeanette Edwards Rattray, *East Hampton History*

Who is "one of us"?
—Homi Bhaba, "Cultural Choice, Cultural Respect"

In his studies of disorders such as epilepsy and depression, the medical anthropologist Arthur Kleinman theorizes that disease possesses a social course, a term that he contrasts with "the biomedical idea of the natural course" of the disease. According to Kleinman, the social course of a condition "is organized as much by what matters for the participants in a local world as it is by the biology of the condition." Although biology sets limits and boundaries, "the microcultural worlds in which patients and families engage in everyday social activities" are "the only valid grounds for understanding illness and treatment." In Kleinman's example of epilepsy in two Chinese provinces in the late twentieth century, seizures shaped the lives not only of the affected individuals but also of their entire families, whose members often found themselves ostracized and stigmatized by others in the community. Whatever was deemed to cause the seizures—anger, fright, anxiety, possession, and head injury were among the most common explanations—applied to the whole family. Stigma, the cultural devaluation of a condition, profoundly shaped their experience.[1]

But in other settings, stigma constituted a much less significant aspect of the affected individual's experience. In one twentieth-century Turkish community, families actively strove to protect their members with epilepsy, and even to reframe their condition as one of mystery and change. And as we have seen, while deafness on the North American mainland was severely stigmatized in the late eighteenth and early nineteenth centuries, in certain communities on the island of Martha's Vineyard, off the New England coast, hereditary deafness during the nineteenth century hardly constituted a handicap at all. According to the anthropologist Nora Groce, the shared background of the inhabitants, along with the high incidence of deafness, helped to create a local culture in which deafness was not a distinguishing mark of identity. Indeed, hearing people as well as deaf ones used sign language along with spoken English, a form of bilingualism. This absence of stigma on Martha's Vineyard, according to Groce, suggests the ways in which "a handicap is an arbitrary social category," not a universal given, and something that can be changed in the future."[2]

While a steadily worsening neurological disorder differs significantly from a stable impairment such as deafness, or from an episodic condition such as epilepsy—with which chorea was historically associated—the perspectives of Kleinman and Groce suggest that the social meanings of St. Vitus's dance and Huntington's chorea may also have differed across time and place. A bit of genealogy is necessary here, but the historical traces of Phebe Hedges, her sisters and descendants, can shed light on how one community addressed this condition, and how members of these families coped. Haunted by the memory of Phebe Hedges, we can follow her two sons and one daughter, her eleven grandchildren and thirty-seven great-grandchildren (those who remained in East Hampton), and the progeny of her sisters, to ask how they lived over the course of the nineteenth century. We can observe their interactions with their neighbors, ask whether they got married and to whom, whether they were elected to town office if they were men, married whaling masters or farmers or day laborers if they were women. We can ask whether they were ever "visited" by a church "committee" for bad behavior, or whether they were part of the committees that did the visiting; whether they showed up in cases at court or came under the jurisdiction of the Overseers of the Poor. We can see what their neighbors may have said about them in letters, memoirs, or diaries. All these traces can help us grasp the social course of St. Vitus's dance in the years before "hereditary chorea" became a recognized disease.

THE HEIRS OF PHEBE HEDGES

As members of the first generation of Americans born after the Revolution, Stafford Hedges, born in 1786, Stephen, in 1790, and Betsy, in 1795, entered a community somewhat removed from the commercial and industrial transformations of the early Republic. On his travels around New England in 1804,

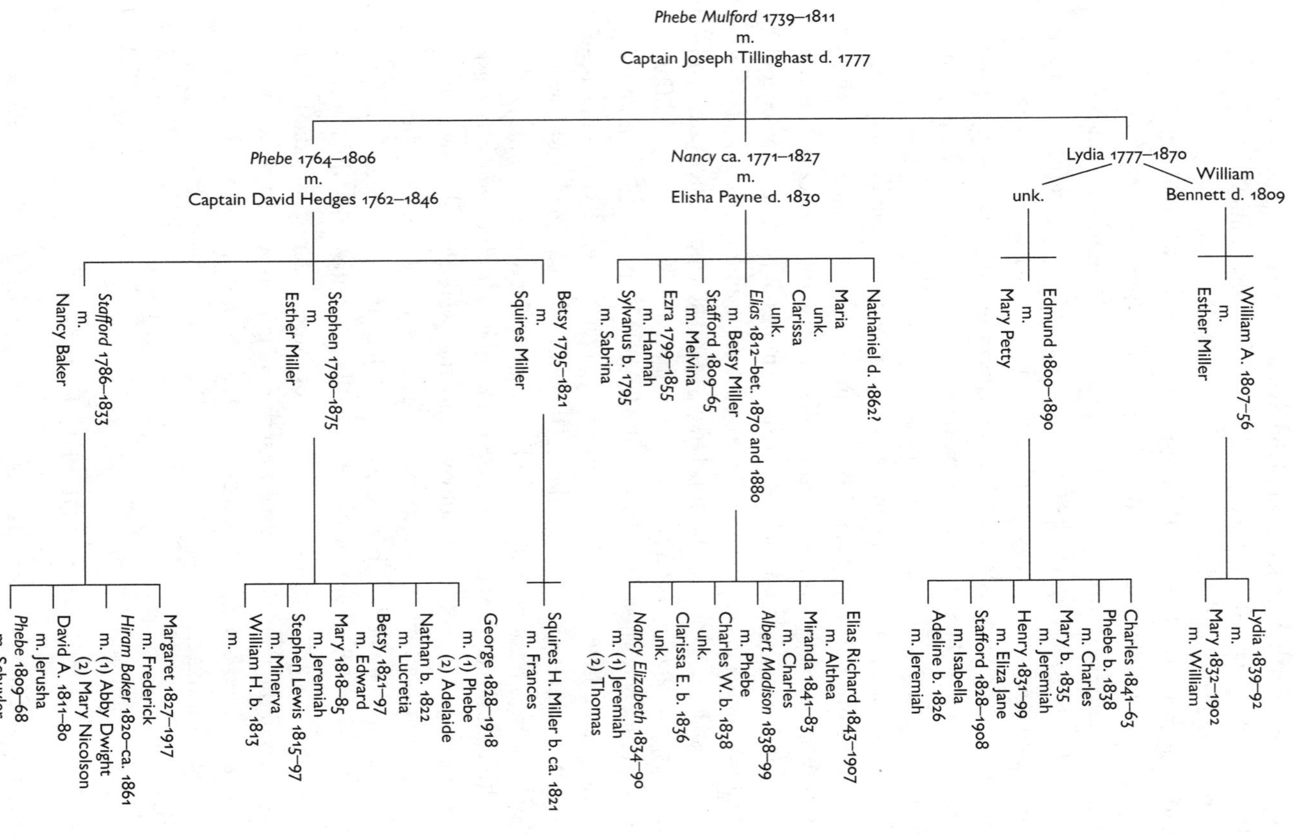

Reported St. Vitus's Dance or Huntington's chorea indicated by italics.

Descendants of Phebe Mulford (1739–1811) and Captain Joseph Tillinghast (d. 1777), East Hampton

Yale University President Timothy Dwight found the people of East Hampton both admirable and insular. "Sequestered in great measure from the world, they exhibit scarcely a trace of that activity which everywhere meets the eye in New England," he wrote. Although there was "no want of the social character," the people here were "more attuned to the customs of their ancestors, and less to the influences of the wider world." According to Dwight, they were "uncommonly healthy," many of them living into old age (sixty years or more). But one disorder stood out in Dwight's report: they suffered to an unusual extent from "the hypochondria," associated at the time with irritability, melancholy, and "restless agitations." This malady "was said to be unusually frequent here, at Bridgehampton, and at Southampton," precisely the places where St. Vitus's dance was later reported to appear.[3]

By the middle of the nineteenth century, steamboats, turnpikes, and the railroad had brought East Hampton closer to the larger world of New York and New England, but the town remained suspicious of progress, "a bit of the eighteenth century in the midst of the nineteenth," according to one native son. Though only a few miles away from the cosmopolitan and commercial whaling village of Sag Harbor, many white East Hampton people still liked to imagine themselves dwelling "where their fathers had dwelt, treading patiently the paths their fathers' steps had beaten, tilling the same fields, sheltered by the same roofs, believing in the same stern creed, worshiping in the same gray old temple, and finally lying down in death almost in the same green graves," as Abel Huntington's literary daughter Cornelia wrote in her roman à clef, *Sea-Spray: A Long Island Village,* published in 1857. Still, they welcomed the summer vacationers from New York City who began to arrive in the 1850s. They beautified their houses and promoted tourism, even while cultivating a romance with the past.[4]

Growing up in this compact community, the three children of Phebe Hedges stayed close to the world of their parents, albeit following distinct paths. Phebe's youngest child and only daughter, Betsy (1795–1821), married a carpenter, Squires Miller, the son of a middling local man. But Betsy died young, probably while giving birth to her only son, who became a carpenter like his father, married, and settled down with his wife to have a family in the neighboring village of Bridgehampton, though not before embarking on at least one whaling voyage, in 1843, as the carpenter on a ship captained by his cousin Hiram B. Hedges, a remarkable figure, as we shall see.[5]

Phebe's elder son, Stafford (1786–1833), lived longer than his sister, long enough in fact to be overcome by his mother's malady, as Henry Hedges later recalled. In 1808, two years after his mother's death, when he was just twenty-two—younger than most men here when they first married—Stafford Hedges married into another old gentry clan (possibly because his future wife was already pregnant, a common occurrence in this town). His first daughter was born seven months later, and eventually three more children followed. While still in his twenties, Stafford Hedges entered the circle of local officeholders: he was elected overseer of highways and twice served as town trustee. But 1817 was the last year he was elected to office, a turn indicating that something was amiss, since he was still only thirty-one, and once elected, men were usually reelected year after year to one office or another at the annual town meeting. Although Stafford fathered children after that date—the youngest of his four offspring was born in 1828, when he was forty-two—at some point he began developing the symptoms of St. Vitus's dance. He died in 1833, at the age of forty-seven.[6]

Because he died before his father had bequeathed the major portion of his land to his sons, Stafford inherited a relatively small proportion of his father's estate, and in turn he left a limited inheritance to his children. This circumstance, along with his illness, may have helped turn his sons toward more adventurous pursuits than farming—an occupation many young people here considered dull and demeaning in any case. Stafford's younger son, Hiram B. Hedges (1820–ca. 1861), who was thirteen at the time of his father's death, went on his first whaling expedition a few years later. While still in his twenties, Hiram Hedges moved up the whaling hierarchy, from greenhand to boatsteerer (harpooner) to first mate to captain. He undertook several voyages to the North Atlantic and the South Pacific as captain on the barque *Monmouth* out of Cold Spring Harbor, and one around-the-world, three-year expedition on a Sag Harbor ship, the *Josephine*, previously captained by the famous whaling master Thomas Welcome Roys. For all his adventurousness, Hiram Hedges was a follower of temperance, enforcing a no-liquor regulation on his voyages, with the exception of the provisions for "medicine."[7]

Hedges became a local celebrity whose arrival back in East Hampton after a voyage was something of an occasion. "Captain Hedges returns from the sea," wrote the local banker J. Madison Huntting in his diary on January 3, 1846, as if this were an event of general importance. Whaling captains enjoyed tremendous prestige in nineteenth-century eastern Long Island, where a whaling voyage was a rite of manhood. As one twentieth-century local historian put it, "a young man in Amagansett had not won his spurs until after he'd gone on his first whale chase and had come back, literally from the shadow of death, covered with the blood of the dying whale." Articulate and self-confident, the dashing Captain Hedges addressed his ship owners as equals and did not hesitate to change course when he deemed it advisable. Those who sailed with him admired him as "a free, open, and thorough sailor" and a man who was "always kind to his men, and highly respected by them," a view that probably described his reputation at home as well.[8]

In 1857 the thirty-seven-year-old Hiram Hedges, his second wife, an Englishwoman, and their young son traveled to the Oregon Territory, where Hiram took out a land claim of 940 acres near Portland and began a new life as a farmer, although according to his son, he continued to "follow the sea." (Hiram's first wife, a teacher from Plattsburg, New York, whom he had married after a six-week courtship, had died of consumption in 1848.) Hiram's elder brother, David A. Hedges (1811–80), a carpenter and active officeholder in East Hampton from the time he was twenty-four, also went west, settling with his wife, Jerusha, in Oregon City, south of Portland, and working as a barrel maker at the Harvey Flour Mill. Nine years older than Hiram, David A. had been twenty-two when their father died, so he would have been especially aware of his father's illness. Although we cannot know just how this affected him, it is worth noting that both brothers married women "from away," and both decided to leave their hometown for the West, suggesting a strategy for escaping the legacy of the three generations before them. (Hiram's commitment to temperance suggests an additional strategy of forestallment.) David A. Hedges evidently lived out the remainder of his life in Oregon, "a prominent and highly respected citizen," according to his obituary. He reportedly died in Portland in 1880 after falling off his horse at the age of sixty-nine.[9]

His brother came to a more dramatic end. Sometime in 1861 Hiram Hedges vanished. According to his son many years later, he had traveled by boat to Shoalwater Bay, near the mouth of the Columbia River, and was on his way back to Portland when he "was caught by a gale, and has never been heard of since. His vessel was finally posted as missing and it is supposed that it foundered." This was a reasonable assumption, as many boats and ships were lost in those waters.[10]

However, Hiram Hedges's niece later told Elizabeth Muncey, the physician and eugenics worker who visited East Hampton in 1912, that Hedges had committed suicide in Oregon, a story that seems unlikely to have been invented. Hiram Hedges was in his early forties when he died, approaching the age at which his grandmother had walked into the sea, back in 1806. Whatever the truth of his death, and of his life, he left behind three young children, a whaling log of several voyages, and memories of "the handsomest captain who made port in the Sandwich Islands [Hawaii] in his time."[11]

Hiram Hedges was clearly an admired, almost a mythic figure in his hometown during his lifetime. His elder sister, another Phebe (1809–68), and her family also left their mark in the community, albeit in a different mode. This Phebe married a man of modest resources from one of the founding Amagansett families, possibly a step down the social ladder for a Hedges from the village of East Hampton. (Although it is difficult to imagine today, Amagansett in the nineteenth and early twentieth centuries was considered déclassé by the "upstreet" gentry of East Hampton village.) Still, the Conklings were a large family with prominent relatives: Schuyler's distant cousin was Alfred Conkling, a judge and congressman from New York. For the first few years of the marriage, in the early 1830s, Schuyler Conkling went off each year on a whaling expedition to the South Atlantic, leaving Phebe on her own. But in 1835 Phebe and Schuyler moved out to Further House, one of the keepers' places on Montauk, six thousand acres of grassy rolling hills where East Hampton's cattle and other livestock were pastured each summer. For the next six years they shared the responsibilities of overseeing the livestock and laborers, as well as maintaining the house, keeping all the outbuildings repaired, and welcoming visitors to the place. After they returned to Amagansett in 1841, Schuyler Conkling held various local offices, including constable, overseer of highways, and town trustee, although in 1843 he decided to go off with his brother-in-law Hiram Hedges on a two-year whaling expedition, leaving Phebe to manage their five young children at home.[12]

But at the age of forty, Schuyler was rather old for a whaler. He was ill on the voyage, and though he was second mate, he had tensions with the crew. On his return home, he stopped attending church, prompting a committee of elders to "visit" him several times for his "neglect of church ordinances." Eventually, though, they excused his absences, suggesting that he may have been sick or disabled. Whether because of hardships suffered at sea or from other causes, Schuyler died when he was only forty-seven, in 1850, leaving his forty-one-year-old widow with six children (one more had been born after his return from whaling), ranging in age from nineteen to three.[13]

Many years later, in a memoir called *Whale-Off: The Story of an American Whaler,* the grandson of Phebe and Schuyler Conkling wrote that his grandmother Phebe had died eight years after her husband, leaving his mother, their eleven-year-old daughter Adelia, to do all the cooking and housework for her brothers, as well as "learning the trade of a tailoress and making all their clothes. Even in those days," he wrote, "this was very unusual for such a young girl, and to-day it sounds incredible." Actually, Phebe lived for eighteen years after her husband's death, dying with St. Vitus's dance in 1868 at the age of fifty-nine. The story Phebe's grandson told seems to evoke the emotional impact of her illness on the family. It was as if she had died in 1858, even though she survived for a decade longer. Instead of being a factual account, the narrative appears to convey the sense of loss in the family occasioned by Phebe's growing disability, and the toll it took on her youngest daughter. It may also have evoked Phebe's disappearance from the community life of East Hampton, marking a kind of social death that long preceded her physical demise.[14]

Stafford's other daughter, Margaret (1827–1917), who was nearly twenty years younger than Phebe, grew up in circumstances quite different from those of her elder sister and her two brothers. Yet she too showed the family's characteristic resourcefulness. She was only six when her father died (and fourteen at the death of her mother), and would have had few memories of him. In 1843, at the age of sixteen—extremely young for this community—she married a whaling captain like her brother, albeit a considerably older man (aged twenty-seven) from a prominent Shelter Island family of whalers. And like her elder sister, Margaret was also widowed at a young age; she was thirty-three in 1860 when her husband, who was then forty-four, died suddenly of a stroke ("apoplexy"). For all the prestige and admiration they enjoyed, whaling captains were not always wealthy, and Frederick Cartwright was among the more modest of means. Though she had little more than a mortgaged house, the enterprising young widow turned her sewing skills into work as a seamstress for other East Hampton families, including the Huntingtons. Her neighbors apparently raised the funds that enabled her to keep the house, and later she took in boarders to support her three children and herself. She never remarried. Margaret Cartwright lived until the age of eighty-nine, a woman "held in high esteem by many friends," according to the *East Hampton Star.* It seems highly unlikely that she could have suffered from St. Vitus's dance.[15]

As we have seen, Stafford's four children met adversity in diverse ways, each following a distinct path, from whaling to barrel making to sewing and taking in boarders to overseeing Further House on Montauk. In contrast, Stafford's younger brother Stephen Hedges (1790–1875) and his children followed a more conventional gentry trajectory, mostly remaining in East Hampton and, in some cases, holding positions of local prominence. From a young age Stephen Hedges was active in town affairs, elected at the age of eighteen to his first post, as swine and sheep pounder. When he was twenty-six, in 1816, he became a town trustee for the first time. After that he alternated the post of trustee with other offices such as overseer of highways and, later, overseer of the poor and tax assessor, an especially responsible position. Stafford's death in 1833 had made Stephen the principal heir of his father's considerable landholdings. Indeed, Stephen eventually became a wealthy man, although he did not receive the bulk of his father's estate until Captain David died at the age of eighty-four, in 1846, when Stephen was already fifty-six years old.[16]

The death of his elder brother in 1833, when Stephen was forty-three, seemed to deepen his commitment to the church. The year after Stafford died Stephen was elected deacon, a position of respect that he held for the next forty-one years. Although he continued to hold town offices, after 1841 he devoted his energies increasingly to religious affairs. Known in town as "a strict Presbyterian," he served on many church committees, occupied the number twelve pew (an indicator of his wealth, since the pews close to the front were more expensive to rent), and held prayer meetings in his house. For some he served as a moral beacon. Fanny Huntting, that self-appointed guardian of the morals of Main Street, was "reminded of my sins" when she observed Deacon Hedges, at age seventy-six, passing "by my window, tottering under the weight of years." But his narrow outlook and extreme conservatism did not endear him to his lively granddaughter, Mary Esther Mulford Miller, who mentioned him dismissively in her 1931 memoir *An East Hampton Childhood*—considered a classic account of growing up here in the 1850s and 1860s—as one of the "old worthies" who had "prayed for 'the dear youth who are going on, Gal[i]leo-like, caring for none of these [traditional] things,'" implying that he himself cared for these things alone.[17]

In his eighties, Stephen began to grow "twitchy" and forgetful. "Last night about six, an alarm was raised that Deacon Stephen Hedges was lost," Fanny Huntting reported in her diary, perhaps recalling the stories of Stephen's mother, who had been "lost" many years before. "He left home about one o'clock to go to some woodland about two miles from home. A large force went in pursuit of him. They found him about ten o'clock, three or four miles from home. He must have walked nearly twenty miles in all. He is 83, and his mind somewhat impaired." Some of the neighbors evidently concluded that he had developed his mother's illness, albeit "not a very bad case." When a descendant of another old family with no history of the malady developed the telltale symptoms, talk went round that Stephen Hedges had fathered an illegitimate son. But George Huntington did not agree. As if to put an end to the gossip, Huntington later insisted that Deacon Hedges had never suffered from chorea, not even when he had become "an old man, insane, and a terror to the boys. Although fully entitled to be a choreic," according to Huntington, "he never became one, and *none of his posterity* have ever developed the disease, nor have they ever become insane."[18]

George Huntington's reassurances, however, came years after Stephen Hedges had died, in 1875, at the age of eighty-four. Stephen's four sons and two daughters had no such certainty about their father's condition while they were young and watching their uncle and cousins becoming affected. Nonetheless, like their father, they too grew up to become prominent figures in town affairs. The most active of the children was Stephen Lewis Hedges (1815–97), who began holding office in his early twenties, elected as overseer and commissioner of highways, an inspector of common schools, overseer of the poor, and then, in 1842, when he was only was twenty-seven, a town trustee. By the time he was thirty-five, in 1850, Stephen Lewis Hedges was called "Esquire," indicating his wealth and high social status.[19]

In 1854, when he was not yet forty, Stephen Lewis was elected supervisor, the highest-ranking position in the town. He was reelected to this position ten times, including during the years of the Civil War—a post that gave him the epithet "the war supervisor"—although as a lifelong Democrat, he had opposed the election of Lincoln. Indeed, before the war, East Hampton had harbored considerable sympathy for the South, and many white people in the town worried more about the consequences of emancipation than about the evils of slavery. Though often credited with raising troops during the war, in fact Stephen Lewis did the opposite: as town supervisor, he participated in town meetings to find substitutes for East Hampton men to keep them out of the Union Army, and even traveled to New York City for this purpose. Main Street, home to gentry families, sent few volunteers to fight, while the working-class neighborhood of Springs sent many.[20]

A few years after the war ended, however, Stephen Lewis dropped out of local governance. He was in his early fifties, and he may have tired of local politics, or found himself at odds with his neighbors' politics and not been reelected. Or possibly he feared for his health. Whatever the reasons, he left local politics behind. For the last nine years of his life he taught school. When he died in 1897 at the age of eighty-two, he had "the distinction of being one of the oldest residents of Suffolk County," according to the late-nineteenth-century *Portrait and Biographical Record* of local worthies, "and one of those who have made much of its unwritten history."[21]

While Stephen Lewis held more elected positions than his siblings, several of the others also played active roles in the community, and all of them married and had children. One of Stephen Lewis's brothers outdid their father by serving as a church elder for fifty-seven years, until his death at the age of ninety. One sister helped her husband, "a man of considerable means" and himself a prominent figure in town, manage a large farm that was locally famous for its hospitality. The other sister married a wealthy whaling captain and lived next door to the Huntington physicians. Two other brothers, one of whom was also a whaling captain, eventually settled in California.[22]

As we have seen, George Huntington insisted that neither Stephen Hedges nor any of his descendants ever suffered from chorea. However, some of them may have been considered so by others, even if only "slightly affected" or "not badly affected," language Elizabeth Muncey recorded in her notes, and even if they lived to be eighty-three or ninety: once the illness was known in the family, any malady was likely to be identified as St. Vitus's dance. Still, almost all of these children and grandchildren of Phebe Hedges married at ages typical for their generations. All had families ranging from one to six children (though for one couple no children survived beyond infancy). Some married into other old East Hampton families and some married spouses "from away" (but mostly from neighboring places such as Southold or Shelter Island). Like their neighbors, some married into wealthier families while others married into more modest clans. Some inherited more land than others. While only a few members of these two generations had landholdings or wealth equal to that of Captain David Hedges, a pattern of reduced property over successive generations was characteristic of old New England and New York towns, where land was divided among sons generation after generation. More important, many of the children and grandchildren of Phebe Hedges—those born from the 1780s to the 1820s—held positions of esteem and respect in East Hampton. Though not every male member of this family was active in local affairs, the election of many of them to town or church office indicates the family's integration within the community. For this family the legacy of St. Vitus's dance was not a cause for exclusion.[23]

THE EAST HAMPTON SIBLINGS OF PHEBE HEDGES

Still, Phebe Hedges's husband, Captain David Hedges, outlived her by forty years. For a long time her children and grandchildren had a prominent father around to keep an eye on them and intervene on their behalf—and even a grandfather to register an "earmark" (distinguishing mark) for his grandsons Hiram and David A., or insist in his will that David A. support his sister Margaret until she married. But what of the former Phebe Tillinghast's two sisters who also stayed in East Hampton (two siblings had married and moved away), Nancy Tillinghast (ca. 1771–1827) and Lydia Tillinghast (1777–1870)—whose marriages were distinctly different? How did they and their offspring fare?[24]

Whereas Phebe Tillinghast had married into one of the wealthiest old gentry clans in East Hampton, her sister Nancy married into a laboring family, considered by some as people "from away," since they came to East Hampton in the early 1700s rather than the 1650s. When Nancy Tillinghast married Elisha Payne in October of 1793, he was working as a handyman on the Isle of Wight (Gardiner's Island)—a manor owned by one of the founding East Hampton families. In comparison with Nancy's father, Elisha Payne was a man of limited means. Still, if Payne belonged to the lower end of the economic spectrum in the town, he was not among the impoverished. In 1801 his property was equal in value to that of Abel Huntington, around $30, and in 1815, his assets were slightly higher, $190 compared with $150.[25]

Nonetheless, this marriage between the daughter of elite parents and a laboring man differed from the typical East Hampton pattern, in which young people married into families of similar social rank. Possibly Nancy was pregnant, as were a good percentage of late-eighteenth-century New England brides, for whom premarital pregnancy was often a way of overcoming parental objections: following the Revolution, more women generally married on their own inclinations, for love and companionship rather than duty. Nancy's marriage may well have been a personal choice, rather than a necessity.[26]

Nancy and Elisha Payne lived on the Isle of Wight through the War of 1812, Elisha shuttling to the mainland to purchase supplies, food, tools, and medicines, and to bring visitors to the island, including the Gardiner family physician, Abel Huntington. After the war they moved across the bay to the mainland, settling in Springs, where other laboring families lived. Nancy Payne died in 1827, having passed on St. Vitus's dance to at least one of her sons. Elisha married again, but he died soon after, in 1830, bequeathing his widow a house, a chest, "sixty-six Dollars and Fifty Cents in money," and the need to petition the town for support.[27]

Of the five (out of seven) of Elisha's and Nancy's grown children whom we can trace, all married and had families. They and their descendants, according to the census, included at various times sailors, "boatmen," a shoemaker, farmers, day laborers in the local fish factories, and one son who temporarily received aid from the town. Two of them evidently went on at least one whaling voyage, that requisite ritual of youthful masculinity. But eventually the youngest son, Elias, developed St. Vitus's dance (according to George Huntington). In 1870, although he had always been a sailor, the census listed the fifty-eight-year-old Elias as "without occupation," a further indication that he was now severely disabled. He died sometime before 1880.[28]

Neither Elisha Payne nor any of his and Nancy's sons was elected to local office, so far as I can tell. But at least two of their grandsons (sons of their son Elias) became officeholders in East Hampton for several years, indicating their status as active participants in the community. Elias Richard Payne (1843–1907) was elected town trustee and served from 1879 to 1883, while his elder brother Albert Madison Payne (1838–99) served several terms as constable. Both brothers married and had children of their own. Elias Richard never developed his mother's illness, although he evidently had other disabilities: at least he told the army surgeon who examined him for pension eligibility following his Civil War service that he suffered from "debility and fits."[29]

Albert M., however, suffered a crueler fate. After receiving bayonet and grapeshot wounds during an assault on Fort Wagner, in South Carolina, and also varicose veins from "hard marching," Albert spent nearly a year in army hospitals before returning to East Hampton in 1865. Soon after his return he married a local woman, and they went to live with her parents in Amagansett while he worked for the next nine years as a day laborer at the John Smith Fish Oil and Guano Factory at nearby Napeague. But he had difficulties with his legs—whether from the varicose veins or developing chorea is unclear—and according to his boss, "He was frequently obliged to quit work sometimes for hours and sometimes for more than a day," and was altogether unable to perform any heavy labor. By the time he was fifty-eight, in 1898, he could no longer sign his name, and marked an X for his signature on his pension papers. He died two years later at the age of sixty. Nearly a decade afterward George Huntington recalled his neighbors "Elias P. and his son Albert, the latter but little my senior and a picture of robust health when I knew him as one of the 'bigger boys,' now dead of the disease."[30]

Another member of this family, one of Nancy and Elisha's granddaughters, who was also named Nancy (1834–90), left behind an especially haunting memory. Neighbors told Elizabeth Muncey in 1912 that as a young woman Nancy Elizabeth had been "counted a great beauty with pleasing manners." She married a "boatman" who was killed in the Civil War, and then married a former steamer captain and fisherman with a talent for storytelling and a gift for handling boats and men, according to the local newspaper. Their sons, in turn, became housepainters and fishermen. But years later, after she developed St. Vitus's dance, Nancy became "the terror of the neighborhood," according to Muncey's report, dying at the age of fifty-seven in an especially gruesome manner, "found on the floor burning to death," apparently because "she was lighting a lamp which was upset by one of her involuntary motions."[31]

And what of Phebe and Nancy's youngest sister, Lydia (1777–1870), who cared for their widowed mother, the elder Phebe, through the latter's long illness? In 1800, as a young unmarried woman, Lydia had had a son Edmund, whom she reportedly gave up for adoption to a wealthy childless East Hampton couple. Four years later she married an East Hampton weaver, William Bennett, from a modest local family, and had a second son, William A. Bennett, who became a whaling captain, married, and eventually died at sea at the age of forty-nine. Edmund, meanwhile, stayed behind in East Hampton, where he married in his mid-twenties, had six surviving children, and held the office of town trustee for several years. He became relatively well-to-do later in his life and died at the advanced age of ninety.[32]

Although Lydia was only thirty-two when her husband died, in 1809, she never remarried. Indeed, three women in this family, all widowed in their thirties, remained widows—not only Lydia but also her mother, the elder Phebe Tillinghast, and Phebe's granddaughter Margaret Cartwright. We may speculate whether their continuing widowhood had anything to do with St. Vitus's dance, such as fear on the part of prospective spouses or their own desire to avoid having more children. But since many widows of this era remained single, this situation does not appear unusual. As it happened, Lydia never developed St. Vitus's dance, nor did any of her children or grandchildren, a circumstance that I believe was crucial to George Huntington's later construction of the hereditary pattern of the disease, as we shall see. Following her husband's death, she lived on for another sixty years. In 1870, just two years before Huntington published "On Chorea," she died at the age of ninety-three.[33]

This picture suggests that, outwardly at least, the children and grandchildren of Phebe Hedges and her sisters lived much as their neighbors lived in East Hampton, as marriage partners, parents, and participants in town and church affairs. While many East Hampton individuals showed up in the church sessions records for such misdeeds as "rumoured intemperance" (October 10, 1854), "leading an immoral life" (March 31, 1856), or having a manner of life and language "not becoming to professors of religion" (March 8, 1885), few belonged to the families of Phebe Hedges and her sisters. I have found scant mention of this family in the records of the Overseers of the Poor, or in minutes of the Suffolk County courts; they do not appear as inmates at the Suffolk County Asylum at Yaphank, although in the 1870s and 1880s there were several residents with "St. Vitus's dance" and "chorea" who came from nearby towns. When one of Phebe Hedges's relatives appears in the town records, it is most often as a trustee or supervisor or holder of another local office. In short, they are notably absent from local records where evidence of social conflict, antisocial behavior and abandonment often turns up.[34]

Of course, elite families were sometimes able to avoid penalties and hush up unwanted publicity: for instance, in January 1860 the town went into "a ferment of excitement" when a young member of (a different branch of) the Hedges family got into a "midnight scrape at the hotel" with the hotelkeeper, who brought charges of "assault with a deadly weapon" and "attempted murder" against his assailant. Although Hedges was arrested, a few days later Mary Huntington noted in her diary that the "court [was] dissolved, prisoner discharged and the business silenced—everybody feeling bewildered—some glad but more mad—." In contrast, three years earlier, when George Floyd, a poor young black man from the town, shot the Huntingtons' neighbor, Captain Jeremiah Mulford, a wealthy white man, in an attempted robbery on the "turnpike" to Sag Harbor, wounding him but "not dangerously," according to George Lee Huntington, who treated the victim, Floyd was arrested, tried, and sent to prison.[35]

In short, official records of social conflict may be shaped by private interests. Archives are incomplete. Evidence of rejection, abandonment, and abuse may go missing. And social integration did not preclude psychic suffering. Caregiving responsibilities alone would have been enormous, especially when relatives reached the later stages of the disease. That family members avoided talking about it or, if it was absolutely necessary, did so with "a kind of horror," refusing to say the name and mentioning it only as "that disorder," as George Huntington wrote, suggests intense anxiety and shame.[36]

And then there were those who began developing the symptoms and found themselves going down the long road of the disease. These individuals are the most difficult to capture in the historical records, as they left no direct testimony and often ceased to act in public roles. We have seen how Phebe Hedges's "extreme dread" of St. Vitus's dance apparently drove her to end her life. However, George Huntington emphasized also that if some ended their own lives, others faced the illness with a stoic and resigned attitude, a stance deeply rooted in East Hampton's Calvinist traditions. These individuals knew the outcome so well that they rarely consulted a doctor, even after symptoms began, working "at their trades long after the choreic features had developed." They "lived on if not content, still seemingly reconciled to Fate, until mind and body both exhausted they fell asleep."[37]

SEEING ST. VITUS'S DANCE

In considering the local meanings of St. Vitus's dance, it is useful to recall that mid-nineteenth-century East Hampton was a town imbued with a deep sense of the precariousness and uncertainty of life. Accidents were frequent, with fingers caught in farm machinery, fatal falls from mills and haystacks, and tumbles from farm wagons with runaway horses trampling people underfoot, drownings, shootings, burns, and axe and knife wounds. While visitors considered the town a "healthy" place, physical illness was ubiquitous, not only in the ledgers of the Huntington physicians but in East Hampton letters and diaries noting cases of the measles, "pleurisies and great colds," dysentery, headache, toothache, "pukings," fevers, smallpox, typhoid, lockjaw, and of course "that dread disease consumption," from which entire families sometimes perished. Except for the fact that consumption typically killed younger people, the analogies between the impact of this illness—which was also considered hereditary—and St. Vitus's dance are striking. Here is Cornelia Huntington mourning the death of a friend in 1824: "Poor Gassner—what a severe disappointment to him—to see his beautiful bride thus gradually sinking to the grave with the sad conviction that he cannot save her—if man could prevent or money purchase relief—Caroline Gassner would not die—but alas hers is a disease which has cut off every member of her family in the prime of life—consumption—hopeless—cureless—and poor Caroline is the last of the race—the final victim—of that fatal constitutional consumption which had previously deprived her of all her relatives."[38]

East Hampton letter writers, diarists, and memoirists also took note of their neighbors with mental disabilities or emotional ills, portraying them with empathy, anxiety, and sometimes disapproval. For instance, in 1855 Fanny Huntting noted in her journal that she had just visited her sister-in-law and "found her comfortable in body and mind. about 4 weeks ago she came home from the Lunatic Asylum in Brattleboro where she has been for 8 years. What greater affliction can befall us," Huntting added, "than to be deprived of our reason." And when Jonathon Parson made a second attempt, in 1856, to kill himself by cutting his throat with a razor, Huntting reflected, as if she too had been tempted, "how much we have to pray 'Lord lead us not into temptation.'" In a less anxious vein, Cornelia Huntington remarked on the loss to the community of a villager known as "Zekial," who had "filled his place according to his capacity," though "denied the powers of mental gifts and graces." Adding that "one of the characters of the place will be lost to us," she implied that he had a recognized position in the town, despite, or perhaps because of, his disabilities. Zekial would be missed, she noted, if not mourned.[39]

In this setting, then, where illness, accidents, and disability were an accepted part of everyday discourse, the paucity of allusions to St. Vitus's dance is striking. Indeed, people referred more to this silence than to the subject itself, as for example when the teenage Frances Sage observed, in 1815, writing to her friend apropos St. Vitus's dance, "I believe it is not much spoken of." This taboo on speech is especially notable since—as we shall see—the evidence indicates that people with St. Vitus's dance in nineteenth-century East Hampton were quite visible in the community, working in their houses or yards, assisting at boarding houses, driving wagons, walking on the paths, and attending church: all places where they would be seen. Moreover, we know that people did talk about it on occasion because they had theories about how it had started. When questioned, they had answers: "John T. Dayton . . . told me some 40 or 50 years ago it was introduced into East Hampton first . . ."; "I have always heard this disorder—chorea as it exists now—came to East Hampton through . . ."; "Mrs. Ludlow . . . says that her grandmother said that St. Vitus Dance was introduced into Bridgehampton from Watermill," and so forth. The silence was not quite as absolute as it seemed.[40]

Those who did mention St. Vitus's dance (whether they referred to the temporary childhood malady or the incurable disorder mainly in adults) were distressed, frightened, and sometimes fascinated. Reporting to a friend that "Mrs. S. appears very dull and melancholy," Frances Sage explained that "her two younger daughters are afflicted with the St. Vitus's dance, which you know is a dreadful disease. I do not think she is sensible how bad they are, always being with them," Sage added, implying that familiarity may have lessened the horror of the illness. "But it disturbed me very much to see them."[41]

In a slightly different mode were the memories of the physician Clarence King, who grew up in the 1860s near Buffalo, New York, but whose father, a physician at the Cattaraugus County Insane Asylum, was from East Hampton and knew the same families as George Huntington. As a young doctor in the 1880s, King recalled "the fear and timidity which possessed me when in childhood I was obliged to pass one of these patients on my way to and from school."[42] Similarly, a great-great-great granddaughter of Phebe Hedges, born in East Hampton in 1903, recalled, some ninety years after the fact, the fear she felt as a small child when a man severely affected with St. Vitus's dance would come to her house to see her father. "We were always scared to death of him, because he shook so, you know," she recalled. "And one day we found a dagger in our shingle in the back entryway, and my father always thought that he brought it there. But you never knew, of course."[43]

If some neighbors responded to St. Vitus's dance with fear, others reacted as if to drunkenness—a common association with the gait disturbances of chorea and one that nineteenth-century East Hampton, with its many followers of temperance, was not likely to overlook. George Huntington probably spoke for many of his East Hampton neighbors when he noted the behavior of "two married men, whose wives are living, and who are constantly making love to some young lady, not seeming to be aware that there is any impropriety in it. They are suffering from chorea to such an extent that they can hardly walk," he added, "and would be thought by a stranger to be intoxicated. They are men of about 50 years of age, but never let an opportunity to flirt with a girl go by unimproved. The effect is ridiculous in the extreme." In her interviews with older people in East

Hampton in 1912—and in other communities as well—Elizabeth Muncey also reported several disapproving allusions to alcoholism, suggesting that observers read the symptoms of St. Vitus's dance in relation to the signs of drunkenness: "the neighbors thought he was drinking excessively"; "he reeled through the streets"; "for years he went about the town jerking, twitching and reeling worse than a drunkard"; "it was impossible to tell whether his gait was controlled by the disease or by the excessive use of alcohol."[44]

Of course, some of those afflicted with Huntington's chorea evidently did use alcohol as part of a strategy of self-medication. In describing someone with Huntington's as "alcoholic," as "a heavy drinker," or as suffering from an "addiction to alcohol," Muncey's informants in East Hampton and elsewhere implied that their symptoms stemmed both from drink and from chorea. The fact that observers linked chorea with drunkenness in their descriptions of men more often than of women suggests that responses to the visual image of chorea may have been gendered, with choreic men more likely than women to be perceived as drunk. On the other hand, men more often reported that they used alcohol as a strategy to alleviate symptoms of chorea. They were also more apt to be out and about in the community, where their neighbors could see them. Women were less visible in general.[45]

In this context, George Huntington's memory of his first boyhood encounter with persons with chorea is striking. "Driving with my father through a wooded road leading from East Hampton to Amagansett," he recalled, "we suddenly came upon two women, mother and daughter, both tall, thin, almost cadaverous, both bowing, twisting, grimacing. I stared in wonderment, almost in fear. What could it mean?" In memory, George Lee's neighborly, sympathetic response—"my father paused to speak with them and we passed on"—helped to mute his son's fear and stir his youthful curiosity and interest. As George Huntington recalled, "Then my Gamaliel-like instruction began; my medical education had its inception. From this point on my interest in the disease has never wholly ceased."[46]

George Huntington reported this event in 1909, half a century or more after it occurred, as part of a presentation to the New York Neurological Society. The meeting on the road soon became an iconic moment and foundational scene in the history of Huntington's disease. Yet it is difficult to believe that the memory of an encounter that had occurred fifty years earlier would not have been altered by subsequent experiences, perhaps compressing many encounters into one emotionally charged scene. Whether or not the memory of his own intense response was literally true, the more neutral background portrait of his father greeting the two women as neighbors probably was, suggesting another of the modes in which East Hampton villagers responded to the "visual disruption" of St. Vitus's dance.[47]

SCRUTINY, SILENCE, AND ST. VITUS'S DANCE

An episode that occurred in the late 1880s further illuminates the feelings of the East Hampton families, both affected and unaffected, in relation to St. Vitus's dance. William Osler, a young Canadian-born physician who at that time was a professor at the University of Pennsylvania School of Medicine, had begun preparing lectures on chorea, based on records of 410 cases at the Philadelphia Orthopedic Hospital and Infirmary for Nervous Diseases, where he had just been appointed as attending physician. While most of these patients had suffered from childhood or Sydenham's chorea, Osler was intrigued by the "hereditary chorea" that he had read about in George Huntington's 1872 paper. In the summer of 1887 he wrote to Huntington at his home in LaGrangeville, New York, a small town in Dutchess County, asking for additional information.[48]

Osler's inquiry came at a time of dramatic change in the United States. Waves of so-called "new immigrants" from southern and eastern Europe, mostly Jews and Catholics, had begun to swell the population, providing cheap labor for the rapid growth of industry, which in turn created new extremes of urban wealth and poverty. In response, workers organized unions and demanded better working conditions while women, now entering colleges and universities, campaigned for the vote and legal equality. The defeat of Reconstruction in 1876 had ended the post–Civil War effort at racial justice in the South, sending many formerly enslaved African Americans and their descendants into northern cities to escape a growing epidemic of lynching and to seek educational and job opportunities. In the face of these changes, white middle-class men grew defensive and anxious, blaming urban slums, crime, economic crises, and labor militancy on the foreign-born and the poor.[49]

In this climate many intellectuals turned to the increasingly popular theory of degeneration as an explanation for social ills. Degeneration theory was first articulated by the French psychiatrist Bénédict Augustin Morel in his 1857 text, *Traité de dégéneréscences physiques, intellectuelles et morales de l'espèce humaine* (Treatise on the physical, intellectual, and moral degeneration of the human race). Morel argued that the problems of modern society caused a progressive deterioration of humans from one generation to the next, through the cumulative impact of environmental, social, and biological assaults. Thus parents increasingly transmitted to their offspring a "neuropathic constitution" that

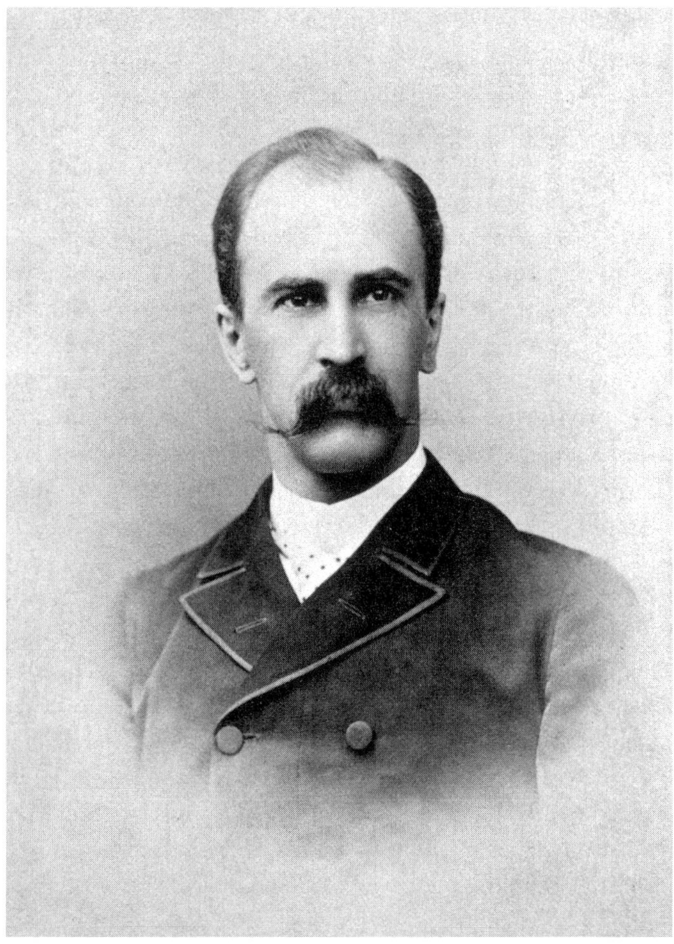

William Osler (1849–1919), 1886. U.S. National Library of Medicine

rendered them vulnerable to a succession of diseases, leading finally to sterility and the extinction of the family.[50]

Degeneration theory achieved its greatest influence in the 1880s, as an explanation for social as well as physical ills. As the historian Daniel Pick has put it, the problems of history increasingly were displaced onto the terrain of heredity. Meanwhile, Darwin's theory of evolution by natural selection, put forth in *The Origin of Species* in 1859, brought questions of heredity to the forefront of biological thinking, especially the puzzle of how random variations in one generation managed to persist in successive generations, thereby contributing to the process of evolutionary change. Darwin's cousin, the English scientist Francis

Galton, added to this dialogue by challenging the almost universally accepted notion that acquired characteristics could be transmitted to offspring. Galton argued that education and other environmental advantages could not influence biological heredity, which alone was responsible for persons of outstanding achievement. Calling for strategies of "improvement" and progress, Galton in 1883 coined the word *eugenics*, by which he meant improving the human race by encouraging the reproduction of the so-called fittest while discouraging or preventing marriage and childbearing among the allegedly unfit.[51]

In this increasingly hereditarian cultural milieu William Osler sent off his letter to George Huntington, inquiring about the East Hampton families with chorea. In reply Huntington urged Osler to visit the town for himself, since there were "several typical and marked cases, at and near East Hampton," whom Osler could personally observe. But as Huntington had moved away more than a decade earlier and had no additional information about these families, he referred Osler to his friend Edward Osborn, who was practicing medicine in his old hometown.[52]

Osborn, born in 1836 to a wealthy long-established East Hampton farming family, was fourteen years older than George Huntington but had come later to medicine, having graduated from the College of Physicians and Surgeons in New York just two years earlier, in 1885, when he was forty-nine years old. He was famous in town for his devotion to the poor, often walking long distances to care for the sick, and making house calls in Springs and in the hamlet of Freetown, where he conducted a Sunday school for black children for twenty years. Though some people said he was a better nurse than he was a physician, "he made up in faithfulness to duty and kind-hearted charity what he may have lacked in skill." He not only doctored "but often clothed, fed, and even buried those people he found in want."[53]

Osborn showed great empathy toward the families with what physicians in the 1880s increasingly called hereditary or Huntington's chorea. He replied to Osler that there were "perhaps four families in which the disorder exists & in which the symptoms are at present more or less manifest." These families were, however, "people whom it would be a delicate matter to approach upon the subject of their peculiar condition," "& whom I should be very unwilling to bring into such notoriety." Osborn offered to help if he could do so "in any other less direct way." It was as if speaking to them about "their peculiar condition" was somehow crossing a forbidden boundary that would acknowledge it publicly and call it to the attention of the community. Even though Osborn was their physician, he too observed the code whereby this malady was not discussed in their presence, unless broached by them. Still, Osborn sent Osler train times and directions, im-

La Grangeville N.Y. July 2nd 1887
My dear Doctor
Your letter making
inquiry concerning Hereditary
Chorea is at hand, and in
reply I would state that
I have no facts in addition
to those published in the
Med. & Surgical Reporter to which
you make refference.—
Since my graduation I have
had no opportunity to study
the class of cases referred
to—much to my regret—and
can only refer you to my
friend Dr Edw. Osborn of
East Hampton, Long Island N.Y.
who may have acquired
facts in addition to those
mentioned in my article

George Huntington (1850–1916) to William Osler, July 2, 1887. "I have no facts in addition to those published in The Medical and Surgical Reporter." Courtesy Osler Library of the History of Medicine, McGill University, Montreal

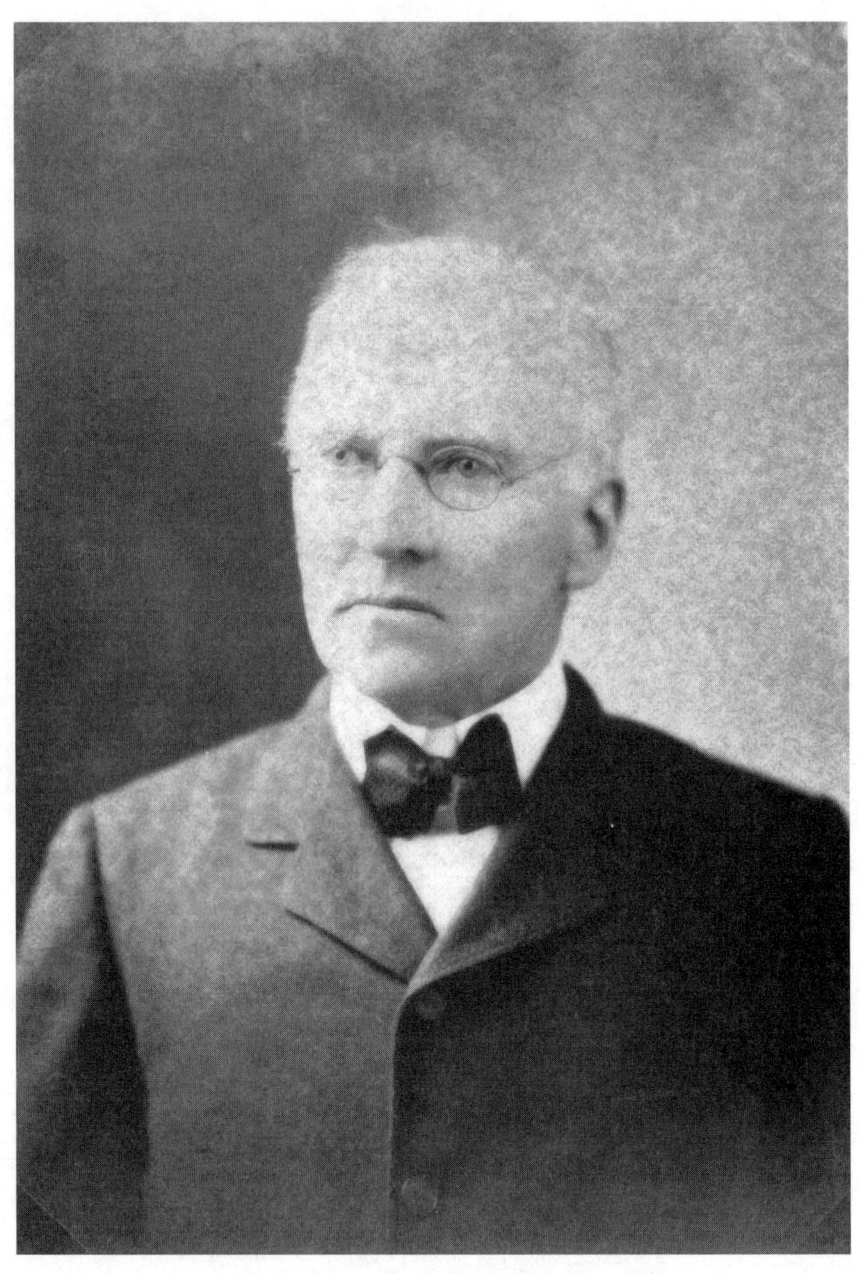

Edward Osborn (1836–1905), East Hampton physician.
Courtesy Pennypacker Long Island Collection, East Hampton Library

East Hampton N.Y.
June 15. 88

Prof. Wm. Osler.

My dear Sir.

Your letter - also the documents came duly. thanking you I would say. that there is no way in which I can bring these people into notice. they are doubtless very sen-sitive upon the subject of their weakness, & they are all friends of mine & it will never answer for <u>me</u> to approach them. The one case now - in which the dis-ease is developing. is that of a young woman about 40 years of age. whose mother died with the malady - also her brother - uncle &c. She lives here in E.H. with her sister - who has no

Edward Osborn to William Osler, June 15, 1888. "They are doubtless very sensitive upon the subject of their weakness, & they are all friends of mine & it will never answer for *me* to approach them." Courtesy Osler Library of the History of Medicine, McGill University, Montreal plying that he expected a visit. Osler, however, did not go. He later reported that Osborn had telegraphed him right before he planned to depart for Long Island, indicating that "it was impossible and not to come." Osborn had told him, he said, that "the subjects were so sensitive that he did not think I could get access to them if I came."[54]

The following year, 1888, Osler again wrote to Huntington, who replied with more direct encouragement to visit, recommending a certain boarding house in East Hampton "which would afford you an excellent opportunity for the study of the peculiar form of Chorea in question." By the 1880s East Hampton had become a "picturesque" and fashionable destination, with artists building cottages in the woods and crowds of visitors arriving to take rooms in the homes along Main Street converted for the summer into boarding houses. Huntington explained that the sister-in-law of this particular boarding house owner "has her home there and, as I am informed, is a victim of hereditary Chorea, a *marked*" case but not "to an excessive degree." Moreover, within a few miles of this boarding house, "in the Village of Amagansett, I am informed there are a number of bad cases," people whom Osler could also visit. Huntington went on to tell Osler that he himself intended to visit his mother in East Hampton the following month, and "I should be pleased to see and become acquainted with you, and aid you in any way possible in the study of the disease."[55]

Osborn too replied to another inquiry from Osler, explaining once again that "there is no way in which I can bring these people into notice. They are doubtless very sensitive upon the subject of their weakness, & they are all friends of mine & it will never answer for *me* to approach them." But Osborn seconded the invitation initially offered by George Huntington. "If you care to you could come to E.H. and take board in the family," he wrote, "& then be able to *observe* the case if no more. You could do this & not excite suspicion because the Sister . . . keeps a house for Summer boarders. & a very good one." Osborn suggested that Osler come around the middle of July "when other boarders get here. You would have a better chance to see her, as I think she assists about the house." Osborn added that the owners were "fine people & you would have a good place with them. You could apply by letter for board & say you have heard of their house as a good one." The family on the side of the owner's wife," he concluded, "have long had victims to the dire malady." Osborn again offered to "gladly do all I can to help you, but I must remain a *silent* partner."[56]

In the end, Osler decided for a second time not to make the trip to East Hampton, for reasons that remain unclear. But ten years after this exchange of letters, in early 1898, he wrote to Osborn for a third time. He was revising his medical textbook, *The Principles and Practice of Medicine*, and probably wished to update the information on Huntington's chorea. This time Osborn was more forthcoming, possibly because Osler was now a famous professor and physician-in-chief of the Johns Hopkins Hospital and School of Medicine in Baltimore. Moreover, Osler had become an authority on chorea, having published a lengthy paper in the *Journal of Nervous and Mental Disease* in 1893, and a monograph, *On Chorea and Choreiform Affections*, in 1894, both of which included discussions of the hereditary disease. Osborn also may have spoken to the affected families about Osler and learned that they were willing, possibly even eager, to see this distinguished physician who was interested in them. In any case, Osborn explained to Osler that there were two "fully developed instances—hereditary—now going on. They are dreadful subjects, the disease at its very worst. Entirely distinct families, one male one female." He promised that, "should you come—at any time to Long Island, there will be no difficulty in the way of meeting one of these present, active cases." Once more, however, Osler decided against it.[57]

The Osler episode illuminates how the affected families and their friends in East Hampton managed St. Vitus's dance in the late nineteenth century. In the first instance, by acting as a gatekeeper, Osborn may have hoped to shield these families from a visit that he believed would only heighten their anxieties. It was as if the families concerned could live relatively "normal" lives within the community so long as the subject was not openly discussed or acknowledged in their presence, so long as it did not cross a certain threshold. Once it was acknowledged—even to a physician, in private, from outside the town—it entered public discourse and was cause for shame and "notoriety." By 1898, however, the severity of the malady suffered by several individuals may have convinced him—and perhaps the family members as well—that a visit from the famous Osler had a potential medical benefit that was worth the possible social cost.[58]

In light of this episode, it is hardly surprising that in 1895, a prominent New York City neurologist, Landon Carter Gray, confirmed the sensitivity of the subject when he complained that the disease was surrounded by "a great superstition" that made it "very difficult to obtain much information about it. I can name at the present moment at least a dozen towns within easy reach of New York," he wrote, "in which it is very prevalent, and yet in which it is nursed as a dark secret."[59]

But as we have seen through Osler's experience, such secrecy in the late nineteenth century appears less superstition than a strategy embraced by the affected families and their friends to avoid embarrassment and public scrutiny, especially at a time when eugenic thinking was gaining in prominence. In 1908 the ninety-one-year-old Henry P. Hedges, who had spent all his life on eastern Long Island, confirmed this view. Though he did not mention St. Vitus's dance

H. P. Hedges
A HISTORY
—OF THE—
Town of East-Hampton, N. Y.,
Including an Address
Delivered at the Celebration of the Bi-Centennial Anniversary of its Settlement in 1849,
INTRODUCTIONS
To the four printed volumes of its Records, with other Historic Material, an
Appendix and Genealogical Notes
—BY—
HENRY P. HEDGES.
"They haunt your breezy hillsides, green vales and thundering floods,
They linger by your gliding streams and mid your moss-draped woods,
They sit beside your green old graves in shadow and in sheen,
And move among your household gods though voiceless and unseen.
Then ye who make your happy homes where once their homes have been,
Deem also this your heritage, to keep their memories green,
To shield within your heart of hearts, the glorious trust ye hold,
And bear unstained the names they bore, those brave, proud men of old."
—Cornelia Huntington.
SAG-HARBOR:
J. H. HUNT, PRINTER.
1897.

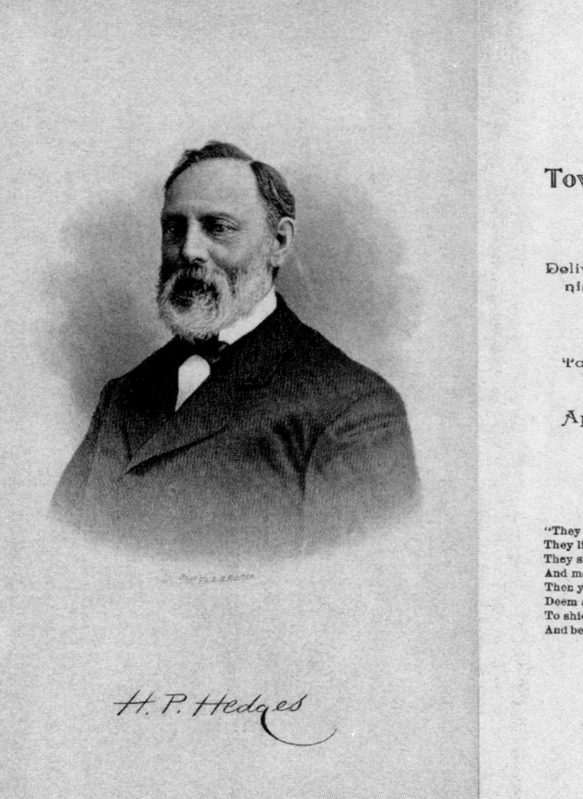

Henry P. Hedges (1817–1911), East Hampton–born attorney, judge, local historian, and friend of George Huntington. Wrote about "chorea, known in my youth only as St. Vitus Dance."
Courtesy Pennypacker Long Island Collection, East Hampton Library

or Huntington's chorea in his history of East Hampton, Hedges knew a lot about it: according to his friend George Huntington, "he is the *only* one on the ground whose memory can easily turn back for three quarters of a century or more, and who, as his name would indicate, has always been more or less interested in 'The Magrums' though his immediate family has never been invaded, I believe." Hedges was willing to discuss chorea with his old friend—"I could tell what I know easier than write," he told Huntington—but he did not entirely approve of such talk. "The subject," he wrote pointedly, "is avoided by most people as distasteful."[60]

WAS EAST HAMPTON AN EXCEPTION?

No doubt the integration of the families with St. Vitus's dance in East Hampton, like those with hereditary deafness on Martha's Vineyard, owed much to the shared cultural background of most of the white inhabitants over many generations, their sense of themselves as interrelated, and the long local history of the malady, going back many generations. A tradition of feeling embattled against outsiders may also have strengthened a sense of solidarity among East Hampton's white Presbyterian inhabitants. In a town with a deep reverence for ancestors and ancestry, organized around distinctions of race, religion, wealth, education, and also length of residence, the fact that the nineteenth-century families in question traced their ancestry to the town's Puritan English founders also undoubtedly played a role: what if the Montauk Rachel Pharoah and her descendants, or the African-American Isaac Plato, the white Methodist John Youngs, or the Jewish-born Aaron Isaacs and his descendants had suffered from St. Vitus's dance? The condition almost certainly would have carried different meanings within this community, shaped by the distinct social locations of those whom it touched.

Surprisingly, the perception that the condition was inherited seems to have muted its stigmatization, perhaps partly because the old families' conviction that they were all cousins "in some degree" made for "tolerance of each other's failings," as Jeanette Edwards Rattray, a local historian and distant descendant of Phebe Hedges, put it. As late as 1999, East Hampton citizens alluded to intermarriage as the origin of the illness. "Almost everyone was closely, maybe too closely, related to everyone else," reported an article in *Newsday*. "If inbreeding brought unanimity, it also brought misfortune. Huntington's disease, once known as Huntington's chorea, first was identified among old East Hampton families, for example." The stability of the community also encouraged forbearance. "Where the characters of fathers and grandfathers are remembered or are handed down by tradition," theorized the English psychiatrist Henry Maudsley in 1889, "peculiarities of character in an individual are often attributed to some hereditary bias, and so accounted for: he got it from his fore-elders, it is said, and the aberration has allowance made for it."[61]

Dense networks of kin were not unique to East Hampton, of course, although few other early New England towns seem to have had clusters of long-established families affected by this malady over many generations. Nor did they have such an enlightened household, over several generations, as that of the Huntingtons, who also helped define the context of St. Vitus's dance in East Hampton. While the evidence for comparison is sparse, it is worth noting that in other old New York and New England towns, perceptions if not practices surrounding families with this condition appear to have been more overtly negative. Dr. Irving Whitall Lyon, a predecessor of George Huntington who grew up in the 1840s and 1850s in Bedford, New York, in Westchester County, described a considerable stigma associated with the magrums (or migrims, as he called it) in his hometown, as well as in the nearby village of Pound Ridge and across the Connecticut border in Stamford and Greenwich, all towns closely related through ties of kinship.[62]

Writing in 1863, Lyon noted that the "migrims" in this locale was "regarded by many as a disgraceful disease," a stigma he attributed to a local "tradition" linking the disease to a curse "upon those who reviled and mimicked our Saviour while undergoing crucifixion," ensuring that they and their descendants were "ever after affected with choreal irregularities." Lyon added, however, that he found the stigmatization of the migrums difficult to understand, implying that not everyone associated it with disgrace. But as he told it, for an individual to admit that he had this "hereditary vice of constitution" was "injurious to his reputation and prospects in life," especially in relation to marriage, since parents in unaffected families "have repeatedly been known to interdict marriage alliances between their children and those believed to be tainted with the migrim diathesis, under the severe penalties of disinheritance and social ostracism."[63]

Seventy years later, as we shall see, Percy R. Vessie, the Connecticut psychiatrist, also reported the stigmatization of families in Stamford and Greenwich, where he practiced. In Vessie's version, those who considered themselves unrelated to the affected clans attributed the disease not to a hereditary curse but to excess intermarriage, which they believed resulted from the affected families' greed and desire to hold on to their "riches."[64]

Vessie did not report the views of those who regarded themselves as related to the families in question. But some of these family members told the story themselves. According to one early-twentieth-century narrator, the disease resulted from consanguineous marriages among the descendants of an aristocratic female ancestor, Anne Millington, who had come to Connecticut in the seventeenth century in search of her lover, who had run away to America. Although she failed to find him, she eventually settled in Connecticut, married and had children. Her carved wooden trunk, which her English family had supposedly filled with fine silks and gold coins, was passed down through the generations, a fetish object and emblem of their aristocratic lineage. "To keep up a relation with gentility," wrote Isabella Ferris, a distant relative, Ann Millington's descendants intermarried. "Somewhere . . . there was a taint in the blood. Magrums or chorea broke out and flourished in all directions."[65]

In this version, the magrums was a condition that affected almost the entire community. "Every member of a family might not have it but very few of the old families in Old Greenwich escaped some of its symptoms," Ferris wrote, "one of which is general all around cussedness—which occasionally I have myself." Joking that "marrying cousins and drinking wine is bad," Ferris recalled that "the query among the old folks was magrums or money, which. If there was money, they married in spite of the magrums."[66]

Significantly, while members of both affected and unaffected families agreed on a narrative of intermarriage in explaining the spread of the disease, the former made allowances and joked about the snobbery of their ancestors while they linked themselves with an aristocratic origin. They also tended to believe that the disease was becoming less prevalent. As Belle Ferris put it, "according to Billy Sunday, sin ends with the third or fourth generation—for *sterility sets* in!" Their unaffected neighbors were less forgiving. They blamed selfishness and greed for motivating the cousin marriages that they believed perpetuated the disease.[67]

A community in southwestern Minnesota offers a sharply different portrait of Huntington's outside the boundaries of the American Northeast and the cultural orbit of New England. The town of Lake Lillian was founded by a Norwegian Lutheran, a Reverend Bomstad, in the early 1860s—much later than East Hampton or the New England towns. He and his family built homes and were active in community affairs, holding many local offices for about thirteen years. Then in 1885 the Reverend Bomstad and his entire family disappeared from the town records. According to interviews, archival research, and oral histories carried out in the 1990s by Jerome Sundin, over the next three decades certain members of the Bomstad family began acting peculiarly. Some were hospitalized. Others committed suicide. Gradually the idea began to circulate in town that "being a Bomstad is a bad thing," and that family members were by definition crazy. Late-nineteenth- and early-twentieth-century local histories erased the Bomstads as the founders of the town. But such efforts at blaming or editing out the Bomstads were not entirely successful. By the turn of the century, a poem in the local newspaper suggested that the family stigma had spread to the entire town, where "'twas said that everybody there, were rascals, sots and rattlers."[68]

However, Lake Lillian was rent from the start by tensions between Norwegians and Swedes. Those who wrote the Bomstad family out of later local histories were descendants of the more affluent Swedish settlers who came to the region soon after the Norwegian Bomstads and acquired considerably more wealth. Eventually the Swedish members of the community gained the upper hand, while the Norwegian Bomstads were ostracized and looked down upon. Thus the social meaning of Huntington's chorea within Lake Lillian was shaped in part by ethnic rivalries, the disease serving as a convenient means for the dominant group to write off their rivals and an excuse for erasing their history. In this setting, fears of the disease appeared to exacerbate ethnic and economic rivalries, while cultural conflicts may also have intensified fears of the disease.

Disability theorists such as Paul Longmore tell us that "the physical effects of illness or injury constitute merely one dimension of disability. At its crux is the sociocultural meaning attributed to physiological conditions." The lives of Phebe Hedges and her sisters and their descendants represent one historical trajectory of St. Vitus's dance/hereditary chorea, in which the malady was a source of dread but was not an emblem of family exclusion. However specific to nineteenth-century East Hampton, their lives underscore the ways in which a disabling behavioral disorder perceived as inherited did not exclude or marginalize the families it touched. Thus a condition that was powerful and damaging in shaping family identity in one community, such as Lake Lillian, was far less significant in another.[69]

Of course, even in nineteenth-century East Hampton, as we have seen, affected individuals did at times experience the fear or ridicule of their neighbors; the fact that by the 1880s the disease was a source of "notoriety" if it was brought to public attention suggests that it certainly was not regarded with equanimity. Furthermore, by the early twentieth century, the illness that had become known in the medical profession as Huntington's chorea had acquired an even more pejorative identity, as an object of eugenic scrutiny and potential target for sterilization.

East Hampton residents whom I interviewed in the 1990s recalled hearing that families in earlier decades had sometimes hidden their affected members with severe symptoms behind blankets or sheets when visitors came to the house, or secluded them in bedrooms or attics so that the community would not know about them, though sometimes the motive was considered more protective: to keep disabled relatives out of danger while the family was away at work. Others recalled neighbors or relatives with Huntington's who stayed out of sight on their own volition, or socialized only with the immediate family to avoid the embarrassment of being seen.

And whether those with visible symptoms were hidden or out in the open, hospitalized or kept at home, the subject of St. Vitus's dance/Huntington's chorea was rarely discussed, within the affected families or outside. All the people with whom I spoke agreed that, like suicide and depression, the topic until recently was taboo. The silence surrounding the malady was so deep that even in the 1990s two men whose wives had died with the disease many years earlier did not know of their common situation, although they lived within a mile of each other and were acquainted. Some descendants of Phebe Hedges did not know of the illness in their ancestry; the disease had vanished in their lineage, and so had the memory of it.

Still, by the early 1970s, this silence had begun to break, at least in the pages of the local paper and in official accounts of the town. News about the advocacy work of Marjorie Guthrie, widow of songwriter Woody Guthrie, who had died with Huntington's in 1967, began to appear in the *East Hampton Star*, with allusions to the historical presence of the illness. One 1973 article acknowledged that George Huntington's paper "was an East Hampton story" and that "Dr. Huntington's Disease [is] Still with Us." An editorial in 1993 announcing the identification of the Huntington's disease gene also admitted that "old-timers here well know why The Star was interested in this genetic abnormality." Published obituaries began including the name of the disease, possibly for the first time since the notice of Phebe Hedges's death in the *Suffolk Gazette* in 1806 mentioned her "extreme dread" of St. Vitus's dance. By 1998, the year of the 350th anniversary of East Hampton's founding, George Huntington had become a figure of pride. During the celebration, a sign posted on the former Huntington home (the "Wickham" house) on Main Street noted George Huntington's contribution to medical science. Missing was the home of Phebe Hedges, which still haunts the maps of this disease.[70]

Community/Medicine

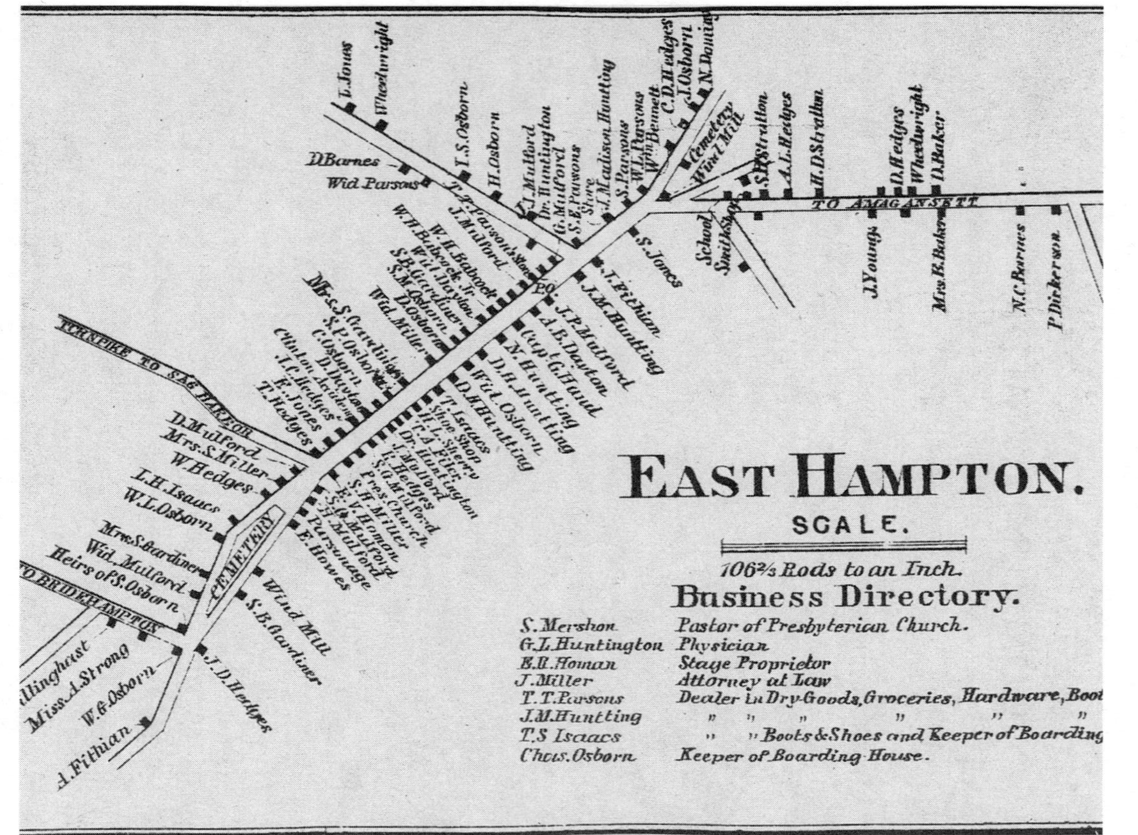

Map of East Hampton Village, 1858. From James Chace, "Map of Suffolk County, Long Island, New York" (Philadelphia: John Douglas, 1858)

3

INVENTING HEREDITARY CHOREA

The whole subject of inheritance is wonderful.
—Charles Darwin, *Variation in Plants and Animals Under Domestication*, 1868

In the annals of Huntington's disease, George Huntington has long been an iconic figure, his photograph featured in books and articles, his 1872 paper "On Chorea" memorialized in a centennial symposium in 1972, his life a topic for papers and Web sites. "In the whole range of descriptive nosology there is not, to my knowledge, an instance in which a disease has been so accurately and fully delineated in so few words," wrote William Osler in his 1893 paper on chorea. "No details were given; the original cases were not even (nor have they been) described, but to Huntingdon's [*sic*] account of the symptomatology no essential fact has been added."[1]

Still, it has long been acknowledged that George Huntington was not the first to describe such symptoms, as several nineteenth-century North Americans and at least one Norwegian preceded him. Indeed, medical writers have speculated that early modern European portrayals of chorea and St. Vitus's dance, as well as of mania, melancholia, epilepsy, and "lunatic ancestery," may well have included cases that would have been diagnosed later as hereditary or Huntington's chorea. So if medical writers before George Huntington described a similar complex of symptoms, why do we today associate it with his name? Why did "hereditary chorea" emerge as a distinct clinical entity only in the mid-nineteenth century if the symptoms were recognized long before? And why did the earliest medical reports appear in the United States, though the malady existed elsewhere as well?[2]

LOCAL KNOWLEDGE AND THE DISCOURSE OF HEREDITY

In the late eighteenth century, chorea in children, though familiar to physicians for centuries, began to attract heightened medical attention, possibly due to an increased incidence of rheumatic fever or "rheumatism," a common childhood malady. Practitioners now began to pay more attention to the episodes of chorea that frequently appeared in the aftermath of such fevers, especially as they became aware that rheumatic fever often led to serious damage of the heart. This eighteenth-century discourse on postrheumatic chorea in children formed the medical background for discussions of chorea in adults.[3]

For the most part, clinicians in the late eighteenth and early nineteenth centuries presented occasional adult cases of chorea as distinctive because of the advanced age of the patients. In his 1774 classic *The Practice of Physic*, for example, the Scottish physician William Cullen described a forty-two-year-old man with chorea. In 1825 Thomas Jeffreys, a doctor in Liverpool, wrote up the case of an attorney who for twenty-seven years, from age fifty-four until his death at eighty-one, suffered miserably from chorea, although evidently without mental and emotional symptoms. Jeffreys believed there were "numerous instances" of chorea occurring beyond the age of puberty, even though such cases were usually considered anomalies. Other clinicians testified that they rarely encountered adults with chorea. "I have been able to find but a single case in the books, of Chorea in so old an individual," wrote one Ohio physician in 1832 of his sixty-nine-year-old female patient with St. Vitus's dance.[4]

But by the 1830s physicians had begun noting certain peculiarities in their adult cases of chorea. For instance, in his 1832 lecture at St. Thomas's Hospital in London, the physician John Elliotson remarked that this malady in adults was "frequently connected with paralysis or idiotism" and was often incurable. "It then appears to arise for the most part from something in the original constitution of the body," he added casually, "for I have often seen it hereditary." These differences from ordinary childhood chorea did not arouse much interest, however. As we have seen, lay and learned people alike assumed that most nervous conditions had a hereditary component, but this was not an important concern. (Note that *hereditary* could mean transmitted from one generation to the next or shared by siblings in the same generation.) Hereditary predisposition was merely one of many malleable influences that determined whether a given individual might develop symptoms of any disease. In the chorea of older people, age, not ancestry, was the point.[5]

In 1842 a lengthy description of the "magrums" appeared for the first time in a medical text classifying chorea, dementia, incurability, and adult onset together

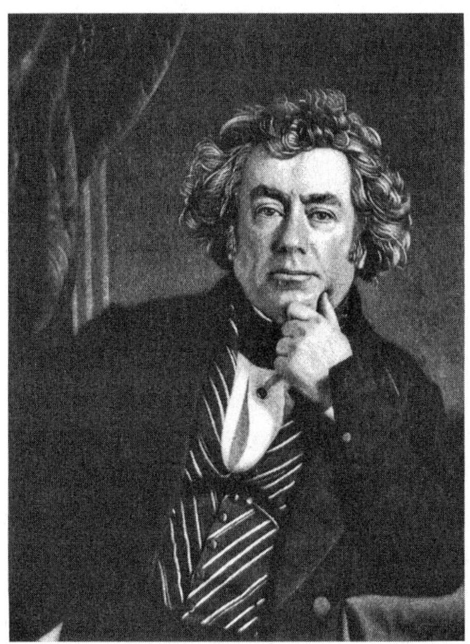

Robley Dunglison (1798–1869), professor of Institutes of Medicine, Jefferson Medical College of Philadelphia, ca. 1846. Engraving by A. H. Ritchie from a daguerreotype by M. P. Simons. U.S. National Library of Medicine

under the sign of heredity. The circumstances of its writing were revealing. The author, Charles Oscar Waters (1816–92), a twenty-six-year-old recent graduate of the Jefferson Medical College of Philadelphia, had asked his professor at the college, Dr. Robley Dunglison, about this malady, which Waters said "prevailed in a part of the country with which he was familiar." As Dunglison had never seen a case, he asked Waters to describe it, and then included the description in his 1842 textbook *The Practice of Medicine.* In his letter to Dunglison, Waters portrayed what he called "a singular affection" that was "somewhat common" in the southeastern part of New York (Westchester County). Waters called it "a peculiar modification of chorea," emphasizing its adult onset, its ending in dementia, and the fact that "when once it has appeared . . . it clings to its suffering victim with unrelenting tenacity till death comes to his relief."[6]

Waters especially emphasized the condition's "markedly hereditary" character. He had "never known a case of it to occur in a patient," he wrote, "one or both of whose ancestors were not, within the third generation at farthest, the subjects of this distressing malady." As nineteenth-century physicians generally assumed that diseases could skip several generations, to reappear in the descendants, a phenomenon known as atavism, a disorder that might skip two at most was unusual. Waters summed up other differences from what he called "ordinary chorea. 1st. It rarely occurs before adult age. 2d. It never ceases spontaneously. 3d. When fully developed it wants the paroxysmal character." Waters speculated that its pathology was "in the main the same" as in ordinary chorea, and that this disease would "probably be found to yield to the treatment most suited to chorea, if to any?"[7]

Despite its publication in Dunglison's widely circulated textbook, Waters's account awakened little interest. But over the next thirty years, at least four additional accounts of the magrums, hereditary St. Vitus's dance, and hereditary chorea appeared in medical publications on both sides of the Atlantic—all of which were written without awareness of their predecessors. Soon after Waters, another of Dunglison's medical students at Jefferson, Charles R. Gorman (1817–79), wrote his thesis on the magrums, having seen it in northern Pennsylvania, where he grew up. Unlike Waters, Gorman emphasized psychological factors—"the sympathy of imitation"—as a cause of the malady, since it "seems to be circumscribed by neighbourhood boundaries," among people interrelated in their social or business relations. (However, since we know of Gorman's thesis only from Dunglison's excerpt in the 1848 edition of his textbook—the thesis itself was lost—it is unclear whether Gorman omitted heredity as a factor in the magrums, or whether he mentioned it as a predisposing influence but Dunglison failed to note it.)[8]

A third account twelve years later, written by a Norwegian district physician, Johan Christian Lund (1830–1906), also described "chorea St. Vitus" as he had encountered it in the valley of Saetesdal, in southern Norway. Lund's report noted that people there called it "the twitches" or "the inherited disease." Although he marked the age of onset as between fifty and sixty—considerably later than other writers—he described a progression of symptoms similar to that portrayed by Waters: the movements that began gradually and increased in intensity, and the mental losses that progressed to dementia "during the last days of their lives." Lund included what may be the earliest published family tree of this disease, showing a familiar pattern of heredity in which a disease might fail to appear in one generation but could reappear in the next.[9]

Lund's account of "chorea St. Vitus" in Saetesdal was published as part of a government report on health and medical conditions in Norway in 1860. It was the only one of the early descriptions to be cited immediately in the medical press, excerpted in the landmark 1862 *Handbuch der historisch-geographischen Pathologie* (Handbook of historical and geographic pathology) by the distinguished German professor of geographical medicine August Hirsch. Unfortunately, Hirsch referred to Lund's report as an account of paralysis agitans, thereby obscuring its connection with other descriptions of chorea. The following year, with no knowledge of Lund or his predecessors, Irving W. Lyon, the physician from Bedford, New York, whom we met earlier, published a fourth account of the magrums, based on several families in and around his hometown. His was the first to use the name "hereditary chorea" and the first full report to appear in a medical journal.[10]

In certain respects, Lyon's portrayal, in *The American Medical Times*, was less complete than that of either Waters or Lund. It omitted any mention of mental disturbance or dementia and suggested that the disease might begin in childhood and continue throughout a long life without interfering "materially" with the person's "general health": a description that has led some authors to conclude that Lyon's cases suffered from benign chorea rather than Huntington's. However, in the 1880s the Philadelphia neurologist Wharton Sinkler diagnosed with "hereditary chorea" a descendant of the Bedford kinships known to Lyon and others as "migrim families," which leads me to conclude that Lyon was discussing the same disease. In fact, Lyon especially emphasized its "hereditary transmissibility," underscoring to a much greater extent than his predecessors the significance and "real interest" of this disease, which was "unlike in its origin to anything described in our standard text books." Since "many physicians are daily observing just what has been described," Lyon urged them to publish additional cases.[11]

Lyon's invitation, however, drew no takers. Like the others, this paper attracted no notice for twenty-six years, until the middle of 1889, by which time Lyon, who had been a twenty-three-year-old assistant physician at Bellevue Hospital in New York City when he wrote the paper, was almost fifty and retired from medicine altogether.

It is tempting to ask why these accounts emerged only now, if the symptoms associated with hereditary chorea had almost certainly existed for decades, if not centuries, before the 1830s. Some have suggested that low life expectancy may have contributed to the relative invisibility of the hereditary factor in chorea even at this time. According to this argument, in an era of low life expectancy, even those who lived long enough to have children were often likely to have died before they themselves became affected. Any offspring who later developed the ill-

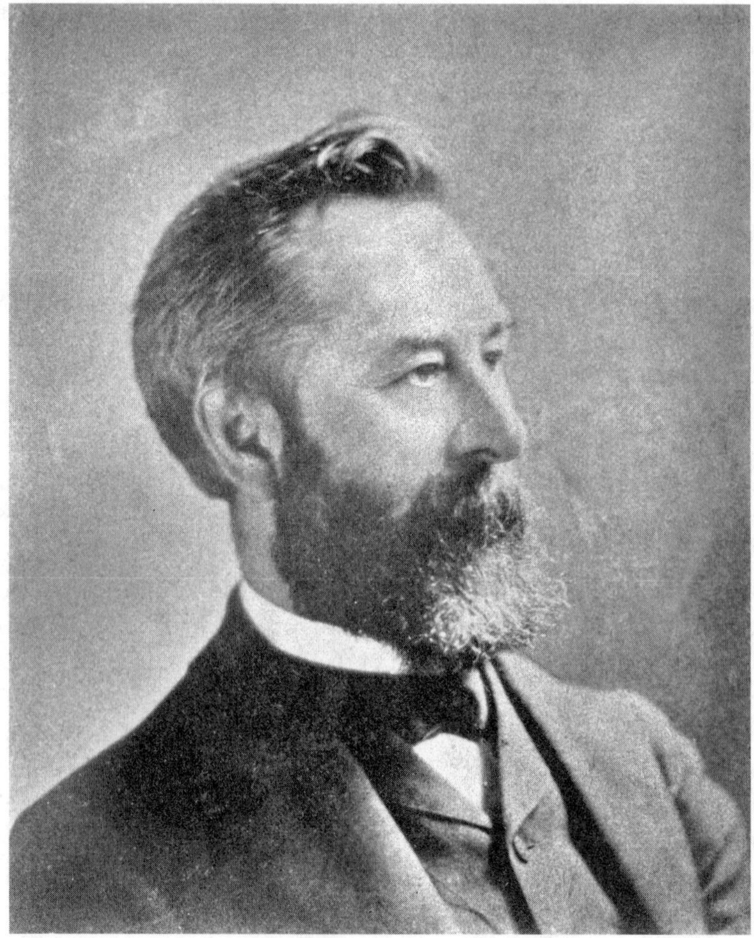

Irving W. Lyon (1840–96), physician from Bedford, Westchester County, New York. Courtesy Winterthur Library: Joseph Downs Collection of Manuscripts and Printed Ephemera

ness would have been unlikely to have a parent with the same condition, "which would tend to conceal the hereditary nature of the condition and would cause the fairly frequent appearance of individuals with chronic incurable chorea, but no apparent family history of the condition." In a population that was relatively young, with the expectation of life fairly low, there would have been many more young persons who were destined to develop the disease in the future if they lived long enough than there were older individuals manifesting symptoms in the present. As the English neurologist David L. Stevens put it, "the gene that causes the disease was no less common then than it is now, but fewer carriers of this gene lived long enough to develop chorea. Thus the chances of this hereditary basis being recognized, let alone documented, would have been small."[12]

This argument fails to explain, however, why the first medical descriptions of the magrums and "hereditary chorea" did emerge in the early part of the nineteenth century, *before* any significant increase in life expectancy occurred. These accounts may have been few and sporadic, but they nonetheless appeared at a historical moment when life expectancy at birth was not so different from what it had been for the previous several centuries, both in England and in New England.

As the demographers E. A. Wrigley and R. S. Schofield point out in their *Population History of England, 1541–1871*, throughout the period 1820–70 life expectancy at birth was only a few years higher than it was in the reign of Elizabeth I, three hundred years earlier. Indeed, infants born in England in 1601, toward the end of the Elizabethan era, could expect, at birth, to live about thirty-eight years, while those born in 1831 might anticipate reaching forty-one. In the United States, life expectancy did not rise substantially until the late nineteenth century.[14]

Moreover, while infant and child mortality was high in early New England, those who survived to age twenty had a greater than 50 percent chance of living to the age of sixty. In mid-seventeenth-century New Hampshire, white colonists who survived to the age of twenty could expect to live to between sixty-two and sixty-seven years of age, about the same age as the citizens of Massachusetts who turned twenty in 1878 or even in 1890. Many children grew up with at least one grandparent.[15]

It seems likely, then, that even before the nineteenth century, a substantial proportion of those destined to pass on St. Vitus's dance or magrums to their children did in fact live long enough to become symptomatic themselves: women like Phebe Hedges's mother, who died a grandmother in 1811 at the age of seventy-one, and men like Hiram Hedges's father, who died in 1833 at the age of forty-seven. While many more gene carriers would have died during the first twenty years of life, those who lived long enough to marry and have children would also have tended to live into the age range of the disease. Even if a symptomatic parent died before a son or daughter showed the dreaded signs, the characteristics of parents and grandparents were handed down in memory and tradition; they would certainly be remembered. In short, the emergence of medical accounts of hereditary chorea in the early nineteenth century cannot be linked to significant increases in life expectancy.

A more plausible explanation points toward the opening of what the historians Staffan Müller-Wille and Hans-Jörg Rheinberger have called a new epistemic or conceptual space of heredity. In a variety of fields, from sheep breeding to horticulture to medicine to biology to popular social thought and politics, biological heredity on both sides of the Atlantic emerged as a powerful intellectual domain. The eighteenth-century movement of animals and plants from their so-called "natural" environments into new ones had raised many questions about the interactions of biological and environmental influences in producing desirable offspring. Motivated by commercial ambitions, breeders and horticulturalists in England and across Europe conducted experiments to explore how to maintain the fine qualities of imported Spanish merino sheep or Arabian horses when these were bred and raised outside their "natural" environments. At a time when most naturalists focused their attention on issues of development—how the embryo develops into a mature organism—these practical breeders were thinking about the transmission of traits from one generation to the next.[16]

The dislocation of Africans and Europeans under slavery and colonialism also heightened preoccupation with heredity, placing it at the center of a discourse on race. If Portuguese settlers in Africa continued to have white children while Africans in Europe and America had dark-skinned descendants, what did these continuities imply about heredity? As Peter Bowler has written, race provided "a model for the subsequent development of hereditarian ideologies," a glaring exception to the almost universally accepted nineteenth-century view that acquired characteristics could be transmitted to subsequent generations.[17]

In medicine, too, heredity was becoming more prominent in accounts of disease etiology, especially in France. Among French physicians, as the historian Carlos López Beltrán has shown, the noun *hérédité* emerged for the first time in the 1830s. By the 1840s in the United States, heredity was increasingly pervasive and popular in explanations of disease and social dysfunction, blamed for everything from poor health to poverty. Whereas hereditary disease had formerly implied such "aristocratic" disorders as gout, now the concept was coming to be associated with "degenerative" maladies of the poor, such as consumption and madness. The meanings of heredity did not change; heredity still encompassed both the transmission of traits and the influences of early development. Until the 1880s almost everyone accepted that acquired influences could be passed on to offspring. But within a few decades, heredity would shift from an important, predisposing factor in many physical and mental conditions to a main (if not *the* main) element responsible for disease. As López Beltrán puts it, "Hereditary transmission had never before been looked at as a subject of special analytical and theoretical interest. Then, in a few years, it was all over the place."[18]

The early medical history of the magrums and "hereditary chorea," then, belongs to this broader cultural history of heredity. However, the emergence of heredity as an important intellectual domain raises yet another question. In light of the growing cultural pervasiveness of heredity, why did these accounts strike no responsive chord among physicians? Why were they greeted with silence?

Certainly these early descriptions were not obscure. Robley Dunglison, as we have seen, was a prominent professor at one of the most prestigious medical schools in the country, a former physician to Thomas Jefferson and a prolific writer whose textbooks and dictionaries were widely used in medical school courses and in doctors' offices. August Hirsch, who had commented on Lund's description, was an eminent German medical professor whose *Handbuch* was considered a major publication. The *American Medical Times*, where Lyon's paper had appeared, was a respectable journal.

Nor were persons with the magrums or St. Vitus's dance entirely invisible to clinicians. A few adult patients with diagnoses of the magrums or St. Vitus's dance had been showing up in North American hospitals and asylums at least since the 1840s, without eliciting much interest. For instance, of a woman who appeared in 1848 at the Bloomingdale Asylum in New York City with "mania accompanied by St. Vitus's dance," the admitting psychiatrist noted that her father, brother, and sister all had the same disease ("chorea"); the father had committed suicide, and the brother and sister both had become "imbecile." Another woman admitted to Bloomingdale the following year was diagnosed as "insane from religious excitement," with "a brother and two maternal uncles having been insane, and several members of her father's family, so says her husband, dying of the *Megrims*."[19]

It is likely that since physicians at this time still assumed that heredity played a role in most nervous disorders, the hereditary dimension of the magrums and St. Vitus's dance did not appear unusual. As the eminent French medical professor Armand Trousseau put it bluntly two decades later in his textbook discussion of childhood chorea: why should not St. Vitus's dance "be subjected to the same law as all nervous diseases in which hereditary predisposition holds such an important place." Still, hereditary predisposition differed sharply from the relatively rare hereditary disease—one that was directly inherited from the parent, apart from any exciting or triggering factors. In general during the mid-nineteenth century, rare conditions such as polydactyly (extra fingers or toes) and color blindness, which were known to be inherited directly, failed to arouse much interest. "Since no one *doubted* that disease and deformity could be hereditary," writes Charles Rosenberg, "these were seen as atypically clear examples of a general and unquestioned truth—too rare and too intractable to serve as appropriate challenges to the physicians' intellectual and clinical skills."[20]

What distinguished those early practitioners who did take an interest in the magrums and (adult) St. Vitus's dance was that all of them had either lived in towns or villages with affected families as their neighbors, or passed through such places on their travels. They had all encountered sufferers in the community, outside of a specifically medical context. They seemed to grasp the subjective psychological and social significance of this malady, its embeddedness in family structures, particularly the repetitions that were less visible to clinicians who encountered the occasional isolated patient in a hospital or asylum setting. They carried with them a kind of community knowledge as well as a clinical appreciation of the symptoms.[21]

Nor does it seem coincidental that all the early North American writers on "hereditary chorea" and the megrims or magrums, including George Huntington, were recent graduates of medical colleges at a time when American medicine was strongly focused on regional variations in health and illness. As John Harley Warner has elaborated, medical knowledge "was necessarily tied to the place where it was generated: it was in essence local knowledge." Medical societies encouraged reports on the diseases prevailing in specific localities, and medical students often chose to write their theses on the medical particularities of their home districts, publishing them in the new medical journals that proliferated in the 1840s and 1850s.[22]

Furthermore, these doctors in their twenties, just starting out, may have been less accustomed than their elders to the ubiquity of heredity in medical accounts of illness. They certainly appear to have been more willing to accord legitimacy to popular knowledge, an approach, the twenty-three-year-old Lyon admitted in 1863, that might be considered "unphilosophical," since many would say that "popular notions of disease should not be accredited by professional men." But because the symptoms of chorea, in his view, were "patent and easy of cognition to all," he believed "the testimony of any intelligent observer of this disease to be valid and worthy of credence, whether he be educated in the medical profession or not." Lyon especially emphasized "the deep-seated popular belief" within the communities where affected families lived that the disease was inherited. Not only the neighbors of the sufferers but also the sufferers themselves "insist upon its hereditary nature," he wrote. If for many older physicians, heredity was something to be assumed, rather than explained, these young men, fresh out of medical school, may not yet have absorbed that lesson.[23]

GEORGE HUNTINGTON IN EAST HAMPTON

In certain respects, George Huntington's 1872 paper "On Chorea" was a culmination rather than a beginning, framing "hereditary chorea" as a local variant of childhood chorea, as his predecessors had done. Yet in one critical dimension his account differed, making his description a significant departure: according to Huntington, this chorea was dramatically unlike most so-called hereditary diseases, which could disappear for a generation or more and then reappear. Once this one was gone, it never returned. Those who had the good fortune to escape the malady of their affected parent would not, and could not, pass it on to their children or their grandchildren. Before considering this point further, let us first take a brief biographical detour to the life of George Huntington in East Hampton.[24]

George Huntington, born April 9, 1850, in East Hampton, was the fourth child and youngest son of Mary Hoogland Huntington and George Lee Huntington, Abel Huntington's youngest son. In his seventies at the time of his grandson's birth, the Honorable Abel, as his descendants called him, looked back on a long life of public service. Besides carrying on a full medical practice and raising four children after his wife died in 1813, he had served as East Hampton's coroner, inspector and commissioner of schools, town trustee, and for several years, town supervisor. In 1821 he was elected to the New York State Senate, and he was soon spending more time in politics than doctoring. He served in the House of Representatives as a Jacksonian Democrat in the 1830s, and was later appointed customs collector in Sag Harbor. In 1846, just four years before his grandson George was born, he participated in the New York state constitutional convention, as one of its oldest members.[25]

As we have seen, Abel Huntington had a reputation as a brilliant, outspoken doctor, noted for his occasional colorful profanity. In contrast, his son, George Lee Huntington, according to one of the neighbors, was "much of a gentleman of the old school," rather dignified and courtly in his manner, although still "full of fun." George Lee, born in 1811, was himself a famous storyteller who spent hours visiting with his patients. Despite training with the eminent surgeon Valentine Mott at New York University's College of Medicine—a superior medical education in the 1830s—he was reportedly not considered as skilled a doctor as his father. And unlike Abel who had participated in state and national affairs, George Lee's sphere was almost exclusively local. Still, within East Hampton he held many prominent positions, such as town supervisor and coroner, an elected post he held for many years. He also continued his father's liberal political affiliations by joining the Republican Party—in the 1850s the party of northern

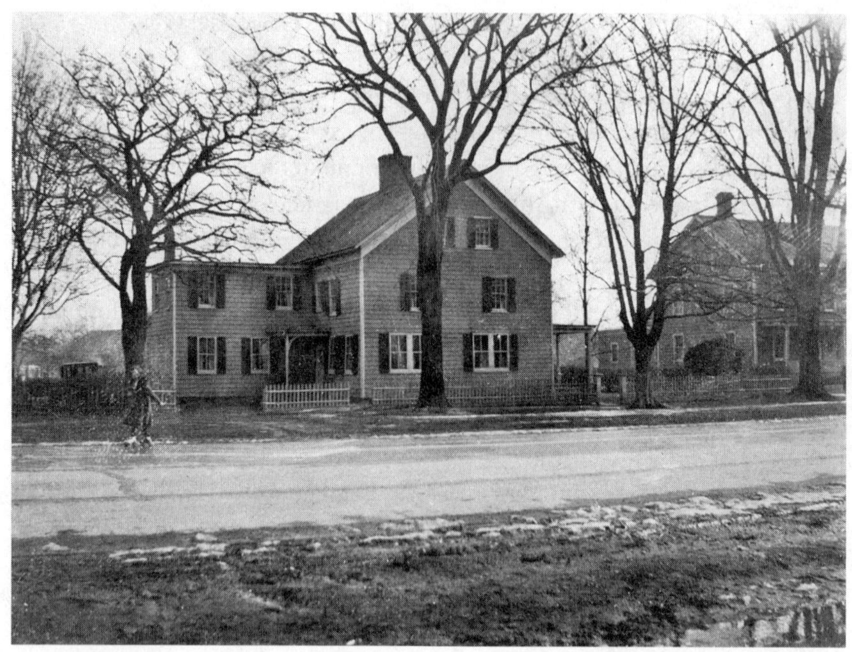

The "Wickham House" at 134 Main Street, East Hampton, home of Huntington family physicians (so-called after former owner Thomas Wickham). Courtesy Milstein Division of United States History, Local History, and Genealogy, New York Public Library, Astor, Lenox, and Tilden Foundations

antislavery elements—in this largely Democratic, conservative and pro–states rights town.[26]

Mary Hoogland Huntington, who had grown up in New York City, was "nice," if "a trifle stiff in her manners" because of being "city born," in the view of a neighbor. She read newspapers and occasionally kept a diary commenting on her work, family affairs, and the visits and gossip of neighbors. She also helped support the family by sewing and quilting for her neighbors. She and George Lee were both progressive minded, affectionate parents—"I don't believe parents the most abused people in the world and aunts and grandparents the cause of all the bad behavior of children," Mary Huntington scoffed in her diary, apropos a disagreement with a neighbor; "I believe kindness and tenderness and unobtrusive influence make better tempers than nasty domineering authority."[27]

By the time of the younger George's birth in 1850, the East Hampton Huntingtons had long been part of the local elite, though they were by no means among the wealthiest. George Lee could not support his family on his "professionals,"

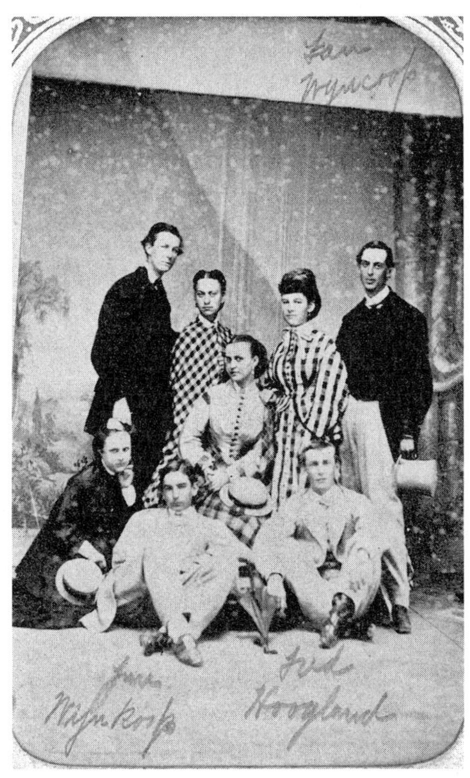

George Lee (1811–81) and Mary Hoogland Huntington (1812–90), standing left, from Mulford album. ca. 1850. Courtesy Pennypacker Long Island Collection, East Hampton Library

as he called his medical practice, and he spent considerable time working his "farm"—the acreage behind the house where the family grew vegetables and kept a cow and some chickens. George Lee was a hands-on father who took great delight in his adventurous youngest son, taking him on his medical rounds, bringing him along on trips, and recounting his son's activities in his medical daybook. "Nothing to do but take care of George who has made himself sick eating grapes," he reported on October 5, 1855, when George was five. "Go back to NY—with Geo—get dinner of oysters at fulton market & take Geo to Barnum's," he wrote when George was twelve. He noted his son's hunting and fishing exploits in an 1865 entry: "Geo quailing first time, got four." By the time George was fifteen he was helping his father plant corn, burn brush, and cart barley, and was even trying to collect bills, all the while attending school at the Clinton Academy across the street. He excelled at his studies, but he also loved parties and performing in "tableux," ice skating, singing, hunting, fishing, and staying out late with his friends. "George has gone to Bridgehampton this Eve. With Lon. Hedges Chet Hornen & some girls," his father fretted in his daybook in 1865. "It is time he was home 11 P.M.."[28]

Typical of an elite East Hampton family in certain respects, the Huntingtons were unusual in others. Certainly they commanded more cultural resources than most families in East Hampton, or in most other rural settings, for that matter. Living in their household on Main Street were two intellectuals who helped educate the young George and contributed to the literary skill evident in his paper on chorea. His aunt Cornelia Huntington (1803–90) came to live with them in 1858 after Abel Huntington died, when George was eight. Cornelia had attended the Clinton Academy in the 1810s and had literary ambitions as a young woman. In her diary she confided her youthful hopes to marry and leave her hometown, "for I want to make my mark somewhere and I stand no kind of chance here." But although she never married nor did she leave East Hampton for more than short visits to family and friends, she did make her mark as a beloved local "poet laureate" and social chronicler of Long Island's East End. Moreover, her East Hampton roman à clef, *Sea-Spray: A Long Island Village,* published in 1857 under the pen name Martha Wickham, centers around a character, Ada Evelyn, whose nervous, fidgety, irritable behavior, unsteady walk, melancholy mood, and growing emaciation suggest the symptoms of Huntington's chorea: "Ada was pacing the house, restless and wretched. It seemed that quiet and peace had utterly forsaken her, and that to be composed and still was impossible. Her health was failing daily, and her nervousness and trembling agitation were becoming too powerful for control. Her pale face was shrunk, and her features were sharpened and shorn of their beauty."[29]

The narrative is full of allusions to bad parental influences passed on to children, as when Ada feels overwhelmed by "the tremendous and crushing thought" of "visiting the sins of the fathers upon the children." The local minister in the novel frames Ada's unhappiness and her toxic effect on her children—two of whom die in the course of the story—as the consequence of the immoral behavior (bigamy) that Ada finally reveals to him. Rather than treat her with understanding, however, he condemns her to exile from the community and, by extension, to her death. But the novel also suggests that Ada's fatal illness and those of her children were the result less of sin than of circumstance: the grief she experienced following the death of her sister, and her numbness after her near-death in a shipwreck. These emotional traumas led her to marry her rescuer,

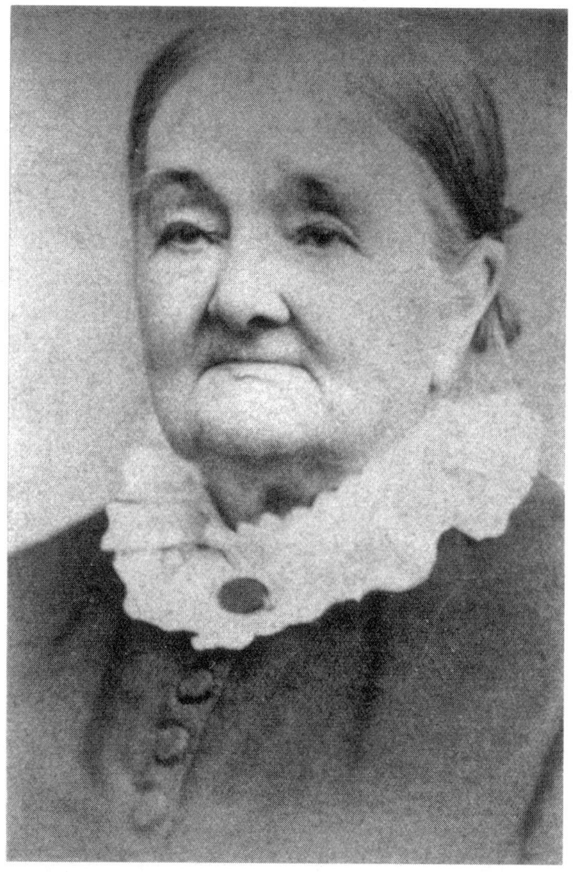

Cornelia Huntington (1803–90), poet, novelist, aunt of George Huntington, ca. 1880. Courtesy Jean K. Lominska and family

although she was already married, thereby precipitating her downfall. Evoking the author's own struggle between the stern Presbyterianism of East Hampton tradition and the more liberal Episcopalianism to which the Huntingtons were drawn, *Sea-Spray* alludes in fictional form to ideas about heredity, family, and illness that Cornelia Huntington's nephew was to address fifteen years later in a different, and more secular, voice.[30]

The second intellectual in the Huntington household was a man known locally as John Wallace. He had arrived with a valet in East Hampton from Edinburgh, Scotland, in 1840, ten years before young George was born. Highly educated, gracious, a "gentleman" in all respects, Mr. Wallace, as everyone called him, never disclosed his background despite nearly thirty years as a boarder with the Huntingtons: a silence that gave him a certain air of mystery. During this period, he founded the local Episcopal church and served as its principal reader. (Mary, Cornelia, and later George converted to Episcopalianism, though George Lee and George attended church only rarely.) Wallace (whose real name was John Wood) also tutored the young George, teaching him Latin, and bringing into the household a knowledge of the classics. Acquaintances later attributed George's "gentlemanly dignity and pleasing address" to Wallace's influence.[31]

With a highly respected literary aunt and a learned Scottish churchman living in their midst, the Huntingtons clearly enjoyed cultural advantages not available to most of their neighbors. As we know from George Lee Huntington's medical daybooks, from the diaries of Mary and Cornelia Huntington, and from their few extant letters, this family read novels and newspapers and attended lectures. They were writers as well as readers. They traveled. They visited New York City and Connecticut as well as Sag Harbor, and George's sister went off with her husband to live in Shanghai. George grew up with a physician father and grandfather, and even an older brother, Abel, who became a physician. In some respects they remained a Connecticut family (one twentieth-century East Hampton historian referred to them as "expatriates") with strong ties to their prominent relatives back in Norwich. It mattered in East Hampton that (the first) Abel Huntington had arrived not in 1650 but in 1797, nearly one hundred and fifty years after the town's founding. After half a century of residence, the Huntingtons were still people "from away." That they were ardent Republicans in a community where many people, for all their New England identification, sympathized with the South during the Civil War, further underscored their difference. In short, the Huntingtons were both insiders and outsiders, standing a little apart from their neighbors. This liminal status, I believe, gave them, and particularly George, a special perspective on the town. As physicians they knew all the local secrets, but they did not share the same taboos.[32]

If George Huntington's upbringing and early exposure to medicine accompanying his father on medical rounds gave him advantages not shared by his neighbors, his formal medical education was more conventional. At the age of eighteen, he enrolled as a student in the College of Physicians and Surgeons (P and S) in New York City, where he followed the typical two-year program of lectures (from September 1868 until March of 1869, and then again from September 1869 to April 1870). As we can see from his notebooks, P and S still emphasized the principle of therapeutic specificity: "an individualized match between medical therapy and the specific characteristics of a particular patient

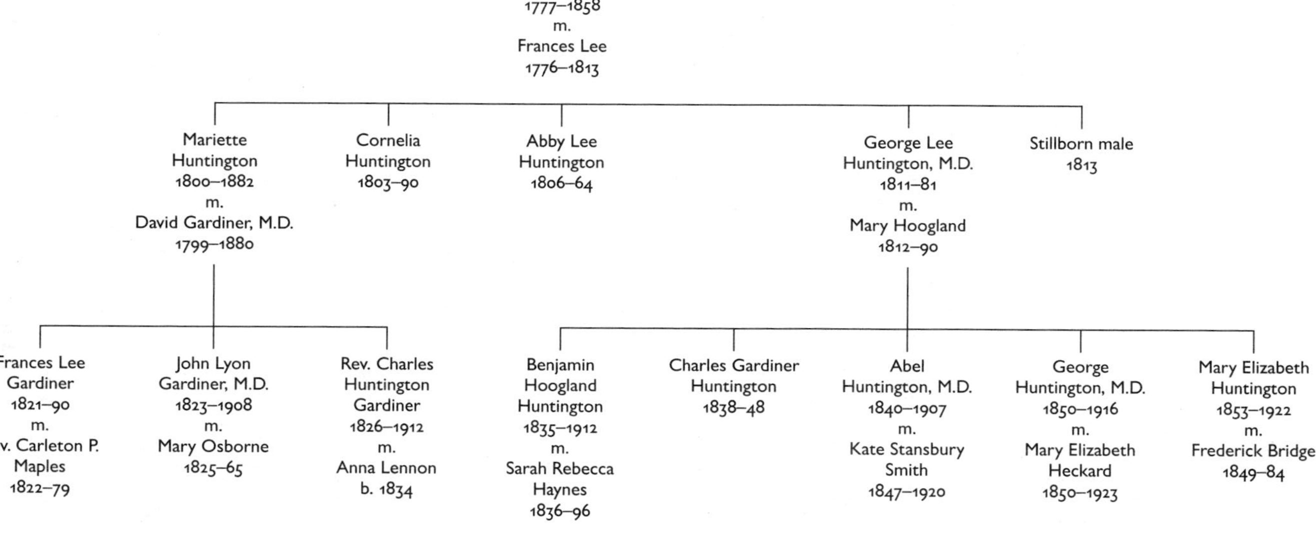

Three generations of Huntington family physicians in East Hampton

and of the social and physical environments" in which he or she lived. George Huntington learned the importance of considering the patient's temperament, whether sanguine, melancholic, nervous, or phlegmatic: ancient medical categories incorporating a general pattern of physiognomy, behavior, vulnerabilities, and therapeutic responsiveness. He learned that the age, sex, race, morals, and locality of the patient affect disease; that "rational" treatment was that given according to indication (meaning that it is prudent and judicious for the individual patient), while treatment that was "empirical" (specific to the disease rather than to the patient, and a term associated with quackery) was equivalent to "treating haphazard"; and that the best instrument for diagnosis is four fingers. He learned that diathesis meant the tendency to a particular malady, such as scrofula, cancer, gout, or rheumatism, if exposed to bad environmental influences. Although experimental science, bolstered by the bacteriological discoveries of the 1870s and 1880s, was about to enter the curriculum, P and S offered few specialized courses during George Huntington's time. The influential American neurologist William Hammond had taught for one term just before George arrived, and Edward Constant Seguin, a student of the French neurologist Jean-Martin Charcot's, arrived just as he was finishing. Although students of George Huntington's generation had some practice in the clinic, they learned primarily through memorizing lectures. Most instructors were practitioners who did not engage in research.[33]

George Huntington later mentioned encountering children with chorea in the clinics of P and S, implying that his observations there as a medical student had awakened his curiosity about the distinct type of chorea he had observed among his grown-up neighbors back home in East Hampton. But during his time in school he did not pursue the subject. Instead, he chose to write his medical thesis on asthma, a disorder closer to his own experience. "Being myself a victim to this most strange and distressing disease," he wrote, "and having suffered some of its bitterest pangs, I very naturally chose it as the subject of my thesis." At some point, however, he abandoned this topic and decided to write instead about opium, a subject with which he was also personally familiar. Like many nineteenth-century Americans, his mother routinely used "opiates" as self-medication, and his father dispensed them in his practice. In describing the uses of opium, George Huntington alluded to another possible reason for his interest in the subject, foreshadowing his later paper on chorea. "Opium is powerfully antispasmodic and there is no drug so efficient in relaxing spasms and allaying nervous irritation upon which irregular muscular action depends," he wrote. "Hence its value in tetanus, in chorea, in cholera, colic, spasm of stomach and uterus, and the bile ducts in the passage of calculi." Indeed, in his view,

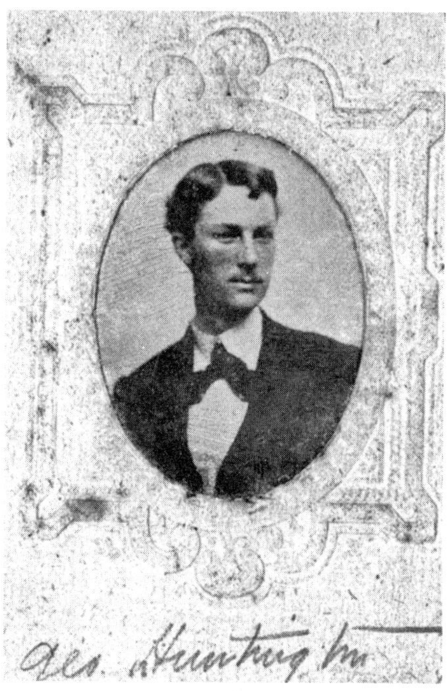

Young George Huntington, ca. 1868; Mulford album. Courtesy Pennypacker Long Island Collection, East Hampton Library

there were so many uses for opium that a complete list would require "volumes." He considered it, in certain forms, "an excellent thing."[34]

WRITING CHOREA

On February 28, 1871, George Lee Huntington noted proudly in his daybook that his son George had "passed his examination & the Degree of M.D. will be forthcoming soon." Four days later, George was home, "having completed his course of studies & rec'd the degree of M.D." Not yet twenty-one, the newly graduated physician seemed in no hurry to begin practicing. As he had in previous summers at home, he spent much of his time, from March to November of 1871, sketching and painting, "gunning," fishing, performing in tableaux, taking violin and singing lessons, picking up books and medical equipment for his father in Sag Harbor and Riverhead, helping around the house and yard, and trying unsuccessfully to collect his father's medical bills. George also accompanied his father on medical visits, and even substituted for him on occasion. Though now a full-fledged M.D., who delivered babies in his father's absence, George Huntington seemingly struggled to establish a grown-up, masculine identity while still engaging in his youthful pursuits and trying to cope with the agonies of asthma.[35]

Did he now begin to sketch the paper on chorea that he would deliver a few months later in Middleport, Ohio? His first biographer, James Winfield, writing in 1908, asserts that George Huntington began making notes preliminary to writing the chorea paper during the summer and fall of 1871 while he was in East Hampton, finally writing a draft that was "carefully revised by his father, and bears the correctional marks of his pencil." Unfortunately, this manuscript has been lost. The fact that George Lee never mentioned this project in his daybook, though he noted most of his son's other activities during these months, also casts some doubt on this claim. Nor have patient notes of the Huntington physicians surfaced, though their descendants have preserved their medical daybooks and ledgers.[36]

Still, the paper itself implies that during these months at home, George Huntington started to reflect seriously on the subject of chorea, comparing cases he had seen in the clinic in New York with those he knew in East Hampton, and discussing the differences with his father. The memories he included in the unpublished notes for his 1909 talk to the New York Neurological Society suggest some additional motives for his interest at this time. Although we have seen a portion of this talk, the omitted section makes the full passage worth repeating. "Driving with my father through a wooded road leading from East Hampton to Amagansett," he wrote,

> we suddenly came upon two women, mother and daughter, both tall, thin, almost cadaverous, both bowing, twisting, grimacing. I stared in wonderment, almost in fear. What could it mean? My father paused to speak with them, and we passed on. Then my Gamaliel-like instruction began; my medical education had its inception. From this point my interest in the disease has never wholly ceased. Then came the hanging of D.H. in his blacksmith shop. He was a victim of incipient chorea, knew it, possibly had been waiting for it, the "Sanctus Invitus," and well knowing the character of the foe he must meet, the so dreaded, the long expected, the conquering, he cut short the taper and his life went out.[37]

The juxtaposition here is revealing, suggesting that the intensity of Huntington's account of his meeting with the two women along the road may have arisen partly from its association, in memory, with a dramatic act of suicide. However, it is unclear whether the suicide occurred during George's boyhood, around the time of his encounter along the road, or later, when he returned home after medical school, precipitating his decision to write the paper about chorea, or even at the time of his 1909 talk, as a kind of screen memory connecting two unrelated events. In any case, I have been unable to identify "D.H.," although the initials suggest a possible relationship with the family of Phebe Hedges.[38]

Sometime in the fall of 1871 George Huntington decided to leave East Hampton. He may not have wanted to compete with his father for patients, especially given George Lee's difficulty in collecting his bills. Asthma may also have been a factor, motivating him to try another location away from the water, in keeping with the medical wisdom of the time. Or perhaps he was feeling adventurous, curious to explore another part of the country. His cousin Frances Lee Huntington, who had married a prominent clergyman and was now living in Pomeroy, Ohio, invited him to come west to visit, with the idea that he might establish a medical practice there. George Huntington decided to accept the offer.[39]

In early November 1871 George Lee withdrew "$90.35 from Sav. Bank for Geo-." Setting up a medical practice was costly, and despite having hoped (according to his granddaughter) that his son would not pursue medicine, George Lee supported his efforts, not only financially but in more hands-on ways as well. "Packing Trunk-box-barrels for George," he wrote on November 8, the day of a "Republican Triumph throughout the State." The following day "George left this AM for Pomeroy, Ohio." George Lee seemed sad and listless. "Wind NW," he noted in his daybook. "Nothing to do professionally."[40]

Had George Huntington not traveled to Pomeroy, and had he not been invited by the Meigs and Mason Medical Academy of nearby Middleport, Ohio, to give a talk soon after he arrived, he might never have written the paper "On Chorea." (His subsequent published papers on the subject were also written in response to invitations to speak.) Perhaps while George was far away from home in Pomeroy, images of East Hampton and Amagansett stood out more vividly in his mind. In Pomeroy, a southern Ohio town across the Ohio River from West Virginia, regarded today as part of Appalachia, George Huntington found himself in a coal- and salt-mining community that was about one-third German and Welsh, dramatically different from East Hampton. Though the people were "genial, frank, warm-hearted, intelligent," and "not at all afraid or suspicious of strangers"—an attitude which contrasted with his inward-looking hometown—George found Pomeroy aesthetically unappealing, for the people cared "but little for the look of the place, not much attention being given to general improvement." Tinderbox houses lined one long street along the river, "waiting only for a spark to produce a conflagration." Raucous, bustling, commercial Pomeroy, with its beer halls and saloons and immigrant miners, presented a startling contrast to conservative, temperate Presbyterian East Hampton. George's letters (published in the *Sag Harbor Express*) could not conceal his chagrin.[41]

Still, his cousin Fanny was here, and her husband, the Reverend Carleton P. Maples. They had connections with the Pomeroy elite, no doubt including members of the county medical society. George began seeing patients in early December 1871 and had a few more patients the following week, but there were long gaps between calls, and in January 1872 he had almost no medical work at all. He would certainly have had the opportunity at this time to write his paper, or, if he had begun it earlier, to complete it between his arrival in November 1871 and February 15, 1872, when he presented it in Middleport. The academy apparently encouraged its speakers to submit their papers to the *Medical and Surgical Reporter,* a prestigious Philadelphia medical journal. But George Huntington decided to send it first to his father, who carefully noted its arrival in his daybook, keeping it for a week and then returning it to his son. The paper, "On Chorea," started on the front page of the April 13, 1872, issue of the journal.[42]

Most of "On Chorea" summarized the etiology, pathology, and therapeutics of childhood chorea to be found in the standard nineteenth-century medical texts, whose authors George Huntington cited in his paper. He implied, in fact, that he personally had seen very few cases. "I do not remember a single instance occurring in my father's practice," he wrote, "and I have often heard him say that it was a rare disease and seldom met with by him." With the exception of an allusion to the young patients he had encountered as a medical student in the New York City clinics, he described no cases he had treated himself. And while he acknowledged that much of the pathology of this disease remained unknown, he felt assured that "science, which has accomplished such wonders through the never-tiring devotion of its votaries, may yet 'overturn and overturn, and overturn it,' until it is laid open to the light of day."[43]

In the final paragraphs of the paper, however, George Huntington adopted a more confident voice as he turned toward his hometown and described a phenomenon that had existed, "so far as I know, almost exclusively on the east end of Long Island." The disease began "as an ordinary chorea might begin, by the irregular and spasmodic action of certain muscles," which "gradually increase[s] . . . until every muscle in the body becomes affected (excepting the involuntary ones) and the poor patient presents a spectacle which is anything but pleasing to witness."[44]

There were several aspects of this form of chorea that, in his view, distinguished it from the more common childhood version. First, it came on later in life, usually between the ages of thirty and forty, and very gradually, "often

George Lee Huntington account book, February 24, 1872: "Recd. from Geo. His Paper on Chorea read before the Academy of Medicine at Middleport this 15th Past." Courtesy Pennypacker Long Island Collection, East Hampton Library occupying years in its development until the hapless sufferer is but a quivering wreck of his former self." Second, "the tendency to insanity, and sometimes that form of insanity which leads to suicide, is marked." *Insanity* was a term that earlier writers on chorea had not previously used, and it evoked considerable discussion among clinicians later on, as we shall see. According to Huntington, in these families, "the nervous temperament greatly preponderates." As he recalled, "in my grandfather's and father's experience, which conjointly cover a period of 78 years, nervous excitement in a marked degree almost invariably attends upon every disease these people may suffer from, although they may not when in *health* be over nervous." Not only those with symptoms but also those without, who merely belonged to an affected family, sometimes committed suicide. Third, most catastrophically, this form of chorea seemed to be "one of the incurables." George Huntington himself had "never known a recovery or even an amelioration of symptoms in this form of chorea; where once it begins it clings to the bitter end."[45]

George Huntington, like Lyon, termed this condition "hereditary chorea," portraying it as "an heirloom from generations away back in the dim past." But he did not merely describe it as hereditary. As we have seen, for the first time in the writing on chorea, he defined a specific pattern of transmission, one that was unlike "the general laws of so-called hereditary diseases, as for instance in phthisis, or syphilis, when *one* generation may enjoy entire immunity from their dread ravages, and yet in another you find them cropping out in all their hideousness." This chorea was distinct: "Unstable and whimsical as the disease may be in *other* respects," he asserted, "in *this* it is firm, it never skips a generation to again manifest itself in another; once having yielded its claims, it never regains them." In other words, only those individuals who developed the disease (usually after they had already had children) were in danger of passing it on to their descendants. Those who escaped it in the course of a normal life span would not and could not transmit it to any subsequent generations. Once it was gone, it was vanquished forever. It would not suddenly reappear.[46]

Actually, the pattern George Huntington described—later called dominant inheritance, in which only those that had a particular condition or trait could transmit it to their offspring—was not unknown at that time in the annals of medicine and science. It does not detract from the beauty of Huntington's observation to note that as early as 1809, a physician in rural Maryland named Ennalls Martin (1758–1834) had published a similar description of a family with many cases of blindness that developed in early adulthood (probably retinitis pigmentosa). In these families, each affected parent almost always had some affected children, but "there has never been an instance, where any of the family, who had fortunately escaped blindness, has had any blind children or that their descendants have been subject to blindness."[47]

Moreover, as such historians as Ernst Mayr and Peter J. Bowler have pointed out, "it is not difficult to find examples of breeders who noticed the occasional instance of dominance from the mid-eighteenth century onward. Men such as the English horticulturalist Thomas Andrew Knight (1759–1863), longtime president of the Royal Horticultural Society in London, and the French agriculturalist Augustin Sageret (1763–1851), had described a pattern of dominance in their experiments with fruit trees and melons early in the nineteenth century, although they did not pursue its theoretical significance.[48]

Nonetheless, nervous disorders differed from eye diseases and the colors of petals. The idea that a nervous condition might abruptly disappear in one generation, never to return, challenged the widely accepted understanding, in the late nineteenth century, of neuropathic inheritance, in which, as we have seen, parents passed on a generalized tendency or vague "weakness" that might develop into any one of a number of ills, or they transmitted a diathesis predisposing to a particular malady. Furthermore, given the belief at that time that hereditary ills tended to accumulate over the generations, becoming increasingly burdensome and deleterious until the family finally became extinct, George Huntington's portrait of the complete disappearance of a disease in one generation represented a radical shift.

The innovation of his interpretation is especially evident when we compare his thesis with the view of his former neighbor Edward Osborn, whose family had lived in East Hampton far longer than the Huntingtons and knew the same local population over many generations. Unlike Huntington, Osborn referred to certain families that "belong to the disease," as if the malady were integral to their identity, whether or not any individuals were currently affected. In two families "in which the disease is hereditary, and in which it appears," Osborn told William Osler in 1898, it was "not at present in active symptoms." But "later there will be cases in these families, as the disease never disappears."[49]

Osborn may have been thinking of young people who were still in danger of developing it as they grew older. However, his claim that "the disease never disappears" implied that it was a permanent attribute of these families, an essential part of their nature, whether it was expressed or not. He was aware that others thought differently. As he put it, "some persons—here—say that when the disease oversteps one generation it lapses forever—but I think not."[50]

THE

MEDICAL AND SURGICAL REPORTER.

No. 789.] PHILADELPHIA, APRIL 13, 1872. [VOL. XXVI.—No. 15.

ORIGINAL DEPARTMENT.

Communications.

ON CHOREA.

BY GEORGE HUNTINGTON, M. D.,
Of Pomeroy, Ohio.

Essay read before the Meigs and Mason Academy of Medicine at Middleport, Ohio, February 15, 1872

Chorea is essentially a disease of the nervous system. The name "chorea" is given to the disease on account of the *dancing* propensities of those who are affected by it, and it is a very appropriate designation. The disease, as it is commonly seen, is by no means a dangerous or serious affection, however distressing it may be to the one suffering from it, or to his friends. Its most marked and characteristic feature is a clonic spasm affecting the voluntary muscles. There is no loss of sense or of volition attending these contractions, as there is in epilepsy; the will is there, but its power to perform is deficient, the desired movements are after a manner performed, but there seems to exist some hidden power, something that is playing tricks, as it were, upon the will, and in a measure thwarting and p'rverting its designs; and after the will has ceased to exert its power in any given direction, taking things into its own hands, and keeping the poor victim in a continual jigger as long as he remains awake, generally, though not always, granting a respite during sleep. The disease commonly begins by slight twitchings in the muscles of the face, w ich gradually increase in violence and variety. The eyelids are kept winking, the brows are corrugated, and then elevated, the nose is screwed first to the one side and then to the other, and the mouth is drawn in various directions, giving the patient the most ludicrous appearance imaginable. The upper extremities may be the first affected, or both simultaneously. All the voluntary muscles are liable to be affected, those of the face rarely being exempted.

If the patient attempt to protrude the tongue it is accomplished with a great deal of difficulty and uncertainty. The hands are kept rolling—first the palms upward, and then the backs. The shoulders are shrugged, and the feet and legs kept in perpetual motion; the toes are turned in, and then everted; one foot is thrown across the other, and then suddenly withdrawn, and, in short, every conceivable attitude and expression is assumed, and so varied and irregular are the motions gone through with, that a complete description of them would be impossible. Sometimes the muscles of the lower extremities are not affected, and I believe they never are *alone* involved. In cases of death from chorea, all the muscles of the body seem to have been affected, and the time required for recovery and degree of success in treatment seem to depend greatly upon the amount of muscular involvement. ROMBERG refers to two cases in which the muscles of *respiration were affected*.

The disease is generally confined to childhood, being most frequent between the ages of eight and fourteen years, and occurring oftener in girls than in boys. DUFOSSE and RUFZ refer to 429 cases; 130 occurring in boys and 299 in girls. WATSON mentions a collection of 1,029 cases, of whom 733 were *females*, giving a proportion of nearly 5 to 2. Dr. WATSON also remarks upon the disease being most frequent among children of *dark* complexion, while the two authorities just alluded to, DUFOSSE and RUFZ, give as their opinion that it is most frequent in children of *light* hair. In every case visiting the clinics

317

George Huntington, "On Chorea," *Medical and Surgical Reporter* (Philadelphia), April 13, 1872. While most of the paper addressed the common (Sydenham's) chorea of childhood, George Huntington turned at the close to an adult form of chorea he considered "an heirloom from generations away back in the dim past." This "*hereditary* chorea," as he called it, "exists, so far as I know, almost exclusively on the east end of Long Island. It is peculiar in itself and seems to obey certain fixed laws."

PATTERN RECOGNITION

How did a twenty-one-year-old just out of medical school come up with a description of the hereditary transmission of chorea so different from most accounts of hereditary diseases at that time?

All writers, starting with George Huntington himself, have emphasized his debt to the collective insights of his father and grandfather, physicians to the affected families in East Hampton for nearly three-quarters of a century. I would add that not only George Lee and Abel Huntington but also George's mother, Mary Hoogland Huntington; John Wallace; and especially George's literary aunt Cornelia Huntington—collectors all of community memory and local knowledge, and lively participants in conversations around the family hearth—no doubt played a role in providing him with crucial insights and information.[51]

Most writers have also emphasized George Huntington's strong aesthetic sensibilities and his practice as an amateur artist, which helped develop the keen eye for observation so evident in his account of chorea. In a local culture that valued killing whales as the highest expression of masculinity, both George Lee and George preferred to spend their leisure hours drawing and painting. Indeed, he once confessed to his daughter that if one were allowed to realize one's greatest desires in the life after death, he hoped "he would be permitted to become the artist he had so longed to be." Certainly his children always regarded him as "an artist at heart." They also recalled his great love of nature. From an early age, he was an amateur naturalist, and later he joined the New York Audubon Society, a membership he maintained all his life. "It was he who told us the names of many different stars; taught us about the trees, and the birds, and the wild flowers," wrote one daughter; "to know that the scientific name of Joe Pye Weed is 'Eupatorium Purpureum'; to watch for glacial scratchings in the rock. In other words, he trained us to go through life with our eyes open." He had a great admiration for the "wonders of science," as we saw in his paper, even if he himself chose not to pursue it.[52]

In this regard it is worth considering that while nineteenth-century physicians generally understood hereditary transmission in vague and hazy terms, farmers and breeders had a practical incentive to study the passage of qualities from generation to generation more precisely. Understanding heredity was not useful to physicians in the way that it was to practical breeders with a commercial interest in learning how to "fix" desirable qualities in their stock and eliminate those that were undesirable. Indeed, Charles Darwin, in his *Variation of Plants and Animals under Domestication,* published in 1868, referred often to his conversations with breeders, whose knowledge of inheritance he greatly respected. According-ing to some scholars, practical breeders in the nineteenth century have a better claim to be considered the forerunners of Gregor Mendel—the founding figure of twentieth-century genetics—than do the plant hybridizers and naturalists who were concerned with more theoretical questions, such as the origin of new species. The biologist Roger Wood and the historian Vítězslav Orel have even speculated that the intellectual milieu of the scientific-minded sheep breeders of early-nineteenth-century Moravia (in the present-day Czech Republic), a major center at that time of woolen cloth production, helped create an "atmosphere of inquiry about heredity" favorable to the conceptual approach taken by Mendel.[53]

As we have seen, since colonial times, besides growing wheat, oats, flax, and corn, East Hampton farmers had raised huge herds of cattle and sheep, driving them onto Montauk each May in the annual cattle drive, and bringing them back to town each November, when some were sold. Town records are full of notations relating to earmarks for animals, as well as notices of fines for damages caused by runaway animals and payments to individuals for various farm-related tasks: inscriptions symbolizing the agricultural identity of nineteenth-century East Hampton. Growing up in this rural agricultural world, George Huntington almost certainly absorbed some of the thinking and the breeding knowledge of the farmers and livestock men who were his neighbors and friends, as well as the patients of his father and grandfather. In fact, some of them were relatives, since his paternal aunt had married into the Gardiner family, one of the earliest East Hampton settler families that, in the nineteenth century, imported and bred merino sheep, fancy cattle, and thoroughbred horses on their private island a few miles offshore. Attending the fairs of the Suffolk County Agricultural Society in nearby Riverhead and listening to discussions about breeding—which, "next to politics," was "probably the most common topic of discussion among the majority of our farmers," according to the popular 1867 *American Farmer's Horse Book*—George Huntington would have been attuned to farmers' ways of thinking about inheritance and noninheritance, ways that may have shaped his thinking about chorea as well.[54]

Missing from this story, however, are the East Hampton families with St. Vitus's dance. While we cannot be certain that George Huntington based his account on the family of Phebe Hedges, several factors argue in their favor: first, the fact that Phebe herself, and many of her relatives and descendants, unaffected as well as affected, were patients—and in one case a next-door neighbor—of the Huntington physicians; second, George Huntington's several allusions to this family, in published and unpublished papers and notes; and third, the presence of several long-lived individuals in different generations of this family who did *not* develop the illness—since those who lived long lives *without* symptoms were critical to George's analysis of the hereditary pattern.[55]

Here is what George Huntington *could* have known, from his own, his father's, and his grandfather's observations, as well as those of the family members themselves: in the first generation with St. Vitus's dance personally encountered by Abel Huntington, there was Phebe Mulford (wife of Joseph Tillinghast), born in 1739, died in 1811. In the second generation, two of her daughters (and possibly others who left town) suffered from the disease. Each daughter, in turn, had at least one offspring with the same malady, and each of these had at least one son or daughter who was also affected. In short, here were cases of chorea in four consecutive generations. Except for Phebe Mulford, whose affected parent remains uncertain, each individual with the illness had a parent identified as a sufferer of the disease. (If we consider that Henry P. Hedges recalled hearing of affected individuals in several earlier generations as well, then George Huntington could have been aware of six consecutive generations in this family in which at least one person had been affected.)[56]

In contrast, Phebe Hedges's son Stephen remained without symptoms at the age of eighty-two in 1872, when George Huntington presented his paper. So too did all of Stephen's six living children, who at that time ranged in age from forty-four to fifty-nine, already beyond the typical age when he thought the symptoms began. Phebe Hedges's sister Lydia was seventy-three when George Huntington was born. She died in 1870 at the age of ninety-three, just two years before he published his paper. She was unaffected, and neither of her two sons was known to be affected, although one, a whaler, had been lost at sea on a whaling voyage at the age of forty-nine. The other one remained without symptoms at seventy-two. None of Lydia's grandchildren—now in their thirties and forties—were affected. In other words, not only did Lydia herself escape her mother's fate; neither of her children or any of her grandchildren showed any symptoms either, at least not so far. Here, then, were three successive generations apparently unaffected by the disease and known to three generations of Huntingtons.[57]

As George Huntington wrote in words consistent with this family's history: "When either or both the parents have shown manifestations of the disease, and more especially if these manifestations have been of a serious nature," he wrote, "one or more of the offspring almost invariably suffer from the disease, if they live to adult age. But if by any chance these children [such as Lydia and Stephen and their children] go through life without it, the thread is broken and the grandchildren and great-grandchildren of the original shakers may rest assured that they are free from the disease."[58]

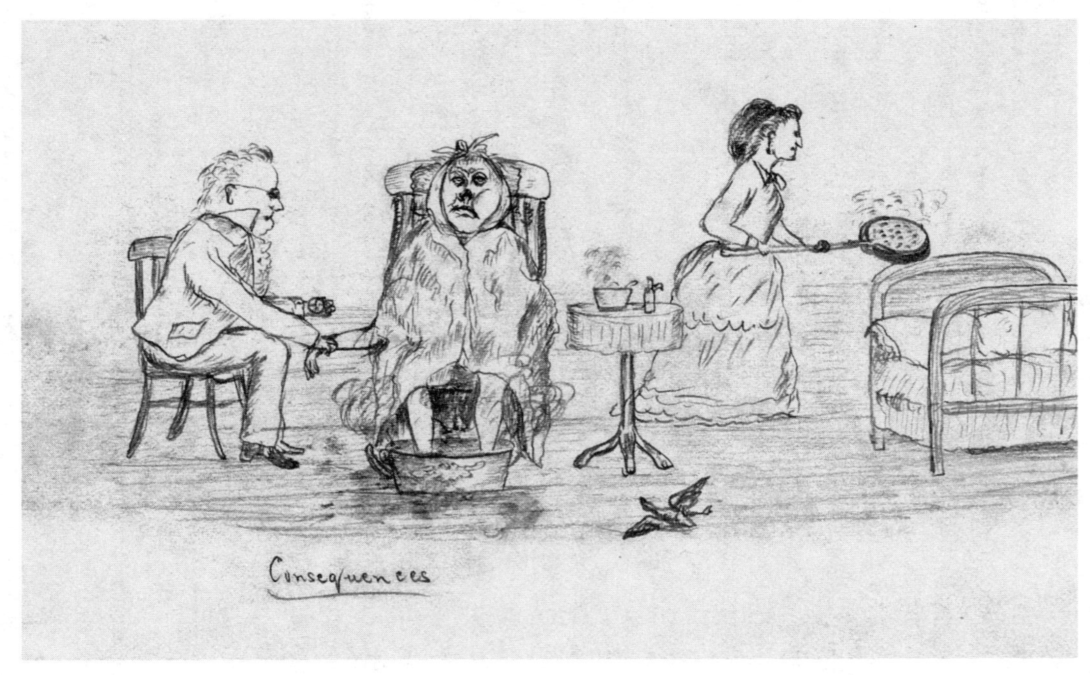

Drawings by George Huntington. Courtesy Jean K. Lominska and family

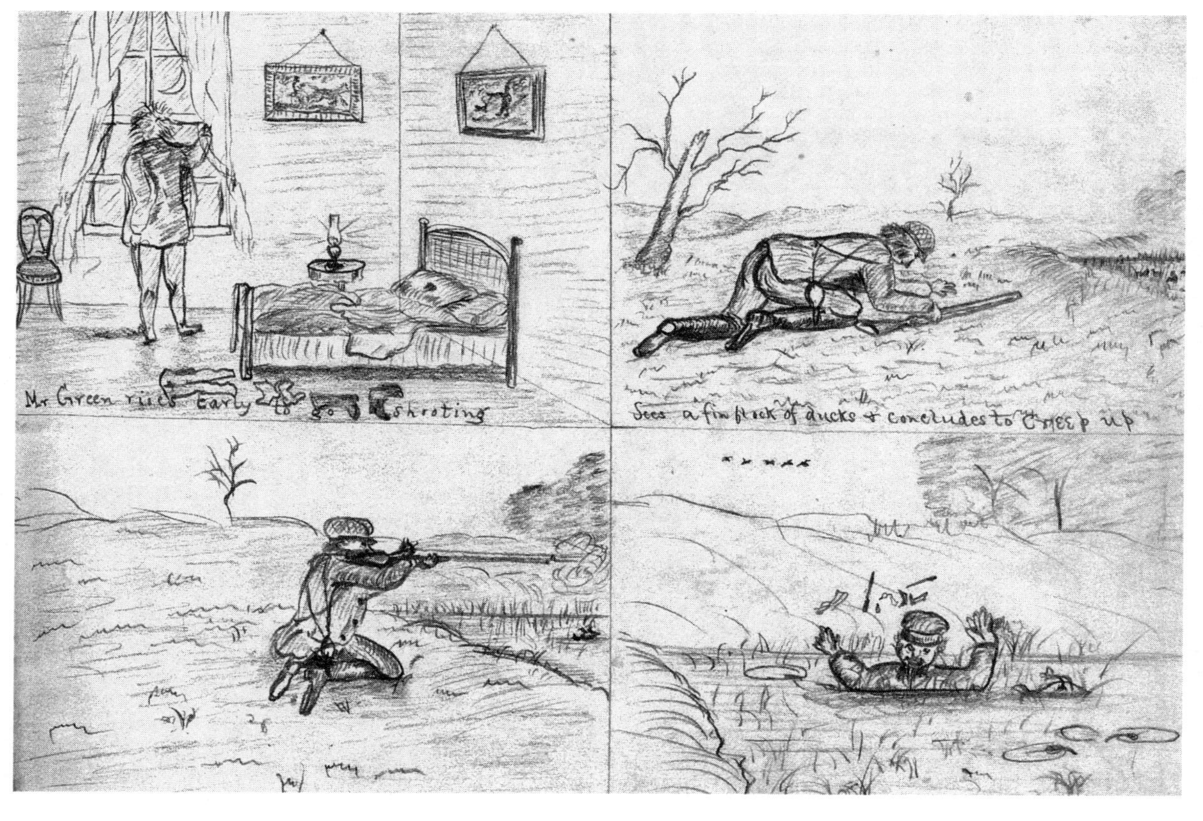
Mr Green rises Early to go shooting
Sees a fine flock of ducks & concludes to creep up

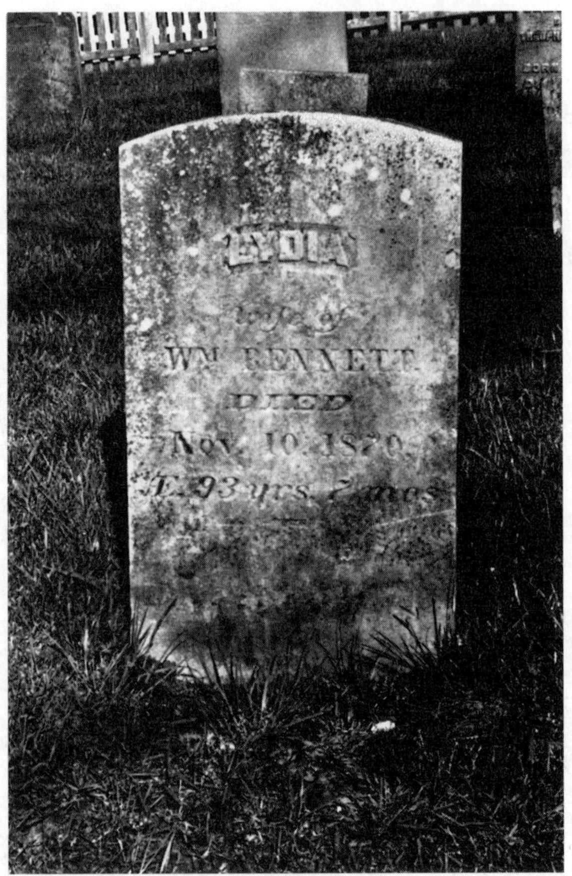

Gravestone of Lydia (Tillinghast) Bennett (1777–1870), who died at the age of ninety-three years and seven months. South End Burying Ground, East Hampton. Photo by the author

THREE QUESTIONS

One: was there an element of youthful bravado, an undercurrent of desire, in George Huntington's claim that the disease could cease in one generation? How could he be so certain that some among Lydia's or Stephen's grandchildren would not become ill? Confidence was certainly part of his youthful performative style. He displayed an almost cocky self-possession in two humorous articles he had published in 1871 in the *Sag Harbor Express*, in which he recounted his trip from East Hampton to Ohio and gave a critical assessment of the town of Pomeroy. With their classical references ("the true Ciceronian's style," the "disciple of Aesculapius") and the style of a Victorian novel—"It was on a bright and balmy day in November 1871, that a solitary traveler might have been seen, rapidly wending his way"—these articles show a young "doc," as he signed himself, who appeared to make his way in the world with assurance, a mode favorable to asserting his claims with confidence, whatever his inner feelings might be.[59]

But I believe there may also have been an element of desire in George Huntington's confident claims, a longing that they be true. For while Osborn's view condemned the affected families to an endless repetition of chorea, George Huntington's interpretation offered the hopeful possibility that a lineage might in one generation break free of the disease. Indeed, he affirmed his wish that this was so when he noted in 1910 that if there were only one individual in East Hampton with symptoms at that time, as he had been told, then "the disease is surely dying out there, a thing devoutly to be desired."[60]

Two: why is George Huntington's account so significant if both dominant inheritance and hereditary chorea had previously been described by others? Clearly his literary ability made this account of chorea more eloquent than most writing on disease. His succinct summation of the symptoms and his vivid description of the families' horror and dread of the disease, their reluctance to name it, and the "quivering wreck" to which sufferers were reduced, evoked the emotional and social impact of the disease more powerfully than any account before his. But most of all, while horticulturalists and even an occasional clinician had described the phenomenon of dominance, no one, to my knowledge, had linked it to a nervous disorder. Certainly no one writing about chorea in adults had made such a connection. Ultimately, it was George Huntington's account that helped to crystallize the identity of "hereditary chorea" as a distinct clinical entity, stirring the interest of psychiatrists, biologists, and neurologists—who were just then organizing themselves in cities such as New York and Philadelphia—in the wide-ranging features of the disease.

However, George Huntington's use of the term *insanity* to describe the depression and weakness of judgment characteristic of the disease may have had the less fortunate effect of associating this form of chorea with an especially frightening and socially stigmatizing diagnosis, one that many practitioners would soon reject as more appropriate to the courtroom than to the clinic. While they accepted most of George Huntington's account as accurate, including his description of the "tendency" to suicide, they noted that many patients in fact retained many mental capacities even in the advanced stages.

Three: was the confluence of elements at East Hampton unavailable anywhere else? It seems that the age and stability of this small community, the relationship of the affected families to the town founders two hundred years earlier, the local worship of ancestors and ancestry, the longevity of many inhabitants, and the local culture of grazing and breeding livestock for the market all contributed to a social and intellectual environment that was favorable to George Huntington's particular construction of "hereditary chorea." While there were affected families with the magrums and St. Vitus's dance in other old communities of New York, Connecticut, Norway, Scotland, Sweden, and Venezuela, to name just a few locales, no other town combined so many of these factors in a single site. That an unusually talented family of physicians, both insiders and outsiders, happened to live in this town for three-quarters of a century made this situation unique.

DISEASE IDENTITY AND PROFESSIONAL IDENTITY

Despite the prestige of the *Medical and Surgical Reporter*, there was no immediate response to "On Chorea" from the medical community beyond two brief references in the European medical press. The first was an abstract in German in the 1873 *Jahresbericht über die Leistungen und Fortschritte in der Gesammten Medicin für 1872* (Yearbook of important writings in the whole field of medicine for 1872), edited by two prominent German medical professors, Rudolf Virchow and August Hirsch; parts of this abstract were translated into English and published a few years later in an abbreviated form in the *Cyclopedia of the Practice of Medicine*. The second, in 1874, was a footnote by the Italian neuroanatomist Camillo Golgi, in a detailed neuropathological study of chorea in an adult male. Unlike the *Jahresbericht*, this one made no mention of Huntington's analysis of inheritance.[61]

Indeed, Golgi and most other clinicians who wrote about chorea in adults during the 1870s were more interested in such questions as whether it was a disease distinct from childhood chorea than in specific patterns of heredity. They continued to stress the advanced age of their patients and the long duration and intractability of the illness. Their passing references to similar symptoms in relatives suggest just how much hereditary influences were still taken for granted. Charcot continued to insist that chorea in the adult was fundamentally similar to ordinary childhood chorea, though he accepted that it was usually incurable and almost always, in the end, associated with dementia. The "exclusive influence of similar hereditary transmission"—the same disease transmitted from one generation to the next, as opposed to dissimilar or transformational heredity, in which a general predisposition might result in distinct symptoms in different generations—was in Charcot's view "a remarkable feature" but did not justify creating a separate clinical entity. For a few authors, however, the incurability and dementia, apart from any question of heredity, made chorea in adults alarming. "The tenacity of late-onset chorea, its debilitating influence on the intellectual functions, make it a much more serious malady than the chorea of children," wrote a colleague of Charcot's, Paul Berdinel, in 1878, foreshadowing later discussions, "and it imposes upon the clinician the need for great caution in making prognoses."[62]

Following his debut performance at the academy of medicine in mid-February 1872, George Huntington grew increasingly depressed. The winter of 1871–72 in Pomeroy had been the most severe in thirty years. When the coal was burning, "a dense black smoke . . . fill[ed] the air and begrime[d] everything," a condition that certainly must have aggravated his asthma. And patients were not forthcoming. He stuck it out through the rest of February and March, and in April he had a few more calls, but in May and June he saw another decline. Not all the patients could pay.[63]

George Huntington had had enough of Pomeroy. Although he had fallen in love with the daughter of a Pomeroy judge, a sociable young woman named Mary Heckard, he needed to find a place where he could live and practice medicine more comfortably. He reconsidered his hometown. In the summer of 1872, he returned, alone, to East Hampton, and in August he placed a notice in the newspaper, announcing that "DR. GEO. HUNTINGTON Tenders his professional services to the people of East-Hampton and vicinity. Having determined to settle permanently in this place," he continued, "a share of the professional work is solicited."[64]

But once again, it seems, patients were not forthcoming. In this town of some twenty-four hundred residents, with several physicians already established, there probably was not enough business for yet another practitioner. The young doctor was spending much of his time painting, quailing, hunting and fishing, in addition to helping his father. His asthma flared up again.[65]

After just six months back in East Hampton, he decided to leave again, this time for Poughkeepsie, a city up the Hudson River in Dutchess County, in the foothills of the Catskill Mountains. A deciding factor may have been the existence, in a nearby town, of a medical practice that was about to be sold. Within three weeks George had written his father "announcing his intention of remaining for the present at LaGrangeville, Dutchess County," a small agricultural community surrounded by orchards a few miles southeast of Poughkeepsie.[66]

After Pomeroy, George Huntington apparently did not consider options other than family practice in a small town. Despite having published a paper in a prestigious medical journal at the age of twenty-one, he expressed no inclination

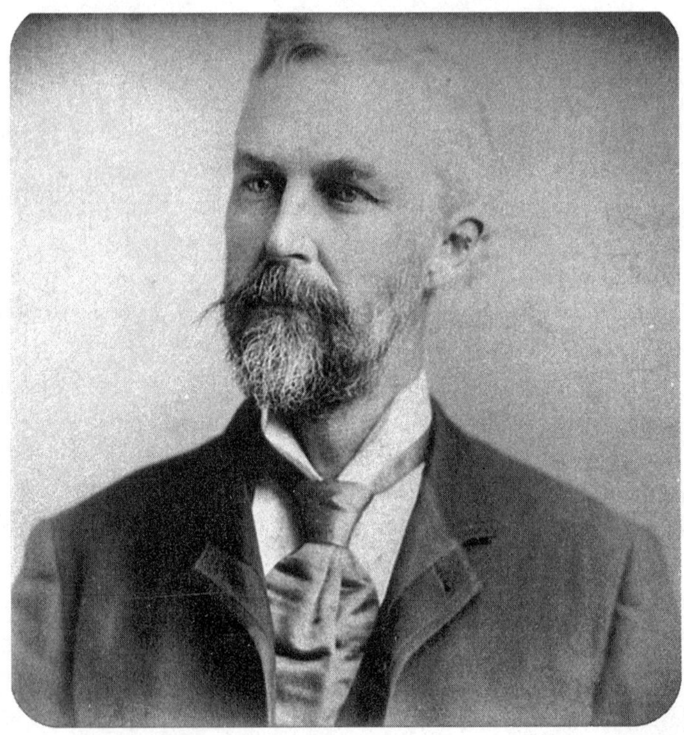

George Huntington, ca. 1896. Courtesy Jean K. Lominska and family

that we know of to seek a hospital affiliation or medical school professorship, the two main avenues of medical advancement at the time. Nor is there evidence that well-connected relatives or influential friends sought to secure such connections. Because the medical community initially greeted his paper with silence, he may have thought it unsuccessful. His claim that he drew attention to hereditary chorea not because it had "any great practical importance" but "merely as a medical curiosity," undoubtedly did not help. Having grown up in a rural environment, with a great love of nature, he may not have wanted to live in a city, a necessity for pursuing a more ambitious career. His later letters show a courtly, somewhat formal style, suggesting that, for all his evident self-confidence, he may have felt uncomfortable with the assertive masculinity needed to get hospital and academic appointments in the emerging world of scientific medicine. In any case, there is no evidence that he considered further investigations of hereditary chorea, though he later published three papers—versions of talks he gave on his original paper—in which he covered largely the same ground, albeit emphasizing a broader age range for the onset of the symptoms (between thirty and forty-five, while earlier he had put the upper limit as forty). While he remained interested in "hereditary chorea," he chose not to pursue research on the subject, devoting whatever free time he had in subsequent years to drawing and painting.[67]

On hearing the news of George's plans, the ever-patient George Lee, back home in East Hampton, packed up his son's trunk and shipped it express to LaGrangeville. Shortly afterward, he himself left for Dutchess County "to adjust Geo in the purchase of Dr. Green's place & practice—concluded on Wednesday the 14 at Poughkeepsie, $40.00—." Seven months later, in early October, George Huntington and Mary Heckard were married in Pomeroy, and the following week they returned to East Hampton for a grand reception at the Huntington home on Main Street. And then the newly married couple were off to LaGrangeville, where they remained for the next twenty-seven years.[68]

4

CHOREA AND THE CLINICAL GAZE

What we call a fact may itself be determined by the theory we happen to hold.
—Lester King, *Medical Thinking*

HEREDITARY CHOREA AND THE BIRTH OF NEUROLOGY

In 1880, eight years after George Huntington's paper appeared, A. Harbinson, an obscure assistant medical officer at the county asylum in the northern English city of Lancaster, published a paper on what he called multiple sclerosis, with some distinctly unusual features for this disease. "A peculiarly hereditary form of this complaint associated with chorea has, during the past few years, come under my notice in three instances," he wrote. Harbinson traced "sclerosis with chorea" through five generations in two related families he had encountered at the asylum. These patients, he wrote, suffered from restless, twitching, jerking motions of the limbs—that is, choreic movements—accompanied by "a vacant look," and a gradual loss of intellectual capacity that progressed slowly to fatuity. "What little intelligence she possessed at first became gradually more clouded," wrote Harbinson of one patient, "until finally she answered 'yes' and 'no' indifferently to all questions." Harbinson summed up the illness by placing heredity at the top of the "interesting features," a point that "by most authors . . . is not even mentioned." Of those who did mention heredity, Harbinson especially cited George Huntington, whose "note" about the cases of chorea encountered on Long Island was "particularly interesting."[1]

Harbinson's paper signaled a new direction in medical narratives of chorea in adults, with heredity shifting from the background to the foreground in a growing number of reports. By the mid-1880s, alongside continuing descriptions of "chorea in the aged," "chorée des adultes," and "chorea at an advanced age of life," clinical reports of "hereditary chorea" began to appear in the medical journals of many countries, some of which cited George Huntington and the other early accounts. Germany produced the most, followed by the United States, France, Britain, and Italy. (It is revealing of the continuing impact of community knowledge that Clarence King, the first U.S. physician after George Huntington to write about hereditary chorea, was also the son of an East Hampton–born physician who had served a medical apprenticeship in that town, and according to his son was "acquainted with choreic families . . . possibly the same that Huntington observed.") By the 1880s physicians from Austria, Brazil, Cuba, Poland, and Russia were also reporting cases. The name *Huntington's chorea* entered medical discourse in 1887, proposed by the Swiss neurologist Armin Huber. A condition that had been defined almost entirely within the context of the patient's age—as a childhood disorder appearing in adults—had suddenly become a function of heredity. In fact, physicians now also described choreic symptoms appearing in children with a family history of adult hereditary chorea. They pointed out that although the clinical picture in juvenile cases often differed from that of adults in the same family since it included rigidity, tremors, and seizures, it was probably the same disease.[2]

By 1892 neurologists were making slightly exaggerated claims that the literature on hereditary, and more often "Huntington's chorea," was "copious," even "voluminous," and that its clinical history was "very thoroughly known." Practitioners even proposed that it was "either endemic to, or at least prevalent in, certain parts of many countries, where its entity is well recognized by the laity, its cardinal signs discussed, and its universally unfavourable termination so proverbial, that members of families in which it is known to exist find great difficulty in securing partners in marriage," although these claims were uncertain at best.[3]

Why should "hereditary chorea" suddenly become accepted as a distinct clinical entity in the 1880s? Why did it now appear "interesting" to medical practitioners and "by no means as rare as we have been led to believe"? The disease itself had not grown in prevalence during the previous decades. Nor had life expectancy risen substantially: average life expectancy at birth (in Massachusetts) had increased only slightly since 1850 (from 38.3 years to 41.74 years in 1878–82 for white men, and from 40.5 years in 1850 to 43.5 years in 1878–82 for white women; for black women and men the figures were starkly lower: in 1900, 35 years for women, 32.5 years for men). Although scientific theories of heredity changed dramatically in the 1880s, as we shall see, most physicians were either unaware of the changes or viewed them with skepticism if not disbelief.[4]

Other social, medical, and scientific transformations had taken place, how-

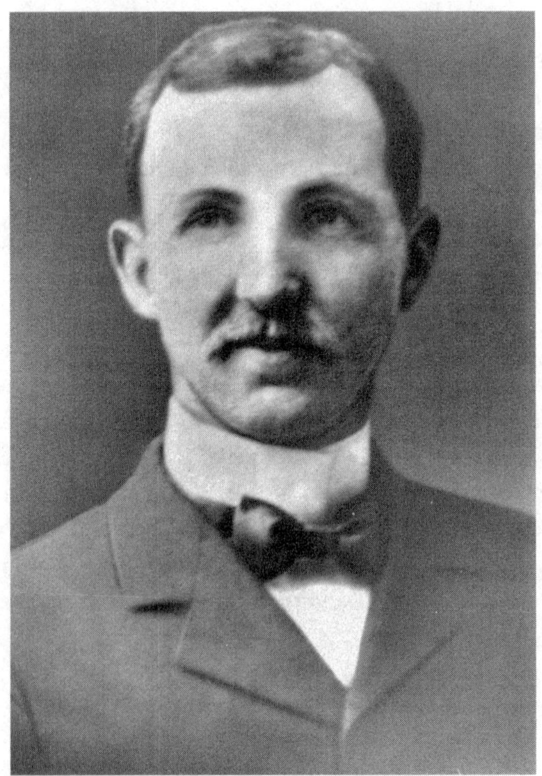

Clarence King (1861–1944), physician and author of five papers on hereditary chorea. Courtesy Cattaraugus Historical Society and King Memorial Library, Machias, N.Y.

ever, altering the lenses through which practitioners viewed this disease. Most important was the emergence of neurology as a medical specialty and the professional ambitions of neurologists to claim scientific and social authority. That the New York Neurological Society, a predecessor to the American Neurological Association, held its first meeting in March 1872, a month after George Huntington delivered his paper in Ohio, symbolizes the linkages between these events. Neurology had developed first in Europe in the 1850s and in the United States in the 1860s, in the context of the Civil War, where the battlefield left many soldiers with severe head injuries. Reacting against the older and more established psychiatrists whom they often dismissed as old-fashioned, young American neurologists in the 1860s and 1870s insisted that nervous disorders of all kinds, including "insanity," were physical maladies like any other and that neurologists were best equipped to diagnose and treat such ills. They fashioned themselves as rigorous and up to date, looking to European scientific ideas as the basis for their practice. As American medicine became increasingly oriented toward science, many young clinicians traveled to Germany for sojourns in German laboratories, the most advanced in Europe in the late nineteenth century.[5]

By the 1870s they had begun to secure medical school professorships and hospital appointments back home in major cities such as Boston, New York, and Philadelphia. They established office practices and sought middle- and upper-class patients, offering fashionable new diagnoses such as neurasthenia and "nervousness." They also organized neurological wards and departments, where patients with these disorders were more accessible to clinicians. They presented papers at meetings of the American Neurological Association, organized in 1875, and published them in the new *Journal of Nervous and Mental Disease,* where many early reports of hereditary chorea appeared. They described other neurological disorders during this time as well, such as Friedreich's ataxia (in 1863), multiple sclerosis (1868), athetosis (1871), and Tourette syndrome (1885).[6]

In addition, as we have seen, by the 1880s optimistic mid-nineteenth-century conceptions of a malleable heredity were giving way to more pessimistic and deterministic understandings, while degeneration theory attributed the decline of advanced societies to the accumulating ills of civilization. "The environmentalism and optimism which had characterized mid-century discussions of heredity," writes Charles Rosenberg, "was gradually replaced in the 1880s by a growing biological reductionism," and an emphasis on authoritarian solutions. In psychiatry, in neurology, and in social thought more generally, leading figures increasingly turned to hereditarianism as a powerful mode of explanation.[7]

Within this context, the expanding population of the older mental hospitals and asylums and the opening of new ones meant that more adult patients with chorea, magrums, and St. Vitus's dance came to the attention of clinicians: in the 1880s the total population of U.S. state mental hospitals doubled, from 31,973 in 1880 to 67,754 in 1890; the figure nearly doubled again, to 129,222, in 1904. (Patients with a diagnosis of Huntington's chorea increasingly ended up in these hospitals for lack of an alternative setting for long-term care.) This meant that several members of one family were likely to come to the same institution, where a single doctor might see all of them, thus offering him or her a clearer window onto the hereditary repetitions of the disease. Since the hospital was coming to replace the home as the principal site for observation and the production of medical knowledge, the growth of the total hospital population was yet

The Journal
OF
Nervous and Mental Disease

AN AMERICAN JOURNAL OF NEUROPSYCHIATRY

FOUNDED IN 1874

MANAGING EDITOR
DR. SMITH ELY JELLIFFE
64 West 56th St., New York

ASSOCIATE EDITORS
WILLIAM A. WHITE, M.D., and GREGORY STRAGNELL, M.D.
372–374 Broadway, Albany, N. Y.

WITH COLLABORATION OF

DR. C. L. ALLEN, Los Angeles, Calif.
DR. LEWELLYS F. BARKER, Baltimore, Md.
DR. B. BROUWER, Amsterdam, Holland
DR. CARL D. CAMP, Ann Arbor, Mich.
DR. C. MACFIE CAMPBELL, Boston, Mass.
DR. LOUIS CASAMAJOR, New York, N. Y.
DR. HARVEY CUSHING, Boston, Mass.
DR. FREDERIC J. FARNELL, Providence, R. I.
DR. BERNARD GLUECK, New York, N. Y.
DR. MENAS S. GREGORY, New York, N. Y.
DR. C. JUDSON HERRICK, Chicago, Ill.
DR. GORDON HOLMES, London, England
DR. J. RAMSAY HUNT, New York, N. Y.
DR. C. ARIËNS KAPPERS, Amsterdam, Holland
DR. GEO. H. KIRBY, New York, N. Y.
DR. ADOLF MEYER, Baltimore, Md.
DR. L. J. J. MUSKENS, Amsterdam, Holland
DR. GEO. H. PARKER, Cambridge, Mass.
DR. SYDNEY SCHWAB, St. Louis, Mo.
DR. PAUL SCHILDER, New York, N. Y.
DR. E. A. SHARP, Buffalo, N. Y.
DR. EDWARD A. STRECKER, Philadelphia, Pa.
DR. OLIVER S. STRONG, New York, N. Y.
DR. WALTER TIMME, New York, N. Y.
DR. FRED W. TILNEY, New York, N. Y.
DR. S. A. K. WILSON, London, England

SERIAL NO. 612

TABLE OF CONTENTS ON PAGE II
2 VOLS. PER YEAR

ISSUED MONTHLY $1.00 PER COPY $10.00 PER YEAR

FOREIGN SUBSCRIPTION $11.00 PER YEAR
Entered as second-class matter at the Post Office at Albany, New York, March 30, 1922. Copyright by Smith Ely Jelliffe, M.D., Publisher, 1932

N. B.: Consult Our Directory of America's Leading Sanitaria

H. K. Lewis, 136 Gower Street, London, W. C. Steiger & Co., 49 Murray Street, New York. G. Stechert & Co., 31 East 10th Street, New York. Paul B. Hoeber, 76 Fifth Avenue, New York. Chicago Medical Book Co., Chicago, Illinois

The first neurological journal in the United States, founded 1874.
Courtesy *Journal of Nervous and Mental Disease*

another element that helped turn what had been a "medical curiosity" into an important disease.[8]

It was during this decade that a German biologist named August Weissman found experimental evidence to contradict long-accepted beliefs in the inheritance of acquired characteristics, laying the foundation for what would soon come to be known as "hard" heredity. As we have seen, Francis Galton had made a similar challenge, but for the first time Weissman provided evidence from the laboratory. Weissman argued that the substance controlling heredity and development was contained in the nucleus of the cell, and that the germ cells—egg and pollen or sperm—were separate from all the other cells of the body—the somatic cells. Thus influences acquired during the lifetime of the parents were not passed on to the offspring as the Lamarckians claimed (so-called soft inheritance), and as almost everyone believed. Inheritance was not created anew with each generation. Instead, each generation transmitted to its offspring only what the parents themselves had inherited from their parents—a phenomenon known as the "continuity of the germ plasm." As Weissman told it, the hereditary material within the cell nucleus constituted a special type of particle he called a determinant. This determinant controlled both the transmission of traits from parent to offspring and the development of the embryo.[9]

Published at a time when the Lamarckians were at the height of their influence, Weissman's ideas encountered great hostility, even from enthusiastic followers of Darwin. According to the historian Ernst Mayr, Weissman's theories were not universally accepted by biologists until the 1930s and 1940s. If physicians were familiar with the new theory at all before 1900, most remained unconvinced. And even many of those inclined to accept Weissman's analysis doubted its usefulness for medicine.[10]

Physicians generally were more receptive to the bacteriological revolution that was also taking place in the 1880s, since the identification of pathogenic organisms responsible for tuberculosis, cholera, typhoid, and diphtheria soon made possible diagnostic tests, antitoxins, and vaccines to combat these scourges. That Huntington's chorea became a recognized clinical category at the same time that many physicians welcomed this environmental turn may appear paradoxical. However, for some clinicians the new bacteriology strengthened their conviction that heredity was critical to understanding disease, since medicine now had to explain why certain people were more vulnerable to germs than others. Moreover, in relation to mental illness, "no really scientific physician denied that heredity was perhaps the most important" etiological factor. Just how heredity functioned, however, the actual mechanisms of heredity, remained entirely unresolved.[11]

NEUROPATHOLOGY, RACE, AND METAPHOR

By the mid-nineteenth century, European neuropathologists had characterized chorea of all kinds as an alteration "of the nervous centres and more precisely of the brain," with several studies by the early 1870s indicating that "a severe lesion or the stimulation of one corpus striatum [the 'striped body' that forms part of the basal ganglia; also called the corpora striata, opto-striate bodies and striatum] can paralyze or excite most muscles on the opposite side of the body." That same decade at least two pathology studies of cases strongly reminiscent of hereditary chorea reached similar conclusions. The first, in 1871—possibly the first such autopsy report—was of a sixty-eight-year-old woman who had died of pneumonia at the Connecticut Hospital for the Insane in Hartford with "chronic chorea," dementia, and "confused delusions" in which she imagined that hospital workers were old friends. Although no family history was available from her prior stay in the almshouse, her residence in Connecticut (where we know affected families lived), her long-term suffering from violent choreic movements, and late-term dementia suggest a diagnosis of hereditary chorea. Her autopsy report emphasized the "very marked flattening of the anterior lobes of the cerebrum [upper part of the brain, including the cortex or outermost layer]," along with "a gaping state of the vessels of the opto-striate bodies."[12]

The second was the autopsy performed by Camillo Golgi in 1874 on a male patient who had died at forty-two of pneumonia at the Hospital for Incurables near Golgi's home of Abbiategrasso, a town near Milan in the north of Italy. This patient had suffered for several years from mental disturbances and choreic movements, and his mother was allegedly a "hysteric," which also make a diagnosis of hereditary chorea likely, although Golgi presented no specific history of other affected relatives. Using his newly developed "black reaction" (a nitrate stain for studying neurons, or nerve cells), Golgi also found dramatic changes, both in the cortex and in the corpus striatum: neurons in the upper half of the striatum were totally altered, with damaged processes (dendrites or nerve fibers) and proliferating glial cells (nonneuronal cells in the brain), "with resulting atrophy of the nerve cells." By the 1880s, many clinical papers included postmortem reports, with general agreement that in this form of chorea, the corpus striatum, and especially that part called the caudate nucleus, was damaged—"wasted," "flat," or "deficient in plumpness." Or as Harbinson wrote in 1880, "all authorities agree in localising the immediate cause of chorea in or in and about this region."[13]

Just what caused the wasting of the striatum—and of other parts of the basal ganglia and cortex that showed damage and atrophy in autopsy studies—was a source of much debate, with arguments centering around two influential interpretations of the etiology of the disease. Golgi had proposed that inflammation was the culprit. In his view, the alterations he had found in the striatum were the results of a chronic interstitial encephalitis, or inflammation of parts of the brain, an interpretation that would have a considerable following over the next several decades.[14]

A second line of interpretation held that Huntington's chorea was a failure of development leading to a process of degeneration. As Wharton Sinkler defined it in 1892, "the pathology of the disease is a degeneration of imperfectly developed cells in the motor tract or in the cerebral cortex and in the spinal cord." He believed that comparisons with hereditary ataxia, "which is now well established as a disease due to defective development of the nervous system," lent support to this thesis. On the other hand, William Osler omitted any mention of defective development, but agreed that "the morbid anatomy of chronic chorea is that of a neuro-degenerative disorder," though he acknowledged that the specific lesions remained unknown.[15]

Several other clinicians also offered hypotheses as to the origin of this degeneration, alluding to older theories about "weaknesses" becoming "entailed" in the "constitution." For instance, Clarence King speculated in 1885 that the initial causes were probably the same as those of ordinary St. Vitus's dance,

> modified, perhaps, by a peculiar disposition of the individual, by some pre-existing malady, or by some unexplainable intellectual influence, self-indulgence, bad education, and the like. And it is even possible that marriages between persons of a weak or deranged nervous organization, continued for several successive generations, may so intensify the original defects as to result in the disease under consideration. And it is in this way that it may first make its appearance, and, finding like soil in the offspring, favored, perhaps, by another improper marriage, the hereditary tendency is developed.[16]

A few physicians, including Osler, attempted to integrate the new bacteriological knowledge with older ideas about etiology. They speculated that the original cause of this disease might be a "choreic virus," "a virus as yet unknown," or a "subtle microbe now lurking in his safe retreat," whose effects were then handed down to subsequent generations—a theory that would be revived for a time in the 1970s. George Huntington himself hinted at his belief in a possible association between chorea and tetanus, which was common on eastern Long Island (possibly due, in his opinion, to the use of a small oily fish called menhaden as fertilizer).[17]

However, by the 1890s, many U.S. clinicians had become convinced, with

Sinkler, that Huntington's chorea was the result of a primary degeneration or "constitutional taint" that led to early deterioration and death. In an influential paper published in 1895 in the *Journal of Nervous and Mental Disease,* Charles Loomis Dana, a professor of neurology at Cornell Medical School and former president of the American Neurological Association, summarized this hypothesis, dismissing reports of inflammation as the underlying cause. In his view, the disease was "a late development of a teratological defect [congenital malformation]. The patient is born with a brain which is abnormal. There is no microbe, no poison, nothing in the environment of the individual or in his general physical make-up that produces this. It is simply a death at the age of thirty of cells which should and do in ordinary people live to the age of seventy." In this process of "decay and death," the disease attacked "the cortex of the brain primarily . . . affecting one region after another until the part is so destroyed that dementia occurs and finally death ensues." Classifying hereditary chorea as "a congenital defect, to be classed, perhaps, with idiocy and due to lack of development of the cortex," Dana concluded that "we have an explanation of the disease which is reasonably satisfactory."[18]

To explain the meanings of teratology, abiotrophy (loss of function without apparent injury), and degeneration in relation to the pathological process of Huntington's chorea, clinicians such as Dana drew not only on scientific knowledge about the brain but also on widely shared stereotypes of race and gender. For example, Dana compared a brain peculiarity in his white male patient—the separation of the parietal (middle) part of the parieto-occipital fissure from the occipital (back) part—to a similar peculiarity in what he called "a low type negress' brain," drawing on assumptions about the inferiority of women and blacks to convey the "imperfect evolution of the brain." (Yet his thirty-five-year-old patient, even after being hospitalized because of chorea and mental losses, would sit in a chair reading Shakespeare's plays or Gibbon's history of Rome, "apparently enjoying them." According to Dana, he later took to reading newspapers "and betrayed his intellectual decay by giving up the classics for the daily news.")[19]

Questions about racial difference in Huntington's chorea also emerged explicitly in clinical discussions in the racially tense 1890s, a decade, in the United States, of lynchings, legalized segregation, and massive immigration. During this decade white physicians questioned whether the disease differed in patients of African and of European descent, in effect using the disease to explore racial difference while at the same time exploiting racist assumptions to construct medical representations of the disease. (As most of the early North Americans with hereditary chorea were either of old-stock English ancestry or recent immigrants from northern Europe, practitioners initially limited their discussions of "race" to questions of distinctions among "Irish," "Germans," "Scotch," "Hebrews," and so forth, since these were considered "racial" categories at the time.) Most writers concluded that there was no evidence of racial difference, though William Francis Drewry, a white physician at the Central State Hospital for the Insane in Petersburg, Virginia, was convinced that "the Negro rarely has chorea in any form."[20]

Other white clinicians, however, read a story about the multiple origins of Huntington's chorea into their African-American cases. The presence of the disease in "a full-blooded negro," as Clarence King put it in 1906, "does not fully conform to our ideas of heredity from a single source." Practitioners such as King could not fathom the idea that whites and blacks with Huntington's chorea may have been biologically related. In their view, these patients proved that the disease could not have come from a single progenitor, as some had believed. Their assumptions about race thus prevented them from taking seriously one of the plausible theories about the single origin of the disease.[21]

Just as clinicians drew on the metaphor of "imperfect evolution" to equate chorea and racial inferiority, they also used the metaphor of degeneration to describe both a disease process in the brain and, through a kind of slippage, the families and sufferers themselves. "A glance at the family history shows the strong tendency to degeneration almost to the point of extermination," wrote the Connecticut psychiatrist Frank Hallock in 1898, using the term *degeneration* to mean the gradual disappearance of the family as a whole. Hallock cited a reduced number of offspring, early deaths of family members, and earlier onset and shorter course of the disease in successive generations as "significant facts" demonstrating the presence of a degenerative process. The distinguished Boston neurologist James J. Putnam in 1904 referred to "the danger of increasing the number of cerebral degenerates," again using a term drawn from descriptions of the disease process in the brain to characterize the person afflicted. Degeneration, as we have seen, was "the ultimate signifier of pathology," but a signifier that was always slipping out of focus and across boundaries.[22]

As a description of the disease process in the brain, degeneration implied a gradual loss of structure and function, a biological process leading eventually to the disability and death of the individual. As a social metaphor, however, degeneration had other implications. It suggested a moral and social deterioration. It also implied the eventual disappearance of these families, and the likelihood that the disease would die out on its own, due to the failure of family members to marry, the tendency even of those who did marry to have fewer children than usual, possibly even no children at all. As Morel had defined it, degeneration as social process moved inexorably toward extinction. And some clinicians and even some eugenicists agreed that families with Huntington's chorea were in fact dying out, "partly due to the debilitating factor that goes along with the disease," as a Vermont "Eugenical Survey" later concluded. But others saw not "degeneration" but degenerates, individuals who had already suffered the process of degeneration but still managed to survive. They were another story altogether.[23]

"INSANITY" OR DEMENTIA?

Disordered movements of the body have a long history of associations with disorders of the mind, and nineteenth-century clinicians sometimes described the physical movements of chorea as if they were an external representation of internal mental states, a sort of "mania of the motor centres," or the "insanity of the muscles" as several writers put it. (Lay people often associated involuntary movement with mental weakness: for instance, in his 1791 biography of the English writer Samuel Johnson, James Boswell noted an episode in which the painter William Hogarth, on observing for the first time Johnson's tics and twitches and not knowing who he was, "concluded that he was an ideot." Hogarth was stunned when the "ideot" began to speak, demonstrating his eloquence and genius. Similarly, when the English physician Thomas Jeffreys recounted in 1825 his case of the fifty-four-year-old attorney with chorea, he noted that observers "when passing, have been known to ask, whether he was not an idiot.") However, whereas Charles Oscar Waters back in 1841 had spoken of "a more or less perfect dementia"—meaning a disorder of cognitive function—and Johan Christian Lund had also referred to dementia, George Huntington had characterized the mental symptoms of hereditary chorea as a "tendency to insanity, and sometimes that form of insanity which leads to suicide," a rather different portrayal. Though nineteenth-century practitioners sometimes used the terms *insanity* and *dementia* interchangeably, they carried distinct cultural resonances. With its evocations of shrieking, incomprehensible madmen and madwomen, of lunatics tied and chained inside prisonlike cells, insanity was a concept with a long history of powerful cultural associations. Popular representations of insanity (along with lunacy and madness) portrayed the insane as wild beasts, frothing at the mouth, shouting nonsense, attacking their neighbors, or sunk into unresponsive melancholy. Insanity, especially hereditary insanity, was a staple of the gothic novel in the nineteenth century, the stuff of thrillers involving family secrets and bitter marriages.[24]

Dementia was also a widely used term within medicine, as one of the four most common diagnoses in mental hospitals, along with mania, melancholia, and imbecility. According to the historian Ellen Dwyer, it was considered the most pessimistic diagnosis that could be made in nineteenth-century North America. But it had fewer cultural connotations. There is no fiction that I know of about hereditary dementia. There were few popular representations of dementia, at least outside of hospital registers and medical texts.[25]

George Huntington's emphasis on "insanity," then, introduced a term that had not previously entered the medical discourse on chorea, and one that may have heightened the social fears and the psychological prejudices surrounding the disease. While it was true that by the turn of the century physicians considered insanity more useful as a legal than as a medical category, as the neurologist Smith Ely Jelliffe would later insist, those outside of medicine continued to use this term well into the twentieth century. Nobody disputed that Huntington's chorea was an organic disorder of the brain, yet the nature of the mental and emotional symptoms was far from certain. Some psychiatrists complained that the neurologist, with his office practice and his focus on the movement disorder and the neuropathology of the disease, was apt to miss "the picture of psychical decay before him." As one Connecticut psychiatrist put it in 1898, "ordinary clinic or private visits, unless very frequent, often fail to reveal the facts of this kind. One must almost live with his patient to fully appreciate the psychical side of many of the so-called neuroses." But those who did "almost live" with their Huntington's patients sometimes emphasized that insane behavior was mainly a response to the social losses entailed by the disease. "Why should not a person become insane who is subject to this distressing affliction," asked Theodore Diller, a compassionate psychiatrist at the State Hospital for the Insane in Danville, Pennsylvania, in 1890. "The embarrassments, the feelings of helplessness and despair, the constant attention to self—the constant dwelling of the mind on the affection—ever present—these, together with the feeling of despondency in the knowledge that his usefulness in life is over, and that he is only an object of pity, charity, and care for his friends would seem to me to be potent factors in bringing about gradually a certain mental impairment or enfeeblement of the mind which would progressively increase, and finally end in dementia."[26]

Some clinicians, both neurologists and psychiatrists, argued that in fact the mental impairment in Huntington's was not always severe. Arthur S. Hamilton, a neurologist in Minnesota who had seen many patients with Huntington's chorea both in private practice and in his state hospital service, declared in 1908 that he had "often been struck with the thought that on close inspection almost all of the well-advanced cases are really much less demented than they seemed at first glance," and that patients rarely became disoriented as to time, place, or persons. In fact, wrote the Yale University psychiatrist Allan R. Diefendorf that same year, while defects of memory were the chief evidence of dementia, memory loss in Huntington's usually progressed very slowly, so that even after twenty-five or thirty years of illness patients still possessed "a very fair memory for both recent and remote events." Diefendorf was often surprised "to observe how well the patients remembered even when speech had become almost unintelligible and when emotional deterioration was profound." Moreover, they continued to grasp what took place around them and remained fairly well oriented until the end stages of the disease.[27]

Clarence King's five papers on hereditary chorea, published between 1885 and 1916, suggest the changing medical representations of the mental aspects of the disease. As we saw earlier, King's father belonged to an old East Hampton family but had left around 1856, later passing on to his son his memories of the affected families in his old hometown. The younger King grew up with the idea that "hereditary insanity was common there," and that "certain individuals in choreic families became insane without having chorea." In his medical school thesis of 1885, King characterized hereditary chorea as "a low form of mental derangement or insanity." In a second paper published the same year, King also referred to "certain strange and insane actions" of a patient with chorea who was considered to have "mental disease." King was even more emphatic in his third paper, published in 1889, noting that "insanity appears to be a quite common termination of the disease." By 1906, however, King had moderated his position. He no longer used the word *insanity* or *insane*, describing instead "marked mental unsoundness . . . which generally takes the form of a slow, progressive dementia." In his paper of 1916 he referred to "mental deterioration" as well as suicidal tendencies—something he had mentioned in all his papers—but he made no mention of insanity.[28]

King's papers reflect practitioners' growing caution in the use of such umbrella terms as *insanity* and a more nuanced clinical understanding of the cognitive and emotional symptoms in Huntington's chorea. By the turn of the century, while those outside of medicine continued to refer to "hereditary insanity," few practitioners were using this term to describe their patients with Huntington's. They spoke of such symptoms as depression, irritability, apathy, and indifference, occasionally using such terms as *nervous* or *hysterical* or *maniacal*, or citing a "weakening of intelligence and of memory" that can advance to dementia, or simply the vague "mental disease." And many emphasized the persistence of abilities in their patients. Dementia might come at the end, but usually not long before.[29]

HUNTINGTON'S CHOREA AND THE MEANINGS OF HEREDITY

By the late 1880s hereditary or Huntington's chorea had largely achieved the status of a distinct clinical entity, recognized as such by practitioners such as Wharton Sinkler, a founder of the Philadelphia Neurological Society and a longtime associate of the city's Orthopedic Hospital and Infirmary for Nervous Diseases. "Hereditary chorea" first appeared as a separate category in the *Index Medicus* in 1889 and in the *Index-Catalogue of the Library of the Surgeon-General's Office, United States Army* in 1898. Although French neurologists such as Jean-Martin Charcot and his student Ernest Huet continued to regard it as a variant of Sydenham's chorea, most clinicians by this time considered hereditary chorea a different disease.

They also paid more attention. Whereas forty years earlier descriptions of the magrums had failed to awaken any notice, now many neurologists and psychiatrists decided that hereditary chorea was "interesting in the extreme, on account of the mystery which at present surrounds its nature and pathology," and because of "the peculiar and unvarying symptoms in every case which is met with." Annual meetings of the American Neurological Association from the late 1880s through the early years of the twentieth century regularly included discussions of hereditary/Huntington's chorea by members of an elite group of present and future leaders in American neurology—among them such medical professors and presidents of the association as Charles Loomis Dana; James Jackson Putnam of Harvard Medical School, founder of the first neurological clinic at the Massachusetts General Hospital in Boston; Landon Carter Gray of the New York Polyclinic Postgraduate School; and especially Sinkler, the North American neurologist who took the most sustained clinical interest in this disorder during the late 1880s and 1890s. Sinkler later became known more for his work on syringomyelia and epilepsy, but during this period he published several often-cited papers on hereditary chorea, including the family tree of a descendant of one of the Bedford families known to Lyon. He also used this disease to explore other "family" diseases.[30]

More psychiatrists in state institutions than neurologists in private office practice probably encountered patients with Huntington's, yet the distinctions between the two specialties were not clearly drawn, and despite the tensions between them, many turn-of-the-century physicians practiced both. In any case, there was no serious disagreement that Huntington's chorea was an organic disorder that fell squarely within the neurologists' terrain. No one denied the presence of visible lesions in the brain, unlike the case with more fashionable

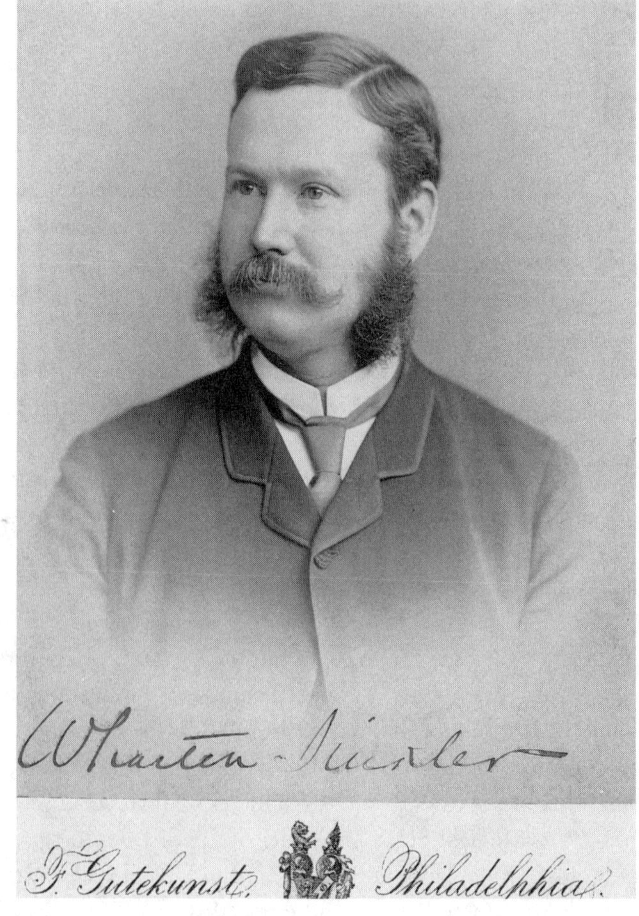

Wharton Sinkler (1845–1910), eminent Philadelphia neurologist. Courtesy Library of the College of Physicians of Philadelphia

disorders such as neurasthenia. Especially in an era in which neurologists faced intense criticism from general practitioners and psychiatrists who accused them of stealing patients and offering exaggerated promises of cures, many neurologists embraced Huntington's chorea as the neurological disorder par excellence, although such patients were hardly in demand.[31]

It is revealing, however, that although many clinicians in the 1880s and 1890s were intrigued by this malady, they made little effort to test George Huntington's claims about the hereditary pattern. They alluded to the intensity of heredity (the high number of affected people in successive generations) rather than to a specific pattern of inheritance. Or they said that it was "markedly hereditary," or "one of the most hereditary of all diseases" or that it had "an extra-strong, predisposing cause"—or, as Osler put it, that "heredity is one of the most remarkable features," and that "the hereditary character of the disease is very striking." Until 1900 few considered what George Huntington's account of the transmission pattern meant for understanding heredity more broadly, nor did they explore his claim that the malady could vanish in one generation. Most accepted his view that once the disease failed to develop in the offspring of an affected parent, it would not reappear, although some, like Sinkler, believed that while Huntington's theory was "generally the case, [it] is not an unvarying rule" (a reasonable assumption, since individuals who might have become affected sometimes died of other causes before any symptoms appeared, thereby potentially masquerading as a skipped generation). Clearly physicians at this time were less interested in the idea that hereditary chorea sometimes stopped—a point of great importance, however, to the families in question—than in the observation that its manifestations often continued unchanged for generations. As Osler put it, "in the whole range of inherited disorders there is scarcely one in which a larger percentage of individuals have been found affected."[32]

Nonetheless, through the 1880s and 1890s, and well into the twentieth century, clinicians disagreed about whether heredity should be foregrounded in the name. Some practitioners argued that the disease should be called *degenerative chorea* to emphasize its worsening course over time and eventual termination in death, an outcome distinctly different from that of ordinary chorea, which tended to resolve by itself. Others proposed *chorea of the aged* as a name that continued to highlight the late onset of the symptoms. *Choreic dementia* or *dementia choreica* emphasized the cognitive losses. Within this nomenclature, the mental symptoms were made primary, and the disorder was classified with *dementia paralytica* and *dementia senilis*, a view that did not, however, find many followers.[33]

The most common alternative was *chorea chronica progressiva*, or chronic progressive chorea, which a number of clinicians preferred as more descriptive of the condition's long, slow course and the occasional cases apparently without familial antecedents. Indeed, some writers continued to use this name even after *Huntington's chorea* became the accepted term in the literature, or to use the two interchangeably. Ironically, while William Osler preferred *chronic progressive chorea*, his prestige and praise played a significant role in legitimating the eponym *Huntington's chorea*, which bypassed the label of *hereditary* altogether, while substituting a somewhat similar-sounding name.[34]

GENDER, CHILDBEARING, AND HUNTINGTON'S CHOREA

George Huntington had speculated that chorea was "*more* common among *men* than women," and later clinicians also raised the question of gender, asking whether the disease affected women and men in equal numbers and in the same ways. Some (such as Gray) insisted that "the female sex are much more prone to Huntington's chorea than the male." Others (including King and Hamilton) asserted that there was "a slight preponderance of males." Family members often generalized from the gender distribution of the disease among their own kin. Eventually, however, clinicians came to the conclusion that men and women were affected at about the same rate, a view that is still accepted today.[35]

What varied, in the opinion of some, was the fertility of those who later developed chorea, in comparison with those who did not, and with men and women in the general population—a continuing debate throughout the twentieth century. By the early twentieth century, anxieties about "race suicide" had begun to circulate widely among middle-class white native-born Americans fearful that the allegedly high birth rate of the poor, the foreign-born, and the "feebleminded," in comparison with their own steadily declining birth rate, would lead to their social demise. Within the context of the Progressive-era emphasis on science, efficiency, and reform, social thinkers began to investigate the differential birth rate of immigrants, the poor generally, and all those considered to suffer from hereditary ills. As early as 1889, Sinkler had asserted that women who developed Huntington's chorea were "especially prolific" during their childbearing years—a position that, as we shall see, became a point of contention and foreshadowed later claims about the heightened fertility of the "unfit."[36]

But knowledgeable clinicians recognized that a history of Huntington's chorea in the family posed difficult dilemmas for women and men in relation to childbearing, since symptoms usually began in the thirties or later, after children had been born but were still young and dependent, but sometimes after the children were grown up, married, and starting their own families. As we saw earlier, physicians since the late eighteenth century had been warning against marriage to those "descended from unhealthy parents," while lamenting that such advice was rarely taken. So it is not surprising that by the early 1900s a few clinicians such as Clarence King were urging their colleagues to advise all members of families with Huntington's chorea not to marry, "at least until the chain of heredity has been broken for two or more generations" (although just how the chain could be broken if there were no children born is unclear).[37]

Few physicians before the 1920s recommended birth control as an option for families with Huntington's chorea. Yet as the historian Janet Farrell Brodie has shown in her definitive *Contraception and Abortion in Nineteenth-Century America*, various methods of contraception were already practiced in the United States in the nineteenth century, methods involving condoms, vaginal pessaries, sponges, tampons, spermicides, douches, and even early versions of the diaphragm. Certainly the dramatic decline in fertility between 1800 and 1900 (from an average of 7 live births per white woman in 1800 to 3.56 in 1900) has been well documented, although the causes of this decline are complex. Securing information, drugs, and implements became increasingly difficult in the late nineteenth century, however, especially after the 1873 passage of the Comstock Law prohibiting the interstate mailing of "obscene" information—including specifically information about contraception. Most early-twentieth-century physicians opposed birth control, not merely disapproving of contraception but, according to the historian Linda Gordon, expressing "a revulsion so hysterical that it prevented them from accepting facts." As for abortion, new state laws passed after 1860 helped drive the procedure underground, "making it difficult, expensive, and dangerous to obtain—a criminalization that lasted until the 1960s."[38]

Under these circumstances, marriage without childbearing was virtually impossible for most women. As states enacted marriage prohibitions for certain conditions such as "insanity" and epilepsy in the 1900s and 1910s, more doctors expressed the position that members of families with Huntington's should not marry. Those family members who did marry but tried to limit their childbearing, or even to remain childless—choices that lay them open to social disapproval—found themselves in a nearly impossible situation, burdened not only by anxiety about the disease but by the criminalization of contraception and abortion that weighed especially heavily on women.[39]

An episode in Boston in 1900 illuminates the dilemmas, for clinicians as well as for patients. A married woman of thirty-five with advanced Huntington's chorea and five young children discovered she was pregnant. Three years earlier she had consulted James J. Putnam, now one of the most eminent neurologists in America. Putnam saw that she suffered from choreic movements, though in his view, these were not yet so obtrusive that they would immediately be noticed by an observer unfamiliar with the disease. He learned from her that her father, paternal grandmother, and two aunts on her father's side had all suffered from the same malady. When she became pregnant for the sixth time, her husband was "overcome with horror at the outcome of his indiscretion," according to his friend, the Boston obstetrician Horace Marion, who later wrote up the case. The husband, and presumably the wife, pleaded with Marion to perform an abortion. Marion, in turn, consulted his colleague Putnam for advice. After careful consideration, the two physicians decided against it. "We were agreed that we had no right to assume that the product of this conception would prove a mental derelict and declined to countenance any interference," Marion reported. Two years after the birth of her child, the woman, now thirty-seven and the mother of six young children, committed suicide by poisoning herself. Underscoring the depth of her determination to end her life, Marion noted that through twelve hours of terrible suffering, she never made a single murmur or expressed any regret.[40]

Both Marion and Putnam were deeply disturbed by this outcome, and addressed it in separate papers published in 1904. Presenting the case as a eugenic cautionary tale, Putnam insisted that unfavorable heredity was important to consider with respect to the family and community, in order to avoid increasing the number of "cerebral degenerates." Although he rejected claims that insanity was increasing or that "civilized races" were in danger of being swamped by a growing tide of neurotic and defective citizens, as some charged, Putnam agreed with Marion that "epileptics" and insane persons should not marry, and that "where either party is burdened with an inheritance like that of the subject of this paper," marriage should not take place.[41]

For both Putnam and Marion, hereditary illness offered new professional opportunities and responsibilities for physicians. Both men emphasized that new knowledge about "the transmissibility of certain brain defects" was dramatizing the need for the medical adviser to play a broader role "preventing unions, the fruit of which tend to the lowering of the scale of intelligence in the coming generation." As adviser, the physician could call attention to "the inexorable laws of heredity." He or she could also stand "ready to consult with patients regarding the conditions for proper prevention of conception." Indeed, Putnam appeared open to birth control, urging that physicians consider "other alternatives" to abstinence. And while he thought that marriage without intent of procreation was mostly unjustified, there might be circumstances where this alternative was acceptable.[42]

Hereditary illness also raised the question of "terminating gestation," but this was a subject that neither physician wished to pursue. Marion's willingness, like Putnam's, to consider "alternatives" to abstinence, and his openness to marriage without childbearing, made him one of the more progressive clinicians of his time on this issue. Moreover, both he and Putnam appeared to accept that their patient's suicide stemmed in large part from her desperate situation, rather than simply from the disease. Still, when presented with a choice between performing an illegal abortion and acceding to the birth of an unwanted child to a mother of five who was already ill with Huntington's chorea, they chose not to intervene. Legal prohibitions on abortion and birth control both prevented this woman from exercising the limited choices open to her and undermined the ability of her physicians to help their patient cope with the vicissitudes of the disease.

HEREDITY AND THERAPEUTICS

The establishment of Huntington's chorea as a hereditary clinical entity had one important practical benefit to clinicians. As Clarence King put it in 1885, "ordinarily the diagnosis is easy on account of the history of chorea in a parent or grandparent; in fact, the patient and his friends are watching with fear for the expected development of the disease." Though Osler, Sinkler, and others acknowledged that there were occasional cases in families with no history, or in which parents and grandparents had died young, the recognition of a specific pattern of heredity gave the clinician a powerful new diagnostic tool.[43]

Furthermore, some clinicians throughout the 1880s and 1890s reported their continuing efforts to ease symptoms even if they could not cure the disease. They repeatedly tried all the long-established antispasmodic and sedative drug therapies used in ordinary chorea, such as hyoscine and hyoscyamine (drugs obtained from the nightshade family of plants), digitalis, belladonna, and opium. They also used tonics such as chalybeates (iron), arsenic, and zinc. They recommended massage and electricity. And they tried supportive therapies such as music at meals, healthful diets, and an environment as free of stress as possible. In 1841 Charles Waters had also reported one patient's claim that his involuntary movements "ceased under the influence of all instrumental music, except that of the common 'Jew's-Harp.'" James MacFaren, at the Royal Edinburgh Asylum in Scotland, reported that his forty-six-year-old male patient who had been affected with chorea for six years actually improved with a "nourishing diet, a small allowance of stimulants, and a dose of bromide of potassium [a salt used as an antispasmodic and sedative] three times a day."[44]

However, by the 1890s most practitioners agreed with Sinkler that "the disease so far has resisted all medication." As Hay wrote in 1890, "I have at different times used full and continuous doses of iron, arsenic, hyoscine, hyoscyamine, the bromides, sulphonal [a sedative] and many other drugs," but "no permanent good resulted in any case under any of the various treatments." Moreover, the drugs that did have some slight effect in easing symptoms, such as hyoscine and arsenic, had to be given at such high doses that they caused gastrointestinal disorder and were therefore not justifiable. For Hay, general hygiene and avoidance of excitement and anxiety, with "tonic and nutritive measures," constituted the best treatment available.[45]

Even after the turn of the century, with many pessimistic reports in the medical literature and the growing influence of eugenics, a few clinicians continued to experiment with supportive treatments for patients. Nicholas J. Dynan, a psychiatrist at the Government Hospital for the Insane in Washington, D.C., proposed wisely in 1914 that "extra and special diet must be given, as usually the appetite is ravenous." And Clarence King, in 1916, recounted hearing of a patient whose choreic movements were quieted "wonderfully" by the music of a violin, "so much so and so promptly that it became a regular practice for a fellow patient to play a few strains of music before he attempted to eat his meals," and also before he went to sleep at night.[46]

But by this time, many clinicians were emphasizing prevention rather than treatment, urging that potential subjects of Huntington's chorea be protected against excitement and mental strain and placed under "hygienic conditions" as prophylactic strategies, as Sinkler had recommended, the same as with those predisposed to insanity. They cited their own experiences to affirm that no remedy offered any hope of halting the symptoms once they began. And increasingly, they urged eugenic measures, calling on doctors to advise their patients from these families against marriage, and insisting that the disease merited "very serious consideration" on the part of all those concerned with "the problem of the socially unfit."[47]

HUNTINGTON'S CHOREA AND "AMERICAN" NEUROLOGY

Around the turn of the century, North American neurologists became increasingly self-conscious about their identity as Americans in a medical specialty until then dominated by Europeans. European neurology was more scientifically advanced and more institutionally established, and before 1910 the majority of papers on Huntington's chorea appeared in the European rather than the North American medical press, with additional papers in Brazilian, Cuban, Russian, Argentinian, and Polish publications. (Of 57 articles on hereditary chorea in medical journals published worldwide in the 1880s, only 8 appeared in U.S. medical journals, while 17 were published in British, 17 in German, 12 in French, and 3 in Italian journals. In the 1890s, of a total of 150 publications, 34 were in U.S. journals, with 59 in German-language journals, 20 in French, 10 in British, and 16 in Italian. From 1900 to 1909, of 197 publications worldwide, around 40, about the same 20 percent as in the previous decade, appeared in the United States, although 12 of those appeared in a single issue of one journal, *Neurographs*, and not all of them were by Americans.

In this decade, 56 accounts, about 28 percent, appeared in German-language journals, 30 in French, 15 in Italian, and 10 in British journals, with 2 each in Cuba and Brazil.)[48]

Still, hereditary chorea was one disease that had been described first by North Americans and had been named after an American. Thus it may have been partly this rivalry with European colleagues that prompted William Browning, a New York neurologist who had attended the University of Leipzig, in Germany, to publish, in 1908, a special Huntington Number of his new journal *Neurographs*, emphasizing the American—and indeed the Long Island—dimension of this disease. In his opening editorial, Browning contrasted the many "operations, methods, and instruments" that were known by the names of their American originators or describers, with the "very few" diseases so designated. Huntington's chorea, then, stood out, since "no single disease of equal importance is so commonly designated and understood by a native's name." Not only Huntington but also the other early describers of hereditary chorea, according to Browning, were comparable to "the pre-Columbian discoverers of America," such as the Norsemen! *Neurographs,* in short, was performing a heroic narrative of Huntington's chorea, turning doctors into explorers and emphasizing the American identity of this disease.[49]

Browning insisted that Huntington's chorea was inherently historical, since "from its most marked feature, heredity, an historical order of investigation comes naturally first to mind." Never mind that clinicians had been writing about hereditary chorea for more than three decades without thinking of a historical orientation, and that there was nothing "natural" about that approach. Now for the first time, neurologists would focus on the history and genealogy of Huntington's chorea. To this end, *Neurographs* included brief genealogical and biographical essays on the malady by such distinguished figures as William Osler, now a Regius professor at the University of Oxford, Frederick Tilney at Columbia, and Smith Ely Jelliffe, editor and publisher of the influential *Journal of Nervous and Mental Disease*, the organ of the American Neurological Association. There were also papers on the neuropathology and psychiatric symptoms of Huntington's by the French medical professors M. Lannois and J. Paviot of the Medical Faculty at the University of Lyon, Adolf Strumpell, director of a medical clinic in Breslau, and Allan R. Diefendorf at Yale.[50]

Browning's approach was almost certainly inspired by Jelliffe, whose interests in genealogy and heredity had led him to begin a genealogical study of Huntington's chorea several years earlier. Indeed, Jelliffe was a critical nexus in the early history of this disease, a neurological entrepreneur who had many connections

HUNTINGTON NUMBER

NEUROGRAPHS

A SERIES OF NEUROLOGICAL STUDIES, CASES, AND NOTES

Editor
WILLIAM BROWNING, Ph.B., M.D.

Associates
R. M. ELLIOTT, M.D.
E. G. ZABRISKIE, M.D.
F. C. EASTMAN, A.B., M.D.
F. TILNEY, A.B., M.D.

Vol. 1, No. 2
Issued
May 25, 1908

GERMANY: TH. STAUFFER, UNIVERSITÄT-STRASSE 26, LEIPSIC
BROOKLYN-NEW YORK
ALBERT T. HUNTINGTON
1908

Neurographs, "Huntington Number," May 25, 1908

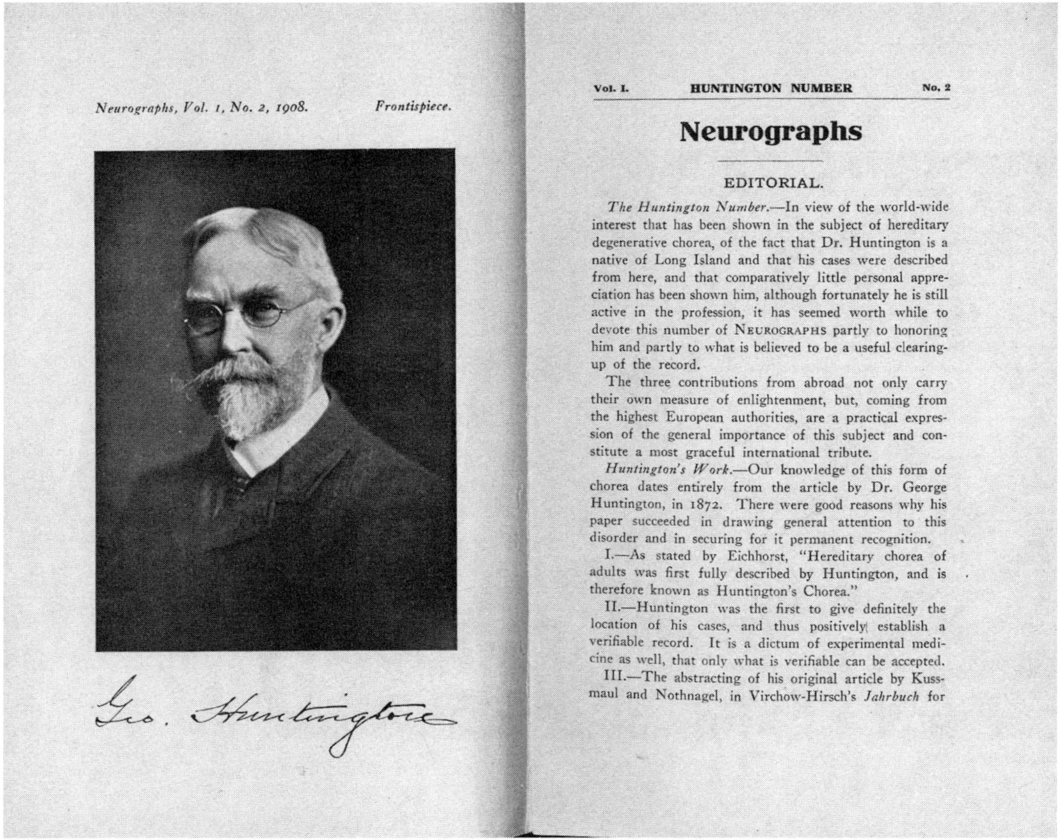

Neurographs, Vol. 1, No. 2, 1908. *Frontispiece.*

Geo. Huntington

Vol. I. HUNTINGTON NUMBER No. 2

Neurographs

EDITORIAL.

The Huntington Number.—In view of the world-wide interest that has been shown in the subject of hereditary degenerative chorea, of the fact that Dr. Huntington is a native of Long Island and that his cases were described from here, and that comparatively little personal appreciation has been shown him, although fortunately he is still active in the profession, it has seemed worth while to devote this number of NEUROGRAPHS partly to honoring him and partly to what is believed to be a useful clearing-up of the record.

The three contributions from abroad not only carry their own measure of enlightenment, but, coming from the highest European authorities, are a practical expression of the general importance of this subject and constitute a most graceful international tribute.

Huntington's Work.—Our knowledge of this form of chorea dates entirely from the article by Dr. George Huntington, in 1872. There were good reasons why his paper succeeded in drawing general attention to this disorder and in securing for it permanent recognition.

I.—As stated by Eichhorst, "Hereditary chorea of adults was first fully described by Huntington, and is therefore known as Huntington's Chorea."

II.—Huntington was the first to give definitely the location of his cases, and thus positively establish a verifiable record. It is a dictum of experimental medicine as well, that only what is verifiable can be accepted.

III.—The abstracting of his original article by Kussmaul and Nothnagel, in Virchow-Hirsch's *Jahrbuch* for

Neurographs, "Huntington Number," May 25, 1908

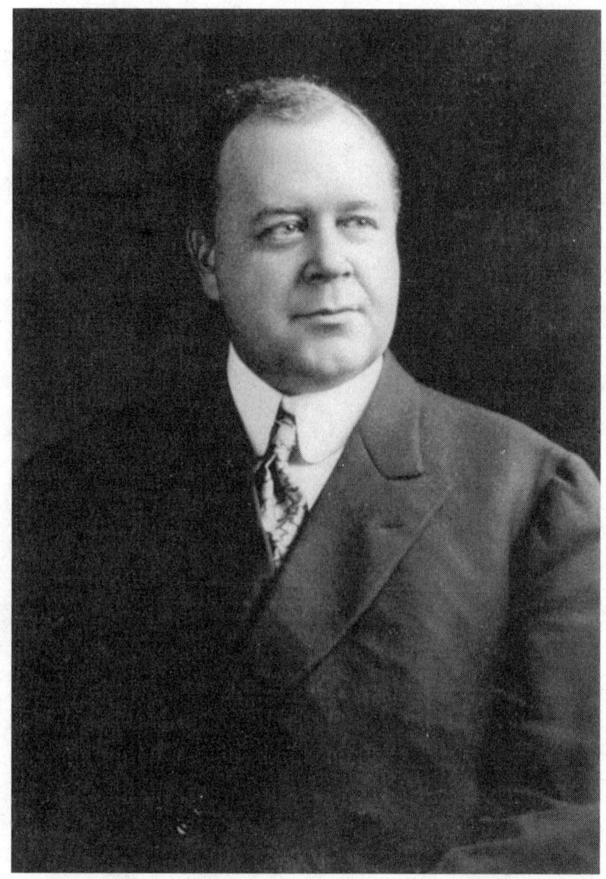

Smith Ely Jelliffe (1866–1945), neurologist, psychoanalyst, and editor and publisher of the *Journal of Nervous and Mental Disease*. Photo by Harris and Ewing. U.S. National Library of Medicine

among neurologists, psychiatrists, and psychoanalysts (including Freud and Jung), as well as with biologists and geneticists on both sides of the Atlantic. Born in 1866 in New York City, Jelliffe attended the Brooklyn Polytechnic Institute, where he graduated in 1886, in the same class as his friend the future geneticist and eugenicist Charles B. Davenport. He later received his M.D. at the College of Physicians and Surgeons in New York, and a Ph.D. at Columbia University. The enterprising descendant of an old New England family, Jelliffe, like George Huntington, was the son of a physician. Unlike Huntington, he traveled to Europe after medical school, pursuing studies in general medicine and pathology at universities in Berlin and Vienna. Back home in New York, he practiced neurology and psychoanalysis, taught at the New York College of Pharmacy and at Fordham University, and attended at several New York City hospitals. He was also active in both the New York Neurological Society and the American Neurological Association, of which he was president in 1913–15. In 1898 he became assistant editor, and a few years later editor and publisher, of the *Journal of Nervous and Mental Disease*, a position he held for more than forty years.[51]

In 1903 or 1904 Jelliffe became intrigued by the suggestions of Clarence King and Wharton Sinkler that many if not most of the cases of hereditary chorea in the United States may have stemmed from one center of origin, perhaps the same coastal region in Connecticut where Jelliffe's own ancestors had settled. With his long-standing interest in genealogy—less in *who* than in *where*, according to his biographer—he decided that a genealogical and geographical study linking various family trees might illuminate the historical origins of the disease while offering "evidence bearing on the question of heredity." He began corresponding with physicians who treated patients with Huntington's, among them George Huntington and Edward Osborn, who was more forthcoming than he had been with William Osler eighteen years before. In 1905 Jelliffe visited Amagansett, where he saw at least one person afflicted with the disease.[52]

In a preliminary paper included in the Huntington Number of *Neurographs*, Jelliffe posited the presence of four clusters of families with Huntington's chorea living in four regions of the northeastern United States—eastern Long Island (the East Hampton group); coastal Connecticut and its inland extension Westchester County, New York (the Bedford group); Wyoming County in northern Pennsylvania; and Massachusetts. He speculated that "an original Connecticut source" had been the origin of the disease in both the Long Island and the Westchester families. Jelliffe included no family trees, but he expressed hope that he might eventually be able to connect the four groups, as "one family tree often ties a dozen heretofore unrelated families together."[53]

Meanwhile, Jelliffe kept in touch with his college friend Davenport, soon to become a leading figure in the North American eugenics movement. Following graduation from Brooklyn Polytechnic, Davenport had pursued graduate study in zoology at Harvard, where he earned his Ph.D. He taught zoology both at Harvard and at the University of Chicago, and in 1898 he also became director of the Biological Laboratory at Cold Spring Harbor on Long Island, with its summer programs for students and teachers. Six years later he left university teaching entirely to become the full-time director of the new Station for Experimental Evolution, a biological research center also at Cold Spring Harbor that was supported by the Carnegie Institution of Washington, D.C. Davenport's own research focused on inheritance in animals—he carried out important experimental work on inheritance patterns in poultry, mice, horses, and canaries. However, by about 1907 he had become increasingly interested in human heredity, possibly through his contacts with Francis Galton, whom he had met in London in 1902, and through the influence of his wife, the biologist Gertrude Croty Davenport, with whom he collaborated.[54]

Davenport soon emerged as an outspoken eugenicist, head of the Eugenics Section of the influential American Breeders Association and founder in 1910 of the Eugenics Record Office (ERO) at Cold Spring Harbor, a combined research institute, educational center, publication office, and archive on human heredity in all its myriad forms. Funded initially by a wealthy donor, Mrs. E. H. Harriman, and after 1917 by the Carnegie Institution, the Eugenics Record Office soon became the nerve center of the eugenics movement in the United States, and, with Davenport as its director, the premier training center for fieldworkers in human genetics and eugenics. Indeed, the two fields were intimately linked; as the political scientist Diane Paul has written, "from the start, human genetics was intertwined with—and sometimes indistinguishable from—eugenics." High school and college biology texts regularly cited Davenport's 1911 *Heredity in Relation to Eugenics*, considered by many as the era's most important text of both human genetics and eugenics, a book "well used in college classrooms" between World Wars I and II. Davenport made no secret of either his conservative politics or his extreme biological determinism. For him "the salvation of the race through heredity" meant preventing the birth of those he deemed "unfit"—a category defined by racial, class, and ethnic identity as well as by physical and mental disability. It also meant halting the immigration of the "actually undesirable," which for Davenport meant essentially those from outside northern and western Europe. Although he always insisted that the ERO was exclusively a research and educational center, his aims were clearly political: to gather data that would help to advance these goals.[55]

Sometime after the publication of the special issue of *Neurographs* in the spring of 1908, Jelliffe proposed to Davenport a collaborative field study of Huntington's chorea. Jelliffe's own resources for conducting such a study were limited, and he hoped that the ERO might undertake such a project. Davenport liked the idea, and in 1911 he recruited a fieldworker for the family study that would help shape the historical and genealogical narrative of Huntington's chorea in America for decades to come.[56]

ENDINGS AND BEGINNINGS

To look back over the forty-five years from Dunglison's first publication of Waters's letter on the magrums in 1842 to the naming of Huntington's chorea in 1887 is to witness a paradigm shift in the identity of a disease, from a disorder considered by lay people and doctors alike as a local peculiarity in scattered geographical settings to a clinical entity recognized worldwide; and from an illness regarded as a peculiar variant of chorea to one that was fundamentally an unusual exemplar of heredity and a "preeminent" neurological disease. By framing hereditary chorea in relation to other so-called hereditary maladies such as consumption and syphilis and spelling out its unusual pattern of inheritance, George Huntington opened up new questions about the nature of biological inheritance generally, a point not appreciated until after the rediscovery of Gregor Mendel in 1900.

George Huntington made this intervention, moreover, at the historical moment, in the 1870s, when the specialty of neurology was becoming established in the United States. Thus the professional interests of neurologists and the emergence of neurological associations, hospital wards, specialized journals, and clinics helped to transform a "medical curiosity" into a visible and "interesting" disease. But despite George Huntington's emphasis on a specific hereditary pattern of transmission, there was no effort before about 1906 to test or verify his hypothesis, not even in the increasingly hereditarian 1880s and 1890s, when the neurological and psychiatric journals in Europe and the Americas carried many clinical and pathology reports on the disease. In this regard George Huntington was unique in attaching importance to a precise pattern of transmission, a point often ignored even by admirers such as Osler. That this pattern might reveal something new about the mechanisms of heredity more broadly was a point that not even Huntington considered.

It hardly seems coincidental that clinicians recognized Huntington's chorea as a "degenerative" disease at a time, in the 1880s and 1890s, when degeneration was a dominant metaphor for thinking about society and history. From the vantage point of a fin de siècle culture preoccupied with decline, the same processes appeared to operate within the nerve cells of the brain as in the larger social world. In this regard, the metaphors of the larger culture informed medical thinking about disease, just as medical thinking helped give "scientific" legitimacy and authority to the dominant metaphors of the society.

Did sufferers and their families benefit from the new knowledge and "the world-wide interest that has been shown" in Huntington's chorea at the turn of the century? On the one hand greater clinical knowledge and a clearer understanding of the hereditary pattern no doubt enabled more clinicians to make accurate diagnoses and in some cases give more sympathetic supportive care. They were able to assure those whose parents had never developed the disease that they were not in danger, since it was now generally accepted that once the malady failed to appear in one generation it was gone forever. The children and grandchildren need not worry.

On the other hand, the representation of Huntington's chorea as an exemplary "hereditary disease" may have strengthened the presumption that it was not only incurable but also untreatable, in part because late-nineteenth-century clinicians increasingly turned to heredity as an explanation for their inability to relieve the condition of patients with intractable ills. In the case of Huntington's, increased knowledge, in fact, appeared to deepen the conviction of many physicians that there was nothing to be done for these patients, that this disorder was a site for surveillance and science rather than therapeutics. Especially in the context of pessimistic turn-of-the-century hereditarian thinking and an emerging eugenics movement, this outlook probably contributed to the harsh practices of some physicians, such as warning healthy young people from affected families not to marry and not to have children, and in general consigning them to a sense of hopelessness and despair. If for the Minnesota neurologist Eugene Riggs in 1901 "cases of Huntington's chorea are always of scientific interest even though they may present no distinctively novel features," for those who actually suffered symptoms, and for their families, the benefits of this "scientific interest" were as yet far from clear.[57]

Medicine/Eugenics/Memory

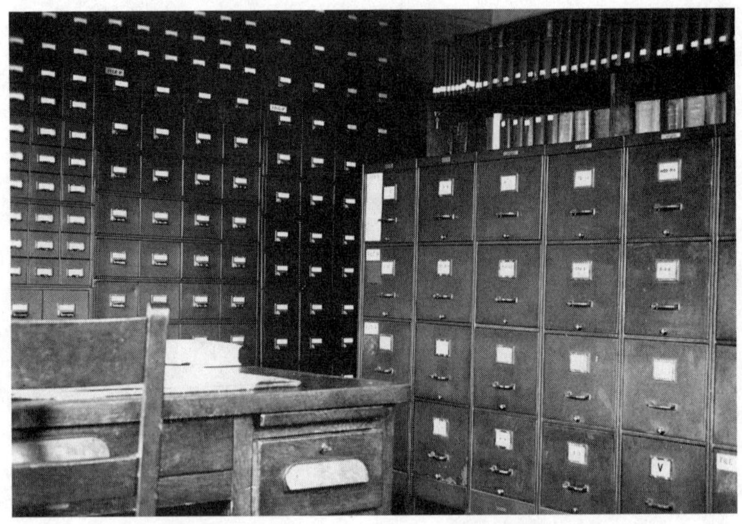

Eugenics Record Office. Courtesy Cold Spring Harbor Library Archives, Cold Spring Harbor, N.Y.

5

The Eyes of Elizabeth B. Muncey, M.D.

The fact that a source is not "objective" . . . does not mean that it is useless. A hostile chronicle can furnish precious testimony.
—Carlo Ginzburg, *The Cheese and the Worms*

HUNTINGTON'S CHOREA AS EUGENIC PARADIGM

How disease is imagined, and how sufferers are portrayed, helps shape the experience of illness. As Susan Sontag famously demonstrated, metaphors have material effects. The association of HIV/AIDS with "sinful" sexuality helped delay the recognition of a global epidemic and still thwarts strategies for prevention. Stereotypes of the old man with Alzheimer's disease as an "empty shell" and images of the old woman who has lost her "self" perpetuate indifference and neglect of the elderly, fanning the dread of those facing a diagnosis. Popular images of the disabled as villains, monsters, and freaks spawn self-hatred and self-doubt among those living with disabilities, while legitimating discrimination and injustice.[1]

But stereotypes of disease and disability arise in specific historical and cultural circumstances. As historians of disability have shown, the era from about 1880 to the 1930s was "a moment of major redefinition" in the United States, when public policies, laws, institutions, and professions either questioned the competency for citizenship of people with disabilities or else flatly declared them unqualified. "The regime fashioned during this era," write Paul Longmore and Lauri Umansky, "continued to shape the lives of many people with disabilities throughout the twentieth century."[2]

For families with a history of Huntington's chorea, these decades also marked a moment of redefinition. Although eugenic ideas of "better breeding" had emerged in the 1880s, it was not until the early twentieth century, the start of the so-called Progressive era of social and economic reforms, that these ideas began to acquire political clout. To be sure, "better breeding" was a flexible idea, spawning different meanings in distinct cultural environments. A belief in the importance of biological inheritance, as Diane Paul and Nancy Leys Stepan have shown, was compatible with a variety of social commitments, ranging from improved education and sanitation to prohibitions on marriage and sterilization for those deemed mentally or physically disabled. Like Progressives generally, most eugenicists in the United States believed in applying modern science to social problems. But by the early 1900s mainstream eugenics in the United States had acquired a socially conservative, restrictionist, racist orientation, aimed primarily at preventing the "unfit" from reproducing or entering the country as immigrants, while encouraging large families among those eugenicists considered the "fittest."[3]

In the United States, much eugenic legislation was enacted at the state level. In 1895 Connecticut became the first state to pass a law, albeit rarely enforced, prohibiting the legal marriage of people deemed "epileptic," "idiot or imbecile," or "feebleminded." Indiana, in 1907, passed the first state legislation legalizing sterilization of the inmates of public institutions as a condition of release, a practice that expanded to other states over the next decades. By 1913, twenty-four states had passed laws prohibiting certain classes of people from getting married on penalty of imprisonment, fines, and annulment. Powerful new groups—for example, the American Breeders Association and the American Eugenics Society—campaigned to translate eugenic ideas into research programs and legislative policies, including the racist 1924 immigration law establishing tiny quotas for southern and eastern Europeans and excluding Asians altogether. Three years later, in the famous *Buck v. Bell* case, the Supreme Court upheld the state of Virginia's program of involuntary sterilization for the mentally disabled, opening the way to expanded practices of sterilization nationwide. By the 1930s, according to Stepan, "the United States possessed the most extensive and extreme eugenic legislation in the world outside of Nazi Germany."[4]

Throughout this period, the new literary genre of eugenic family studies helped popularize hereditarian ideas. The first such study had appeared in the United States in 1877, with the genealogy of the "Jukes"—poor, native-born rural whites of English ancestry, living in the northeastern United States—whose poverty and alleged prostitution, criminality, and feeblemindedness had multiplied over the generations. The author had intended this "cacogenic" family saga to highlight the devastating impact of poverty and the need for social reforms. But after the turn of the century, the Jukes became an emblem of bad biological inheritance, used by eugenicists as evidence that biology trumped education and environment. Eugenic family studies proliferated, with Charles Davenport's cowritten *Hill Folk: Report on a Rural Community of Hereditary Defectives* in 1912, and the all-time best-seller in this genre, *The Kallikak Family: A Study in the Inheritance of Feeblemindedness*, also in 1912, a book that, in the words of the historian Leila Zenderland, encoded the notion of "troublemaking families of dubious lineage" in the very phrase "the Jukes and the Kallikaks."[5]

Coincident with the growing acceptance of eugenics, however, the new science of genetics emerged, opening up an entirely new way of thinking about heredity. With his long-standing interest in the biology of inheritance, Charles Davenport became one of the earliest scientists in North America to promote and publicize Mendelian genetics.

An Augustinian monk and scientist in Brno, Moravia, Gregor Mendel spent years studying flowering pea plants in the garden of his monastery. His method involved tracking the transmission of certain variable traits or characters in pea plants over several generations. Mendel focused especially on traits that came in two alternative versions—for instance, roundness or wrinkles in the seeds, tallness or dwarfness of height, and white or grayish-brown color of seed skins, which correlated with white or purple petals. Breeding thousands of plants over several generations, he showed that the first-generation offspring (F1) of pure-breeding (later called homozygous) tall with pure-breeding dwarf pea plants were all tall. Tallness, then, was what Mendel called a dominant character. However, the offspring (F2) of this first generation of tall plants, produced through self-fertilization, yielded some tall and some dwarf plants. Mendel inferred that although dwarfness had not been expressed in the tall plants of the F1 generation, it was nonetheless present, since it appeared in some of the next generation. The F1 tall parents were hybrids (heterozygous), carrying factors (later called genes) for tallness and dwarfness, although only the dominant character, tallness, was expressed. Dwarfness, then, was a recessive character. Unlike his predecessors, who had also occasionally observed these patterns, Mendel counted the numbers of tall and dwarf plants in each successive generation, coming up with precise calculations. He observed that when the hybrid F1 tall plants were fertilized with pollen from pure-breeding dwarf plants, their offspring, the F2 generation, were approximately half tall and half short: a 1–1 ratio. However, when the hybrid F1 generation plants were self-fertilized (with pollen from identical hybrid F1 plants), then the ratio of tall to dwarf plants in the F2 generation was about 3 talls to 1 dwarf, the famous 3–1 ratio.[6]

From these observations, Mendel theorized that tallness and dwarfness derived not from many factors, as biologists had thought was the case for most traits, but from two, and only two: one inherited from the female, and one from the male. When the germ cell or gamete formed (egg, or ovum, and pollen or sperm), it had half the usual number of factors, and just one factor for height. Then, when the ovum and pollen came together during fertilization, they formed a zygote (fertilized ovum) with a full complement of factors, half from the male, half from the female, including one for height from each parent. Mendel argued that the factors inherited from each parent did not combine or blend, as many naturalists believed, but remained separate from one another, reassorting themselves into new combinations different from that of either parent. He referred to this process as the independent assortment of characters.[7]

Mendel's theories, first published in 1866 (six years before George Huntington's paper on chorea) stirred little interest among naturalists at the time, for reasons that historians continue to debate. Most scholars agree, however, that Mendel's conceptual framework differed radically from that of his contemporaries, in ways that may have made his papers seem opaque to those who read them. As we have seen, while most naturalists thought holistically, in terms of the overall character of species, Mendel looked at discrete isolated traits. While his contemporaries, in the wake of Darwin, were interested primarily in variation and difference, Mendel focused on continuities and sameness. Most important, nineteenth-century naturalists generally conceived of heredity as part of the larger process of growth and development. They were far more interested in the developmental question of how an embryo grew into a fully formed organism than in the narrower question of transmission from one generation to the next, the focus of Mendel's experiments. Certainly transmission was a subject that few naturalists in the mid-nineteenth century considered a separate domain of study. Thus scholars have noted that Mendel's way of thinking was more like that of a farmer, breeder, or horticulturalist seeking to perpetuate desirable traits than a naturalist interested in the origin of species.[8]

By 1900 "heredity," in the narrower sense of transmission from one generation to the next, had emerged as a legitimate focus of scientific investigation, partly due to questions raised by Darwinian evolutionary theory, to advances in embryology and cytology (the study of cells); perhaps also to the emergence of eugenics within a world of colonial expansion and massive immigration. While biologists since midcentury had accepted the notion that material particles in the cell nucleus controlled transmission and development, they lacked a theory explaining how these particles functioned. The work of August Weissman and Francis Galton rejecting the theory that acquired characteristics could be inherited also made Mendel's theories appear more plausible than they had thirty years earlier. Mendel's "laws," as they became known, seemed to confirm Weissman's and Galton's claims that parents transmitted to their offspring only what they had inherited from their own parents. These laws also helped to elucidate statistically the patterns of dominance and recessiveness previously observed by plant breeders. Mendel's mathematical results seemed to promise a new measure of prediction and control, at least in the breeding of plants and animals. But what about people? Did Mendel's laws apply to humans as well?[9]

"THESE MELANCHOLY HUMANS"

This was a burning question for the English biologist William Bateson (1861–1926), then a researcher at Cambridge University, and the most influential early defender of Mendelism in Britain. Bateson had long been interested in human variation, and in 1905 he began collecting medical pedigrees—standardized genealogical diagrams indicating particular conditions over several generations. "We do know cases in man where the rules of inheritance traced in other animals and plants must certainly apply," Bateson told a meeting of the Neurological Society of London on February 1, 1906, "but those cases are very few."[10]

As it happened, Huntington's chorea had come to Bateson's attention that very day. "Yesterday I collected Huntington's Chorea at the R.C.S. [Royal College of Surgeons]," he wrote his friend the ophthalmologist Edward Nettleship on February 2. "The transmission through affected only seems to be almost universal," he told Nettleship, "but the ratios are hopelessly wild. Either there is in these descents some quite novel element and disturbance, or as seems more likely, it is not heredity in our sense at all. I can't help suspecting," he added, "there may be a pathogenic organism passed on." A few months later, he felt even "less sanguine of the regularity of the inheritance" in "nervous diseases." "The more cases I go through, the more I doubt whether they are genuine heredity at all," he told Nettleship. By the following October he was "more than ever inclined to think that the transmission in some of these at least depends on processes quite distinct from what we ordinarily find in the heredity of variations." Even "after making evident allowances for errors and misstatements of all sorts," he added, "it seems to me most unlikely that these nerve diseases can be fitted" to the Mendelian rules. In early 1907 Bateson was still feeling frustrated, since "there are, as always, among these melancholy humans, too many persons affected—and this is despite of the fact that all the experts seem to hold that a provocative [triggering or proximate element] is generally necessary."[11]

As he continued to collect pedigrees for Huntington's chorea, however, Bateson found the offspring of affected parents dividing roughly into two groups, half affected and half unaffected, fulfilling Mendel's definition of a dominantly

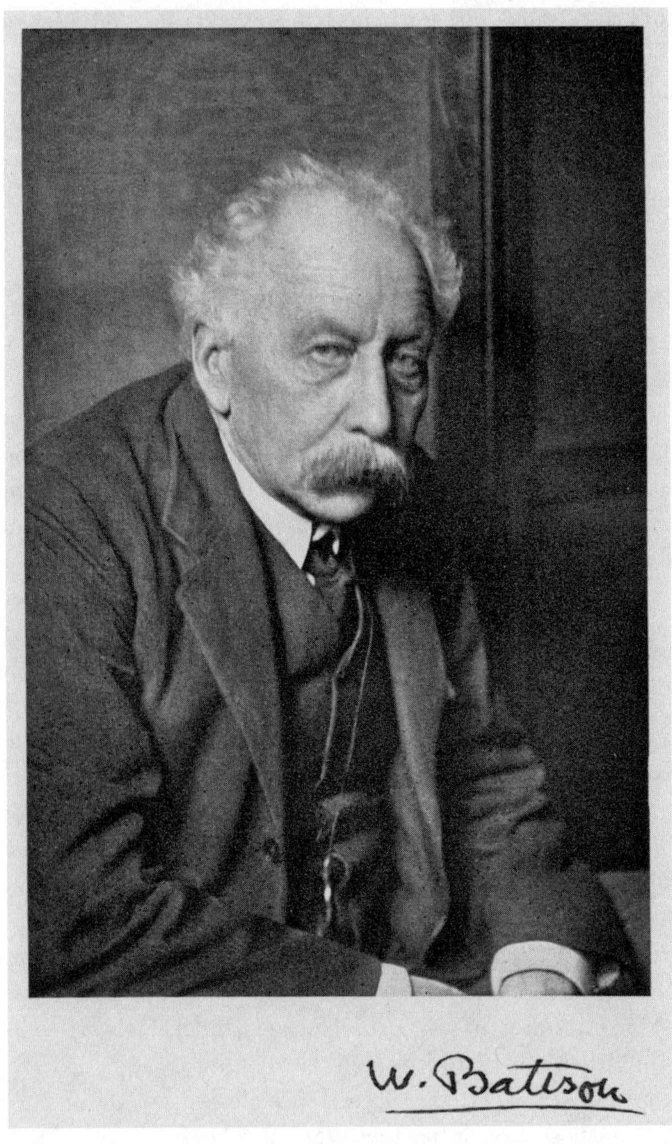

William Bateson (1861–1926), English biologist and early promoter of Mendelian genetics. Courtesy Library of the American Philosophical Society, Philadelphia inherited condition. By the spring of 1908 his collaborator Reginald Punnett felt confident enough to speculate publicly that hereditary chorea might indeed behave as "a simple Mendelian dominant to the normal"—a reference that the up-to-date Smith Ely Jelliffe immediately referenced in his *Neurographs* essay two months later.[12]

Did Bateson read George Huntington's 1872 paper? If so, he did not cite it. Moreover, Bateson's method of collecting as many pedigrees as possible differed from that of Huntington, who had drawn on observations and oral accounts of the relatively few affected families in East Hampton. While George Huntington had tracked the disease through multiple generations in the same families, Bateson counted cases in many different families, comparing his figures with Mendel's predicted ratios for dominant or recessive inheritance.

By the end of 1908 Bateson had arrived at a conclusion. In discussions on "The Influence of Heredity on Disease," held in London at the Royal Society of Medicine in November and December, he listed hereditary chorea among eleven human conditions—and the only neurological disorder—for which there was "no reasonable doubt" as to its Mendelian dominant transmission. Indeed, Huntington's chorea stood out for Bateson as an especially powerful example of Mendelian heredity in humans. In his influential textbook *Mendel's Principles of Heredity*, published early in 1909, Bateson emphasized both the complex transmission of most nervous disorders, in which the element inherited was "evidently the liability, not the developed condition," and what appeared to be the direct transmission of chorea. "The peculiar form of insanity known as Hereditary Chorea is exceptional," he wrote—using the term *insanity*, to which Jelliffe took such strong exception—"in that it very clearly follows the course of an ordinary dominant with few complications." In counting the offspring of at least one affected parent in the pedigrees that he and Punnett had collected, he tallied "117 affected, 99 unaffected, as nearly approaching the normal equality as we can expect when the nature of the evidence is remembered."[13]

FROM GENEALOGY TO GENETICS

William Bateson and Charles Davenport had met several years earlier, and Davenport read *Mendel's Principles of Heredity* over several days on board a ship to Europe in May 1909, noting his reading in his diary. The two men kept in touch during this period, exchanging letters and personal visits in England and at Cold Spring Harbor. Working mainly on poultry, Davenport corresponded with Bateson about "balds" and breeders, but he too was starting to think about

Mendelian inheritance in humans, examining, for instance, the phenomenon of Mendelian dominance both in poultry and in human hair and eye color. With the establishment of the Eugenics Record Office in October 1910, his focus moved almost entirely toward humans. Although it is unclear whether Davenport and Bateson ever corresponded about Huntington's chorea, Bateson's evidence persuaded Davenport. In his book *Heredity in Relation to Eugenics,* published in 1911, Davenport stated that Huntington's chorea was "a typical dominant trait," though he did not credit Bateson with this insight.[14]

Still, the available pedigrees for Huntington's were small. So when Smith Ely Jelliffe proposed a large-scale project, he was eager to begin. A field study and larger pedigrees could strengthen the claim and shed light on heredity more generally. Davenport's argument in the 1911 text that "many of the rare diseases of this country can be traced back to a few foci, possibly even to a single focus," suggests another research aim as well. Although clinical case reports published in United States medical journals over the previous three decades included persons of German, Irish, Scottish, Scandinavian, and African as well as English ancestry, Davenport excluded them from the study. Since Jelliffe believed that many of the older families with Huntington's could be traced back to the New Haven colony (which included Stamford and Greenwich, Connecticut), Davenport decided to emphasize these specific lineages. This investigation would focus on the descendants of English settlers, who would thereafter be considered the progenitors of Huntington's disease in America.[15]

THE PHYSICIAN AS FIELDWORKER

In the histories of Huntington's disease, Charles Davenport, the principal author on the influential 1916 paper that came out of this study, "Huntington's Chorea in Relation to Heredity and Eugenics," has always had more prominence than Elizabeth Muncey. Yet as the physician who carried out the fieldwork and compiled the field notes on which the paper is based, Muncey deserves more attention than she has received.

Who, then, was Elizabeth B. Muncey? Born in 1858 in Bucks County, Pennsylvania, Elizabeth Bailey grew up in the borough of Bristol, an old manufacturing center of some six thousand people on the Delaware River, about twenty miles northeast of Philadelphia. Unlike many professional women of her generation, whose families of origin were middle or upper class, she came from an artisan background. Her father, Thomas Bailey, was a master house carpenter who took young male apprentices into the family home to learn his trade. While her mother ran the household, Elizabeth and her two older siblings attended the local high school. Elizabeth eventually left home to enroll at the State Normal School in Millersville, in western Pennsylvania, returning after graduation to teach at the high school from which she had graduated.[16]

Sometime in the early 1880s she married Daniel T. Muncey, son of a schooner captain in Bristol. Two years older than Elizabeth, the ambitious and energetic Daniel was a reporter for several local newspapers, and by 1882 a publisher and editor as well. The couple moved in 1883 to Washington, D.C., then a center of scientific, educational, and cultural activity attracting many women seeking careers and advancement in the capital. Here Daniel continued to work as a reporter while Elizabeth encountered a vibrant community of professional women, both white and black.

With her normal school training, Elizabeth may have taught school over the next decade. She also gave birth to two children. However, in 1894, at the age of thirty-six, she enrolled at the Howard University Medical College, one of 8 white women among 142 students, 15 of them women, who entered Howard's medical programs that year. Howard had opened after the Civil War as a university that admitted black and white women as well as black men, including especially the formerly enslaved. The Medical Department too began as an interracial program open to blacks and women at a time when most medical schools discriminated against or entirely excluded both.[17]

By the time Elizabeth Muncey enrolled, however, this promise of equality had considerably narrowed. Not all the predominantly male faculty welcomed women, while the opening of other medical schools with more resources—notably Johns Hopkins in 1893—drew many white students elsewhere, both male and female. According to the historian Gloria Moldow, Howard's Medical Department suffered from a lack of resources, declining enrollments, and loss of status. Still, at a time when the increasingly scientific and specialist orientation of American medicine tended to exclude women and black doctors (through denial of clinical and consulting privileges), Howard offered opportunities available almost nowhere else.[18]

Elizabeth Muncey left no record of the impact of this interracial educational experience on her thought. We know that she graduated in 1898, secured a license to practice medicine in 1899, and belonged to one of the state or county medical societies, and possibly to one of the organizations for professional women that flourished in Washington. From her later letters to Davenport, we also know that she valued the social and cultural resources of the nation's capital, including its music, literature, and art. Her interest in tracing what she called "the genealogy of the insane" suggests that she became interested in psychiatry during these years. She may even have worked with William Alanson White, superintendent of the Government Hospital for the Insane (St. Elizabeth's), whom she cited as a reference when she applied for a position at the Eugenics Record Office.[19]

By 1911 Muncey had been practicing medicine in the capital for fourteen years. Her ability to call on two prominent physicians as references, not only White but also the dean of the Georgetown Medical School, George M. Kober, suggests that she was successful and well connected. Why, then, did she want to leave her practice in Washington for the low-paying position of a eugenics worker? The increasing pressures and heightened discrimination against women doctors in the early twentieth century may have been part of the reason. Success in the new scientific medicine depended increasingly upon integration in a wide range of postgraduate professional institutions, such as internships and faculty and hospital appointments, all of which tended to exclude women and blacks. Barriers were increasing instead of decreasing, and many professional women saw the doors that they had opened closing behind them. There were only forty-two regular women doctors practicing in Washington in 1900, about 6 percent of the total corps of practitioners.[20]

Muncey's family situation at this time had also changed. She had more geographical mobility now that her seventeen-year-old daughter had graduated from high school, and her son, now twenty-one, was working as a clerk in a government office. Perhaps most important, eugenics fieldwork was one of the scarce arenas available to women for "scientific" research. For a woman interested in "the genealogy of the insane," it was one of very few options.[21]

MAKING A EUGENIC FAMILY STUDY

Begun at the Eugenics Record Office in the spring of 1911 (with another fieldworker, who resigned and was replaced by Muncey in the fall), the Huntington's chorea study differed from most other eugenic family studies in that Huntington's—unlike, say, feeblemindedness or criminality—was a well-defined clinical entity whose dominant inheritance Bateson had demonstrated. For such a condition, biologists and physicians at the time agreed that pedigrees were a useful and appropriate methodology for illuminating Mendelian inheritance and documenting variations in expression.[22]

Nonetheless, the methodologies of this project—and its difficulties—were similar to those of other eugenic family studies. Like many other fieldworkers, Muncey had to cover a huge territory. Jelliffe and others had identified families living in five states—namely, Connecticut, New York, New Jersey, Pennsylvania, and Vermont. Muncey visited towns in all these places, not only to speak to in-

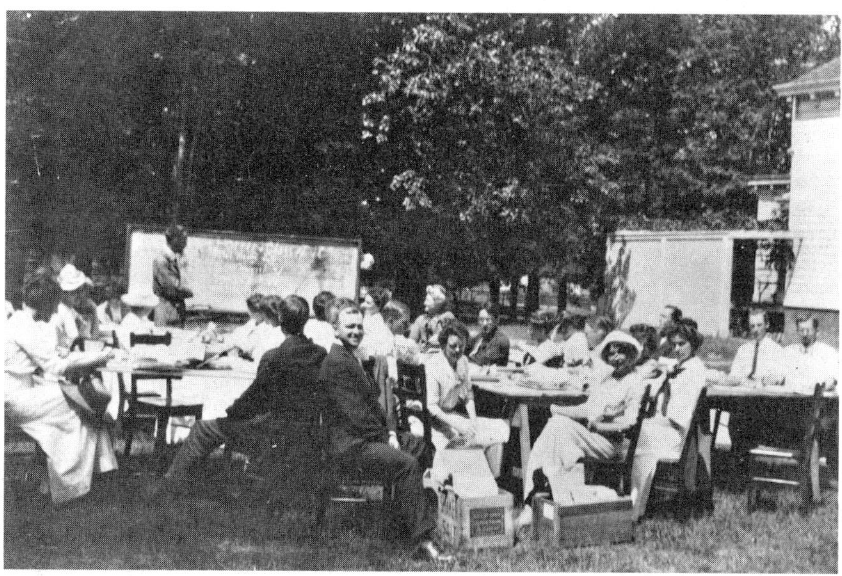

Summer training class for eugenics fieldworkers, 1913, Eugenics Record Office, Cold Spring Harbor Laboratory. Courtesy Cold Spring Harbor Library Archives

formants but also to locate records to supplement the oral testimonies. Besides constructing pedigrees, she also jotted field notes, ranging from a few words—"choreic; history unknown"—to a brief biographical paragraph. She counted some 4,529 individuals in her pedigrees, an enormous number of records for one fieldworker on her own to assemble. But actually, there were even more: in a reanalysis of this data in 2007, geneticists at the Hereditary Genomics Division of the Department of Medical and Molecular Genetics, Indiana University School of Medicine, gave a figure of approximately 5,524, an additional thousand persons. As the historian Amy Sue Bix has observed, Davenport treated his fieldworkers as human research machines, expecting them to work long hours each day, demanding that they report to him constantly, and in general requiring that they maintain an extremely grueling pace. It is not surprising, then, that Muncey's genealogies are often inaccurate, as she sometimes misrepresented information in published sources, miscopied data given to her by Jelliffe, and conflated or confused individuals with the same name in different generations.[23]

If constructing genealogies was difficult, making diagnoses was even more challenging. Even using the kind of neurological examination that pioneering neurologists such as Jean-Martin Charcot and William R. Gowers had developed in the 1880s and 1890s, an experienced neurologist in Muncey's situation would have encountered obstacles. First, nearly three-fourths of the 949 individuals Muncey diagnosed as "choreic" were deceased. (Muncey added up 962 "choreics," but the Indiana geneticists found 949, a more reliable count of her diagnoses, although not of persons that a neurologist at the time might have diagnosed with the disease.) Of the 949, fewer than 250 individuals appear to have been alive in late 1911, when she began her fieldwork.[24]

Of course, relatives and neighbors were often sensitive diagnosticians and witnesses to the deceased. Family memory and community gossip were frequently useful indicators of illness, as good or better than the assessment of a physician in a brief, isolated clinical encounter. Indeed, physicians in hospitals and asylums often accepted the diagnoses made by relatives when patients entered. At the same time, such community diagnoses were highly variable. There was no way for Muncey herself to evaluate local assessments, and death records only occasionally recorded St. Vitus's dance or magrums or chorea as a cause of death, since sufferers usually died of some other cause, such as pneumonia; in any case, medical records were rarely available.[25]

Terminology also posed a problem. As we have seen, lay people in New York and New England (Muncey's bailiwick) used a variety of terms to describe what physicians called hereditary or Huntington's chorea—besides St. Vitus's dance and the magrums or megrims there were "the shakes," "the shaking disease," "nervousness," and also names associated with certain families, as in "Brown's Noddle" and the "Washington Wriggle." But all these terms referred to other conditions as well, including Parkinson's disease and benign tremor. They did not necessarily mean what a knowledgeable early-twentieth-century neurologist or psychiatrist would have diagnosed as Huntington's chorea. Even medical practitioners used terminology variably. Muncey noted in the introduction to her field notes that "whenever in the early records 'palsy' has been assigned as the cause of death for successive generations, and wherever chorea has been found in the descendants of these families, Huntington's chorea has been assumed." But palsy too had a variety of meanings, including paralysis resulting from a stroke.[26]

Even when subjects were living, there were diagnostic difficulties. Members of these families were not always willing to be interviewed. People who were willing to talk to her were often vague and unspecific. As Muncey complained on more than one occasion to Davenport, "the details are meagre as my chief sources of information were old ladies and men who thought they had told all when they said a person was badly affected." Her descriptions of the symptoms of "choreic" individuals sometimes differed considerably from contemporary clinical accounts of patients with this malady. For example, a fifty-four-year-old woman with five children, whom Muncey diagnosed as "choreic," told her that "she does not remember when it [her face] did not twitch. She says that sometimes she gets so tired that she becomes desperate." Was this Huntington's chorea, exhaustion, Tourette syndrome, a tic, or something else entirely? A man who Muncey claimed developed chorea between fifty and sixty years of age lived to be almost ninety-five, and "his mind remained good until the day preceding his death" in 1900. Nor were his choreic movements "pronounced except when under great excitement." None of his children were demonstrably affected. Was this really the dreaded disease of Huntington's chorea as it was understood by clinicians, or the St. Vitus's dance that evoked a sense of horror in those whose families were stricken? It is hard to know.[27]

And then there was the impact of the interview situation itself. Muncey's questioning, as she indicated, sometimes heightened the anxiety of her informants, eliciting behavior that could confirm the presence of chorea (which tends to increase under the influence of anxiety), but could also merely reflect normal nervousness in a situation of unwanted scrutiny by a stranger. "When seen by the writer [Muncey], there was no noticeable tremor at first," she wrote of one Connecticut woman whom she diagnosed as choreic, "but as she continued to give the family history, her head and hands twitched almost constantly. She denied the existence of any nervous trouble in her family." When Muncey visited this woman again eighteen months later, she refused to discuss the subject. "Said she told me all there was to tell last year." Some family members refused to talk to Muncey at all, barring her access to their affected relatives, and actively resisting her inquiries, a response Muncey occasionally denounced as "neurotic" or even "degenerate." On the other hand, she acknowledged legitimate reasons why people might refuse to see her. As she wrote of one Bedford man whose father had Huntington's, "When not drinking he has considerable family pride and resents inquiry into family history."[28]

Finally, Muncey appeared to misunderstand the dominant-inheritance pattern of Huntington's chorea, further compromising her ability to diagnose. (She claimed, for example, that "the admixture of new blood" was reducing the prevalence of the disease, a situation that could have applied to a recessive disorder, for which transmission from both parents was necessary, but not to a dominant one, where a single affected parent could pass it on.)[29]

In short, Muncey based her diagnoses of "choreic" on a wide range of variable criteria that make them useless from a clinical or genetic perspective.[30]

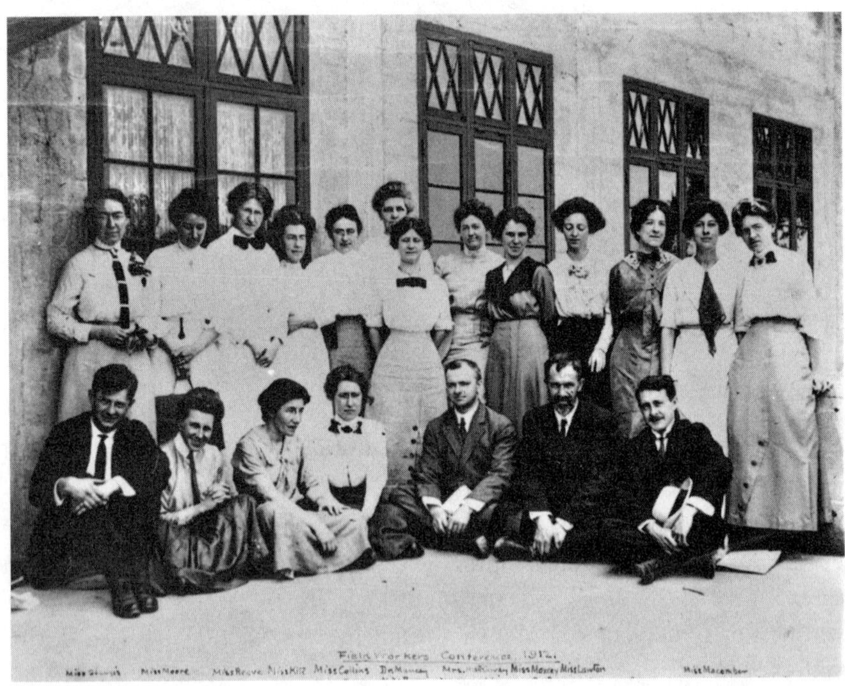

Fieldworker conference at Cold Spring Harbor, 1915. Dr. Elizabeth B. Muncey, standing, sixth from left; Charles Davenport, second from right; Harry H. Laughlin, third from right. Courtesy Cold Spring Harbor Library Archives

HUNTINGTON'S CHOREA AND LOCAL KNOWLEDGE

What makes Muncey's field notes unreliable from the point of view of early-twentieth-century neurology and genetics, however, makes them valuable as documents of local knowledge, especially when there is corroborating evidence from other sources. For instance, Muncey indicated that neighbors had definite opinions about which families in their communities had a history of chorea, in East Hampton and elsewhere. "As far back as can be remembered, chorea has existed in the mother's [or father's] side of the family" was a frequent refrain in Muncey's field notes. (The term *chorea* was probably Muncey's, not that of her informants.) Similarly, "every one spoke of her as belonging to the 'magrum' family," or "it is said that her family have been affected with chorea for many generations," or "it is reported that chorea has existed in his family for generations." As we have seen, such statements show that people in these communities had long acknowledged hereditary illness, and believed that particular conditions ran in certain families. They suggest also that the affected families themselves sometimes passed down an awareness of the hereditary nature of their affliction from generation to generation, even tracking the illness back to the late eighteenth century and debating the original source of the disease. "Throughout the southeastern part of Connecticut the opinion prevails that the Peck family were the original source," she reported. "In the Peck family however the Ferris family is made responsible and they in turn say that either the Lockwoods or Pecks are responsible." If Muncey's informants often disagreed about which side of a family had transmitted the malady, their arguments illustrated how families managed the historical memory of the disease, using it to assign blame and innocence—or, as we shall see, to link the family with prominent or wealthy ancestors.[31]

Muncey's notes also conveyed the keen responsiveness of some relatives and friends to the early signs of the disease. One man reported that though his father's symptoms were slight, "he is going like all the rest." Neighbors described a forty-year-old man who was "just beginning to twitch. He still attends to his business," reported Muncey, "but the neighbors, knowing the heredity, say that 'he is doomed.'" Relatives sometimes offered a searing portrait of a ruined life—for instance, that of "a pretty young girl with a good disposition who married . . . when she was only 20 years old" in 1861: "Shortly after her marriage she became irritable or she would have spells of great depression. While her children were very small, when she was 30 years of age, she began to twitch and these movements soon extended over the entire body. As the disease developed her husband deserted her and as she was not in condition to care for her family she and her three children were in the Stamford poorhouse for a while. She died in 1890 aged 49 years old. The last few years of her life she was unable to walk without assistance, choreic movements over entire body, and her mind was a blank; she did not know her children." Reflecting the difficulties of gathering this information, however, Muncey added: "Everyone speaks of her being so badly affected, but when pressed for details can give none."[32]

Although neighbors and relatives sometimes disagreed in their interpretation of behaviors—"the family says that he is simply nervous, but several friends say that he is beginning to show signs of chorea"—Muncey indicated that families were often repositories of considerable knowledge about the disease, keen observers of onset and outcome. "They are taken with a great nervousness," an informant told her about the clan into which she had married, "which gradually affects their minds so that they imagine everybody ill-uses them, and everything they eat is poisoned. At times they are very violent. They can live a good many years, but when the end comes it is usually with a paralytic shock. They were treated by the best doctors, but nothing helped them, and all of the doctors said the disease was incurable."[33]

Speaking with individuals who had a parent with Huntington's, Muncey reported numerous expressions of anxiety and fear for the future. She described one married East Hampton man, a descendant of Phebe Hedges, who "fears the onset of chorea, and has made his best friend promise to tell him when he sees any signs of the trouble." Though he showed no symptoms, "his friends fear that the mental anxiety will induce the disease." His brother was also "quite nervous over the possibility of heredity," though Muncey noted that he had nevertheless married his second cousin once removed, who also had chorea in her family. The theme recurred throughout Muncey's field notes: "worried greatly over her mother's condition," "is quite nervous over the possibility of heredity," "they are both very anxious about the heredity of chorea." Muncey also recorded several instances of (male) suicide—for example, a man "who was beginning to shake and threatened suicide before he would go round with that d . . . disease," another man who committed suicide "because he recognized that he was growing helpless," and a third who "committed suicide by drowning himself in Taunton Lake" because "he realized that chorea was developing." In this regard, Muncey's portrait of these individuals was consistent with that of George Huntington, who had also noted those who took refuge in drowning or hanging themselves if they felt the disease coming on, or even if they had no symptoms but belonged to a family that did.[34]

While Muncey's informants understood St. Vitus's dance/magrums as hereditary, they also frequently described a precipitating or triggering cause for the onset of symptoms. In one case, Muncey reported that the family attributed the disease "to wounds received in the army" during the Civil War, a common explanation for this generation of male sufferers. Another family noted that the sufferer "fell on the sidewalk fifteen years ago; onset of chorea five years ago, said to be the result of the fall." Similarly, a former state senator "fell from a wagon. A short time afterward tremor developed, the cause of which is assigned to the fall." Occasionally "a complete nervous breakdown" was cited as the beginning of the symptoms. Or a stroke was said to elicit the symptoms, as when one man's choreic movements began "after a slight paralytic attack, which kept him in bed only two weeks." As Muncey told it, these families shared the view of most nineteenth-century medical practitioners that a predisposition to a disease still required a precipitating or proximate cause for symptoms to actually emerge; they did not consider that heredity alone was sufficient to bring on the disease.[35]

Muncey did not specifically address the issue of how those unaffected by the disease regarded their neighbors with the magrums or St. Vitus's dance in the family. Her notes, however, suggest a wide range of responses. "According to reports, the members of this family were so badly affected with chorea that no one would allow his children to marry them," she wrote of one Connecticut kinship. Of another she reported that "they were shunned by the neighbors" and "seem to have degenerated [possibly meaning that they were dying out] more than any other branch of the family." In a third case, "There was much opposition to this marriage on account of heredity of chorea." Muncey also described a few instances of symptomatic individuals inspiring fear or disgust in the community. For instance, one man, a peddler, "would travel all over the country" although he "was so badly affected that the children in the villages were afraid of him." In the case of another severely affected peddler, racism as well as fear of disability provoked a harsh response. "He drove around the country with a colored man without legs," she reported, "and the combination was appalling to the people."[36]

But Muncey also drew portraits that suggested relative social integration and acceptance. Many persons, before they became ill, were active participants in local and professional life. Such remarks also recur throughout Muncey's notes: "he was a man of great business sagacity and enterprise"; "she was a woman of fine character and good poise"; "has had an extensive [medical] practice until 1910"; she married "a man of wealth and high standing." As Muncey told it, in the nineteenth century and the first decade of the twentieth, a history of St. Vitus's dance, magrums, or Huntington's chorea did not preclude a family's acceptance and respect.[37]

Muncey began most of her genealogies, in fact, with a respected male ancestor, often of elite status, who had come to America in the seventeenth century, usually with a wife who accompanied him from England. One was a merchant and an original proprietor of the New Haven colony; a second was a lawyer, whose widow and son had a reputation for wisdom in the law; a third was "a prominent man in his day." Others were farmers or lacked specific occupational identification. Muncey did not, for the most part, attempt to determine who in the earliest generations may have actually suffered from chorea, or who may have been the earliest progenitor. She did, however, identify two women of the emigrant generation in her pedigrees as possible sufferers from the disease.[38]

One was the aristocrat, "Lady Ann Millington," as we have seen, a figure of pride in family stories told by her descendants. The other was a woman named Elinor Knapp, whose alleged conviction for witchcraft Muncey interpreted as an indication that she too may have suffered from chorea. Muncey came up with this hypothesis when she traced the ancestry of several twentieth-century individuals with Huntington's back to Knapp and her husband, Nicholas Knapp, an emigrant from England (Elinor's origins are unknown) who eventually settled with Elinor in Stamford, Connecticut, sometime in the 1630s or 1640s. According to Muncey, Elinor Knapp had been "hanged as a witch in 1658." Furthermore, her "violent temper, convulsive movements, and supernatural powers," supposedly witnessed at her trial, and the fact that many of her descendants suffered from Huntington's, led Muncey to conclude that Elinor too may have been choreic. Muncey also claimed that Elinor and Nicholas had a granddaughter, Elizabeth Knapp, of Groton, Massachusetts, whose "mental moods and violent physical actions," supposedly leading to a conviction for witchcraft, also indicated possible chorea. Muncey did not elaborate on the implications of these speculations. However, her claims about Elinor, Huntington's, and witchcraft, soon became material for a sensational but specious origins story that would resonate in the medical literature on Huntington's for decades to come.[39]

SOCIAL CLASS AND HUNTINGTON'S CHOREA

Suggestions that colonial New England women accused of witchcraft may have suffered from Huntington's chorea or St. Vitus's dance were new in the twentieth century. Questions about the link between chorea and social class, however, had been raised in the earliest medical reports on the disease. As far back as 1841 Charles Oscar Waters had noted that the magrums was "most common among the lower classes, though cases of it are not unfrequently found among those, who by industry and temperance have raised themselves to a respectable rank in society." In the late nineteenth and early twentieth centuries this issue again arose, as the total populations of state hospitals quintupled, and more persons with Huntington's were institutionalized. As patients in these institutions tended to come from impoverished backgrounds, some doctors began to question whether Huntington's chorea was especially characteristic of the poor and uneducated: an inference that perhaps also reflected the eugenic idea of the poor as inherently diseased and genetically inferior—heirs to the burden of neuropathic inheritance. C. M. Hay, a physician at the Asylum for the Insane in Morris Plains, New Jersey, asserted in 1890 that Huntington's chorea chiefly attacked people "in the lower walks of life, and at least it cannot be said to show any selective tendency for highly educated nervous systems." In this regard, then, it was unlike neurasthenia, which fin de siècle Americans considered a malady of the elite. But C. R. McKinniss, chief physician at the State Hospital for the Insane in southeastern Pennsylvania, emphasized in 1914 that Huntington's chorea "was not necessarily a disease of low mentality, and the members of some of our families have held positions of trust and respect, not to be obtained without some intellectual achievements."[40]

By including in her study the families of those who remained at home as well as of those in institutions, Elizabeth Muncey cast a much wider net than was possible for most practicing clinicians. Certainly her pedigrees included the poor and marginal, such as the Pawling, New York, family, who according to their doctor lived together in a filthy hovel with a dirt floor and a mountainside as one wall; a Vermont man who was a fisherman and tramp; and others who were itinerant peddlers. But Muncey's pedigrees also included small businessmen and shop owners, a school principal, a professor of surgery at a New York City medical college, the wife of an elite physician, the president of a shipping line, several teachers, members of a family of "lawyers, high school teachers and successful businessmen," a member of the New York legislature, a town supervisor, several justices of the peace, a physician, several clergymen and deacons, the editor of a popular magazine, a university professor, several town clerks, and a wealthy farmer who was "greatly respected in the community for his 'integrity and common sense.'" Among the earliest generations in Muncey's pedigree, high status was not uncommon, nor was it rare in their descendants. (Muncey did not claim all of these individuals had Huntington's chorea, but all belonged to families considered to be affected by the disease.)[41]

Muncey's pedigrees, then, differed from those of most eugenic family studies, which were inhabited by "paupers," the "feebleminded," and other marginal figures. There were so many accomplished individuals in her pedigrees that Charles Davenport later complained that her study "has been made on three or four high-class families," implying that they were somehow superior to the population of families with Huntington's chorea generally. Yet he was willing to concede that there was even "genius in families with chronic chorea," a reflection, he believed, of the manic symptoms in these kinships that were often associated with productivity.[42]

It is not surprising that Muncey warmed to these families, and to all her middle- and upper-class informants, expressing undisguised admiration for the more educated, affluent and accomplished individuals—of two daughters of an affected father, she wrote that they were both Vassar graduates, "moved in the best social circles, and have considerable wealth." She could be brusque and dismissive toward those of lower social standing, calling one Vermont man "an ignorant laborer" who was married to "a French-Canadian woman with a glass eye" and had three children, "stolid, dirty, uneducated."[43]

But Muncey's diagnoses of chorea did not align with her assessments of low-class status, nor did her judgments of lower-class status equate with chorea. There were some educated, even well-to-do people whom she classified as choreic, while there were poor or marginal members of what she called "the submerged class" whom she did not. For instance, she wrote of one woman (aged eighty) that "she has a fine personality and has been much loved and respected. She has had the best care, a devoted husband, and good medical attention; but these have not prevented the development of chorea, although they may have been factors in retarding its onset." The man whom Muncey called "an ignorant laborer" did not, in her view, have chorea, nor did any of his children. There were also individuals whom Muncey described as peculiar, eccentric, neurotic, insane, or even degenerate, but not choreic, as, for example, "Susy, very peculiar, writes poetry but can find no publisher. Brags of her authorship; talks of nothing else. She is unmarried." But not choreic.[44]

The class status of affected families continued to inspire debate in the medical discourse on Huntington's chorea throughout the twentieth century. One of the most impassioned statements came from a Connecticut physician whose two patients descended from a family in which he counted a total of eighteen cases, all descended from one woman. "Mark you, this is not a family of degenerates," he wrote in 1914, as if expecting his readers to assume that they were,

> but on the contrary they have all been noted for their high mentality. Many of them have made a mark in the professions and all of them have shown great business ability, and even at the present time the patients are of the middle class, that is, none of them are laborers and those who have been committed to the insane asylums of our state have not been state charges, but have been maintained by their own estates. None as far as I have been able to learn have been addicted to drugs or to alcohol, and it has been difficult to even find a tobacco user amongst them. In fact, all are of exemplary intelligent New England stock, who have lived quiet, well ordered lives, until they reached middle life, when the sword of Damocles fell.[45]

A decade after Muncey's project, Estella Hughes's often-cited 1925 study of thirty-two Michigan families with Huntington's chorea drew a slightly different conclusion. Hughes observed that most of them were "respectable and industrious," and "approximated the average in good rural communities," although few were professionals or college educated. Just three families were in "affluent circumstances." Yet the progenitors of these families included prominent early New England settlers, according to Hughes, and many of the families had furnished "excellent Michigan pioneers." Even the California eugenicist Paul Popenoe observed in 1930 "that the families which are best known in the United

States for the presence of Huntington's Chorea are intelligent, superior families." And in 1958 a Michigan study concluded that while there was "a definite suggestion" that "choreics" had a lower occupational status (before the onset of illness) than their siblings without chorea and lower than the general population, the difference was not great, and the siblings without chorea did not differ significantly from the general population. In the absence of the disease, argued these authors, affected families were indistinguishable from the general population.[46]

Nonetheless, the notion persisted during the 1930s, 1940s, 1950s, and even 1960s, that Huntington's chorea was specific to the lower classes, in part because some researchers doubted "that the presence of affected individuals in a kindred for several generations would have no effect on the social behavior and economic status of unaffected members of the kindred." As late as 1968 the Belgian neurologist George Bruyn, in an influential survey of the literature on Huntington's worldwide, claimed that the disease was "particularly frequent among the lower socioeconomical strata of the population." Other clinicians in the 1960s argued more compellingly that the disease "courts a lower-class existence" since it usually begins its destructive influence in the prime of life, just when young adults are establishing occupations and families. From this perspective, the status of the families was incidental to the disease, rather than the disease being indigenous to their social class.[47]

COPING AND CAREGIVING

By the 1890s, with more people living in cities and with more women, the traditional caregivers, working outside the home, more individuals with advanced Huntington's chorea were ending up in state mental hospitals, though they still represented a tiny percentage of the total state hospital population: 1 patient per 425 first admissions to the hospital, according to one 1890 estimate. (Later estimates gave figures between 1.1 and 2.3 cases per thousand first admissions.) In 1922, 26 men and 24 women with diagnoses of Huntington's chorea were admitted for the first time to state mental hospitals in the United States. The following year, according to the U.S. census, there were 146 men and 171 women with Huntington's in state hospitals, 317 individuals out of a total hospitalized population of 229,664, far less than 1 percent.[48]

Muncey's data also showed a low percentage of those affected with Huntington's who were institutionalized at all: of the 949 alleged "choreic" individuals in her study, both living and deceased, I have identified about sixty, or roughly 6 percent, as having been institutionalized at some period of their lives, whether in a hospital, asylum, private sanitarium, or poorhouse. These figures suggest that the major responsibility for caregiving rested with the local community, and especially with the families of those affected, particularly women. Some of Muncey's informants pointed with pride to the home care of their affected relatives. "None of the Crabbes have ever been a public charge, nor have they ever been in any institution," one family boasted. But Muncey also reported the financial and emotional costs of such domestic caregiving, usually by a daughter who cared for an affected parent while worrying about the danger she, her siblings, and her own children faced. In one case, a young woman who cared for her affected mother, sisters, and brother subsequently developed the illness herself: "She was the most intelligent member of the family, and was greatly respected. The other members of the family were immoral, sexual and dissipated [as Muncey reported them]. At the age of 39 she began to show symptoms of the disease, and after her sister was taken to the hospital, she attempted suicide by jumping from the window. From 39 to 45 years there was great depression. As her mind failed, the choreic movements became more marked. She died in 1903–4."[49]

Sometimes a spouse cared for a husband or wife, and later for their affected children as well. In Sagaponack, a village near East Hampton, a woman born in 1784 cared first for her husband and later for four adult sons who developed their father's disease. She buried her husband and three of her children (who died in their late thirties or forties) before dying herself in 1861 at the age of seventy-seven.[50]

But caregivers were not always women, as Huntington's chorea, like other chronic maladies, sometimes led to the reversal of traditional gender roles. Muncey reported several instances of men who took care of affected wives or parents, though usually with economic support rather than the hands on, day-to-day caregiving reported by women. Wealthy men especially had options not available to those with fewer resources, often going to great lengths to make satisfactory arrangements for their affected kin. When one woman developed symptoms at around the age of forty, her husband hospitalized her, "but she was so unhappy that she was removed to a sanitarium. This was equally unsatisfactory and she was taken home for a while. It was impossible to live with her so a private house was rented; a nurse and servants secured, and this institution was kept up for fifteen years. The son said that during that time his father did not miss seeing her for one day." Her husband, however, told Muncey that "he went through hell for twenty years," but he cared for his wife and other choreic members of her family because "he thinks it is his religious duty."[51]

In many respects, the caregiving and coping strategies reported by Muncey resembled those of women and men facing other chronic family illnesses. As the historian Emily Abel has shown, "caregiving dominated women's lives throughout the nineteenth century." However, caregivers for those with Huntington's chorea faced one difficulty that most other caregivers did not: they were frequently grown offspring who felt highly vulnerable to developing their parents' illness themselves, and of passing it on to their own children. Even in the nineteenth century, persons tending to affected parents or siblings were constantly reminded of the fate that they understood might await them and their children as well. Moreover, the inexorable advance of symptoms, all too familiar to the affected families, deprived caregivers, as well as sufferers, of any hopes for remissions. And then, by the time of Muncey's study, the rewards that domestic caregiving sometimes conferred in the mid-nineteenth century, such as the satisfaction of making medical decisions, deepening the caregivers' own religious faith, and even restoring health through empathy and solace, were eclipsed by the growing prestige of professional and scientific medicine. In this setting, institutional care at the turn of the century may have offered some respite for women whose lives would otherwise have been consumed by this disease.[52]

AMBIGUOUS LEGACIES

In March 1913 Elizabeth Muncey finished her work on Huntington's chorea. She had spent nearly ten months, from October 1911 to July 1912, carrying out the fieldwork, and another eight or nine months, from July 1912 to March 1913, at Cold Spring Harbor compiling the results. She had drawn up four large pedigree charts and turned her handwritten field notes into several hundred pages of typed, annotated genealogies, each of which portrayed a lineage stemming from one emigrant English couple or individual who had come to New England in the seventeenth century. The largest lineages extended back ten generations to the New Haven colony, and to a set of three (alleged) brothers and their wives. Several other lineages stemmed from additional sets of emigrant brothers, including two pairs of brothers and their wives who came to East Hampton: the great-great-great-grandfathers of Phebe Hedges and of her husband. And as we have seen, Muncey identified two other Connecticut women in the emigrant generation as possible progenitors—Elinor Knapp, the supposed witch, and Ann Millington, the alleged aristocrat. Although Muncey herself did not elaborate, her data provided the materials that others would rework into a widely accepted genealogy of Huntington's chorea in the United States.[53]

Clearly Muncey managed at moments to capture the feelings and opinions of her informants, conveying the anxieties, fears, expertise, and coping strategies of families with St. Vitus's dance/magrums/Huntington's chorea and their neighbors. Her brief biographical narratives and clinical descriptions often exceeded the parameters of her project, allowing us a glimpse of the humanity of her subjects; their voices penetrated her text. Although she cited some families who were said to have been ostracized by their neighbors, she included many more who were not. If some individuals who began developing symptoms were abandoned by their spouses, ridiculed and shunned, or blamed for their bad behavior, others received sympathy and sorrow from friends and relatives who cared for them over many years.

As Muncey told it, Huntington's chorea crossed class boundaries, affecting the elite as well as the impoverished. It was also a disease of wide variability, destroying the lives of some people in their young or middle adulthood but causing only minimal movements and few mental symptoms over the course of long lives in others. (Of course, since her diagnoses are always open to question, in some cases the persons she called "choreic" probably would not have been diagnosed as such by a knowledgeable neurologist of the time.) Though sometimes triggered by trauma or loss, the disease in her portrayal seemed impervious to all efforts at forestallment.

For many of Muncey's informants, however, she herself, in the context of the eugenics movement, may have changed the experience of Huntington's. Take East Hampton, for example. Her intervention appears especially problematic when we recall Edward Osborn's ambivalence toward William Osler's request to visit, back in the 1880s, and Osborn's fear of calling attention to the affected families in a way that would bring them "notoriety." Although Osborn was more welcoming twenty-five years later when Smith Ely Jelliffe contacted him, it seems clear that by the late 1880s the subject of Huntington's had become extremely delicate within this community. No doubt the emergence of eugenics at the turn of the century heightened this taboo: in 1910 the newspapers of eastern Long Island reported regularly on eugenics, "race suicide," and the "survival of the fittest." The *Sag Harbor Express* carried front-page items on "The Problem of Eugenics," explicitly praising the Eugenics Record Office in 1913 for its work of promoting "the best strains" while fostering "methods of restricting the defective and delinquent classes." Newspaper readers would have been familiar with these themes.[54]

At this time, then, a stranger coming into town under the auspices of the ERO and asking questions about people with Huntington's chorea was bound to raise fears. Muncey was doing science, but also surveillance; she was scrutinizing certain families, diagnosing and labeling them, and in this manner, setting them apart from their neighbors. In this environment, her questioning, not only of the affected families but of their neighbors, ministers, and physicians, as well as town officials, inevitably put the families on display in a way that they had never experienced before. One cannot help wondering whether Muncey's presence sometimes produced the fears and anxieties she claimed merely to report.

Progressive-era charity workers used similar techniques in assessing the need for social services. But however well meaning, such questioning often had unintended consequences, such as driving potential clients deeper into silence and heightening their sense of secrecy and shame. At a historical moment when marriage prohibitions and sterilization were becoming enacted into law, calling attention to the families with Huntington's had consequences Muncey apparently did not acknowledge. If some people welcomed her as a scientist, her research nonetheless targeted and publicized a condition that, within a growing national discourse on the "unfit," potentially framed those affected by it as undesirable citizens. Even when Muncey herself did not express such views, the very fact that a fieldworker appeared in town asking questions about certain families would certainly, in this context, have raised suspicions and heightened the anxiety surrounding the disease.[55]

For Elizabeth Muncey personally, the Huntington's chorea project was sufficiently satisfying that she wanted to continue her eugenics work. If she worried about negative fallout from her research on the families she investigated—other eugenics fieldworkers did express doubts, as the historian Amy Sue Bix has shown—she left no record of her thoughts. She remained at the ERO, acting as an instructor at the 1915 summer training course, undertaking several other field studies (of twins and of pellagra), and eventually taking a position as an archivist at Cold Spring Harbor. Davenport thought highly of her, praising her ability to analyze data and citing the "unusual accuracy and industry in her work."[56]

But Muncey also found her experience with the ERO frustrating. The pay was low, the travel exhausting. During the fifteen months of the Huntington's study, according to an ERO report, she spent an average of fifteen days in the field and nine days in the office, traveled an average of 389.3 miles, interviewed an average of 85 people per month. Every month according to the report, she also drew up pedigrees comprising approximately 361 individuals. Yet if travel was onerous, staying at Cold Spring Harbor was dull and dispiriting. "I spent nine years in that attic most uncomfortably," she wrote Davenport from her home in Washington, D.C., in 1920, "and the only thing that made it at all bearable was the intermittent trips abroad. There are four months in the year when those attic rooms are not fit for human habitation." She missed a stimulating social and cultural life. "Here I have the companionship of my friends and access to

Mr. Muncey [who was living in a rest home] . . . also access to music, literature and art," she told Davenport. "There complete isolation from everything that makes life worth living except the actual work."[57]

Muncey's "actual work" has been considered one of the few worthwhile studies to come out of the Eugenics Record Office, "the foundation for much of the future work [on Huntington's chorea] that was to come." I, too, have argued that Muncey's data have value, but not as the foundation for work in genetics. Her diagnoses are doubtful, her genealogies unreliable, her figure of 962 "choreics" highly arbitrary. Nonetheless, her field notes offer valuable glimpses into the social world of Huntington's chorea, heredity, and eugenics at the turn of the twentieth century. Her archive remains one of the few early-twentieth-century efforts to record, however briefly and inaccurately, the voices, outlook, and activities of families with this disease.[58]

Muncey's typed notes and pages of pedigrees, deposited at the ERO and later at the Dight Institute for Human Genetics at the University of Minnesota in Minneapolis, were never published, although they were available to clinicians and researchers who requested them. In the early 1960s the geneticist Sheldon Reed, director of the Dight, a former president of the American Society for Human Genetics, and a pioneer in genetic counseling, decided to reprint her notes in toto under the title *Classical Huntington's Disease (Huntington's Chorea) Families.* He did so to enable physicians and geneticists "to counsel the descendants of the three unfortunate brothers regarding their adjustment to the facts of this disease." For this purpose, Reed concluded, "its proper use could be most helpful." He did not indicate, helpful for whom?[59]

6

Myths of Origins and Endings

The interesting question is how and why some findings become facts. How are the facts and artifacts created?
—Joan Fujimura, *Crafting Science*

Among all the papers to come out of the Eugenics Record Office, "Huntington's Chorea in Relation to Heredity and Eugenics," published in 1916, stands almost alone in retaining its reputation as a worthwhile scientific contribution, for its analysis of dominant inheritance in nearly a thousand alleged "choreics" and its documentation of the variability of symptoms and age of onset. While Davenport's "flawed" conclusions have been criticized, the data on which these conclusions rest have largely gone unquestioned. Yet this lack of scrutiny may say more about geneticists' and clinicians' lack of historical memory than about the scientific merits of the paper. It may reflect the power of a conceptual model that separates "objective" data from "subjective" conclusions. Although the Davenport and Muncey study shares many of the methodological problems and ideological assumptions that made the eugenic family studies in general "worthless from a genetic point of view," the fact that this paper, and especially Muncey's data, remain mostly uninterrogated—by historians as well as by geneticists and clinicians—suggests these problems and assumptions have yet to be fully addressed.[1]

BIOTYPES, DOMINANCE, AND "CLASSICAL" HUNTINGTON'S CHOREA

By March 1913 Elizabeth Muncey was done with Huntington's chorea. She had completed her fieldwork, drawn the pedigrees, typed her field notes, and delivered everything to Davenport. Now Davenport wanted Smith Ely Jelliffe to

HUNTINGTON'S CHOREA IN RELATION TO HEREDITY AND EUGENICS.

By CHARLES B. DAVENPORT,

Station for Experimental Evolution, Carnegie Institution of Washington.

BASED ON FIELD NOTES MADE BY

ELIZABETH B. MUNCEY, M.D.,

Eugenics Record Office, Cold Spring Harbor, N. Y.

CONTENTS.

1. Introduction.

In the course of the work of the Eugenics Record Office our attention was called to a peculiar disease that found its home within a hundred miles of the Office. Dr. Elizabeth B. Muncey,

From the *American Journal of Insanity*, October 1916

help him analyze these data. But the overextended Jelliffe kept postponing their collaboration. Finally Davenport decided to undertake the analysis on his own, possibly with help from Muncey, working out the ideas in several preliminary articles published in the *Journal of Nervous and Mental Disease*, *Proceedings of the National Academy of Sciences*, and *Science*. The final paper, "based on field notes made by Muncey," with Davenport listed as the author, appeared, in 1916, in the *American Journal of Insanity*, and in Davenport's own *Bulletin* of the ERO.[2]

Although concerned more with variability than with similarities in the expression of the disease, Davenport emphasized that Muncey's data supported the claim of dominant inheritance. As he put it, the disease "does not ordinarily appear in the children whose parents have been free from chorea unless those parents died before the age of incidence." Whenever the offspring of apparently unaffected parents became ill, one supposedly nonchoreic parent either had died before the age of onset or came from a family with Huntington's, and was likely to have been affected even if the illness was never recognized.[3]

Davenport argued further that while it appeared that each successive generation developed symptoms at a younger age than their forebears—a phenomenon called anticipation—this appearance was a statistical artifact, reflecting the fact that those who died young in earlier generations or failed to have children were more apt to be forgotten and left out of the pedigrees, thus making the average age of onset appear greater in the past than in the present. In addition, Davenport calculated from Muncey's data that approximately one-sixth of the cases of chorea developed in people aged twenty or younger, more than a quarter developed symptoms in their thirties, and another quarter became ill either in their twenties or forties, with the remainder becoming affected in their fifties or later—a considerably wider variation in age of onset than George Huntington had described in 1872.[4]

Indeed, the variability of the disease between families was central to Davenport's portrait, part of his effort as a geneticist to delineate the specific smallest units of inheritance, and also an expression of the larger concern of eugenics with identifying superior and inferior lines of descent. In her field notes, Muncey recorded many descriptions of family differences, taken from her conversations with the family members themselves. "There was a lack of mental balance throughout this fraternity," she wrote of one family. Of another, "the peculiarity of chorea in this family is its limited extent," and "early onset is noticeable." A third kinship was characterized by a large number of early deaths, the severity of symptoms, and the number who became "public charges." A fourth commonly had onset between forty and fifty years of age, "and the development of mental trouble occurs late in life—if it occurs at all—and it is not a marked feature."[5]

Drawing on this perspective, and on Muncey's observations, Davenport now theorized that "the four elements of 'classic' cases of chronic chorea"—involuntary movements, mental losses, emotional disturbances, and early or late onset—"are not necessarily associated" and that each might be inherited independently: one individual diagnosed with Huntington's might have severe chorea but few mental symptoms, while another might develop minimal choreic movements late in life with considerable mental loss and a third might become affected at a very early age. Whether an affected individual had both chorea and mental symptoms, such as "manic depressive" behavior, depended upon whether others in the same family, choreic or not, were also subject to manic depressive symptoms, quite apart from whether they were affected with Huntington's.[6]

In attempting to explain these variations, Davenport drew on the concept of biotypes put forth a few years earlier by the Danish geneticist Wilhelm Johannsen, who defined a biotype as "only one single 'sort' of organism," as opposed to "a multitude, or a few." Although Davenport initially implied that all families with Huntington's belonged to a single biotype (he defined *Huntington's chorea* as "a name applied to a group of traits shown by certain persons, who belong to a special race, strain or biotype"), he argued more centrally that the concept of the biotype might explain differences in the pattern of symptoms shown by members of different families. "In general," he wrote, "the symptomatology of chronic chorea is dissimilar in different strains of families." For example, in Muncey's data the Connecticut families had an average age of onset of thirty-three, while affected members of the families on Long Island became ill on average when they were ten years older. These different patterns also constituted distinct "species" or biotypes of the disease.[7]

This analysis of family similarities, and of biotypes generally, failed to persuade many clinicians or geneticists, who documented considerable variation in the symptoms experienced by individuals within the same family as well as among those in different families. Davenport made no attempt to demonstrate quantitatively either the inheritance pattern of a distinct choreic biotype, the separate inheritance of familial biotypes, or the individual inheritance patterns of specific symptoms. Unlike Bateson, he did not count the number of affected and unaffected individuals within the pedigrees, nor did he quantify the appearance of separate traits. Whether all families with Huntington's chorea belonged to a single biotype, families with common patterns of symptoms constituted separate biotypes, or different combinations of symptoms formed biotypes of the disease remained altogether unclear. Still, as late as 1991, geneticists continued to valorize the contribution of the Davenport and Muncey paper to documenting the variability of Huntington's chorea, even if the theory of "biotypes" no longer sufficed as an explanation.[8]

HUNTINGTON'S CHOREA AND NEUROPATHIC INHERITANCE

Davenport touched on more familiar terrain with his claim that choreic families were "characterized by a general nervousness and a liability to a great variety of mental troubles." Muncey had tallied up instances of other disorders in the families within her Huntington's pedigrees, noting that in some of them, chorea had disappeared while other conditions remained or had taken its place (the so-called dissimilar or transformational heredity). In her pedigrees of 4,529 (or 5,524) persons, Muncey counted 39 "epileptics," 73 cases of "feeblemindedness," 37 individuals who were "insane" but not "choreic," 35 who were "alcoholic," 6 criminals, 5 imbeciles, 25 with rheumatism, 74 who were "tubercular," 12 addicted to drugs, 38 who were "eccentric," 26 "deaf mutes," 9 who were blind, 21 suffering from cancer, 9 affected with migraine, and 118 who were "neurotic undefined." Twenty people had committed suicide. There were also 342 cases of infant death, including 19 who died of convulsions, 47 of meningitis, and 41 of hydrocephalus.[9]

Were these numbers exceptional? It is impossible to say, since Muncey offered no comparable figures for a population unaffected with Huntington's chorea. Nor did Davenport when he came to analyze these data. He merely concluded that the frequency of these other troubles was "striking" and "probably" greater than that of the general population.[10]

This claim was hardly surprising. As we have seen, the idea that so-called unfit families were susceptible to a wide range of maladies—the legacy of a neuropathic inheritance—was a central claim of late-nineteenth-century degeneration theory, and a key trope of early-twentieth-century eugenic discourse as well. Even George Huntington had implied that not only the people stricken with chorea but also their unaffected relatives—people "who belonged to families in which the disease existed"—were abnormal in some degree, psychologically if not physically, since they too had a tendency to suicide. Wharton Sinkler, in 1889, explicitly attributed abnormality to all the relatives of the patients he described, pointing to "the marked neurotic taint through their families." He also claimed that "insanity, epilepsy, intemperance, and vice are prevalent in the family history," although he presented no evidence to support these claims beyond an acknowledgment from one patient that her "entire family is nervous."

Davenport's interpretation, then, continued a line of argument that had begun several decades before and, indeed, would continue as a theme in many subsequent studies.[11]

What is surprising is that Davenport faced a number of critics who presented evidence to the contrary, both before and after the 1916 paper appeared. Arthur Hamilton, a psychiatrist and neurologist in Minnesota who wrote up a series of twenty-seven cases in 1908, had been struck by "the relative absence of other forms of mental and nervous disorder" among the relatives of these patients. Acknowledging the claims of many authors regarding the "more or less intimate relationship between chronic chorea, epilepsy and other nervous diseases," Hamilton was more impressed by the "conspicuous" absence of "ordinary nervous and mental diseases" in the families of his patients, a finding he believed was the experience of "the great majority of writers" on the subject. In 1914 Nicholas Dynan of the Government Hospital for the Insane in Washington, D.C., also noted "the absence of other nervous affections or other forms of insanity," although he considered that those affected by this type of chorea came from "a varied ancestry, usually of a neurotic type."[12]

In what may have been the most careful evaluation of Davenport's claims of related disorders, the English geneticist Julia Bell wrote in 1934 that her own review of the published case histories of families with Huntington's failed to indicate a high incidence of these conditions. She observed that while it was "frequently reported" that the siblings of a patient were all "very nervous," in her sensible view "it would require a peculiarly stolid person to live with a choreic parent and choreic siblings without acquiring some degree of nervousness, particularly if the individual be aware of his own liability to develop symptoms." Ultimately, she found "no hint of any defect or disease definitely associated with Huntington's chorea, either in the affected individual or in unaffected members of the stock."[13]

And even Davenport, despite his emphasis on the "liability" of those in families with Huntington's chorea to "mental troubles," highlighted the "surprisingly large number of effective men and women who have done important work in the world," individuals whose presence in Muncey's pedigree he seemed to find especially troubling. If a full professor, or a man "of highest standing in the community," or the son of an eminent physician, could turn indifferent and careless as a result of this disease, with passions "beyond control," then anyone could—including himself, a point that clearly did not escape him, since he noted some (unrelated) Davenports in Muncey's pedigree. Framing Huntington's chorea in terms of "lack of muscular control," the "loss of inhibition," the "loss of emotional control," and "a loss of control of the sex-impulse," Davenport echoed the anxieties evident in his other eugenic writings and in the American eugenics movement generally. For Davenport, Huntington's chorea seemed to embody the loss of restraint and self-mastery so central to turn-of-the-century ideals of middle-class American manhood. It was as if the disease held up a mirror to the American male's most deeply held fears.[14]

FICTIONS OF FERTILITY

Nineteenth-century degeneration theory had held that "degenerate" families would eventually die out, due to increasing infant mortality and ultimate sterility. Degeneration would culminate in extinction. Eugenicists of the early twentieth century tended to reverse the equation, warning that the unfit were reproducing at a rate much higher than the fittest, and would soon overwhelm the best elements of society. They cited the allegedly high fertility of the unfit to strengthen calls for eugenic legislation. It was in this context that the fertility of families with Huntington's chorea became a subject for research.[15]

Actually, neither Jelliffe nor Davenport had envisioned a study of fertility or the related issue of prevalence. But since Elizabeth Muncey specifically claimed in her unpublished notes that the disease was becoming less prevalent—due to the allegedly high rate of infant mortality in these families; "the admixture of new blood," which, as we saw earlier, she implied would inhibit transmission; and, finally, what she claimed was "the public sentiment that has existed for years against marriage into the affected families"—Davenport took on this argument as well.[16]

Calculating the numbers of individuals in successive generations who failed to marry by the age of thirty, Davenport explained that while Muncey's data showed that a higher percentage of Huntington's family members remained single (and presumably childless) in the later generations than in the earlier ones, these figures were misleading. They were partly a reflection of broader population trends but also an artifact of memory: those from the earlier generations who did not marry and leave descendants were more likely to be forgotten and omitted from the data than the unmarried individuals from recent decades whom informants could still remember. Thus, according to Davenport, these data gave the false impression of a great increase in single people over time. From his perspective, "chorea is dying out very slowly, if at all, through being selected against in marriage."[17]

Available statistics largely support Davenport's claim. Figures published in 1925 by the social worker Estella Hughes for men and women hospitalized with Huntington's at Michigan state mental hospitals indicate that women with

Huntington's married at about the same rate as white women in the general population, while men with the disease married at a significantly lower rate: of the 118 women in this study, 106, or about 90 percent, had married, while of the 100 men, 77 percent had married. Another study in 1958 comparing 203 individuals diagnosed with Huntington's from Lower Michigan families (85 men and 118 women) to the general population of the state—using the 1940 Michigan census for comparison—showed a similar result. Moreover, men from these affected families who did not themselves have the disease, a total of 100 in this study, also married at a slightly lower rate than men from the larger society: of those between thirty and forty-four years of age, 83 percent had married, compared with 85 percent in the general population, while of those forty-five or older, 84 percent had married, compared with 89 percent in the Michigan population as a whole. In this study, women with or without Huntington's from the affected families did not differ significantly from women in the general population.[18]

Curiously, neither Muncey nor Davenport commented directly on the size of families with a history of Huntington's. Davenport never claimed that women who developed the disease had exceptionally large families—a claim that had appeared in the literature on Huntington's as early as 1889. Indeed, he did not analyze the fertility of women in Muncey's pedigrees at all. (In 1925 Estella Hughes's figures on the fertility of 218 men and women with Huntington's in Michigan State Hospitals in 1923 showed 2.76 children per individual with Huntington's, also well below the national average in 1920 of 3.17 children per family in the general population.)[19]

Nonetheless, by focusing on six or seven members of the first generation in Muncey's pedigrees as the "probable" sources of "962" cases of chorea, Davenport dramatized the idea that from a very few progenitors had come an enormous number of affected descendants. "All these evils in our study trace back to some half-dozen individuals," he wrote, "including three brothers, who migrated to this country during the 17th century. Had these half-dozen individuals been kept out of this country much of misery might have been saved." To emphasize his point about the spread of Huntington's, he included in the 1916 paper a map of the United States showing the migration of three "choreics" from Long Island and Connecticut to California and Oregon. Whatever the statistics, here was a strong visual image of the cross-country expansion of the disease.[20]

It is not surprising, then, that some subsequent writers continued to claim that families with Huntington's were exceptionally large. A psychiatrist from the New Hampshire State Hospital, for instance, wrote in a 1932 issue of the *New England Journal of Medicine*—alluding to the Davenport and Muncey paper—that "a field study of choreic families" found that "in a great majority of instances" these

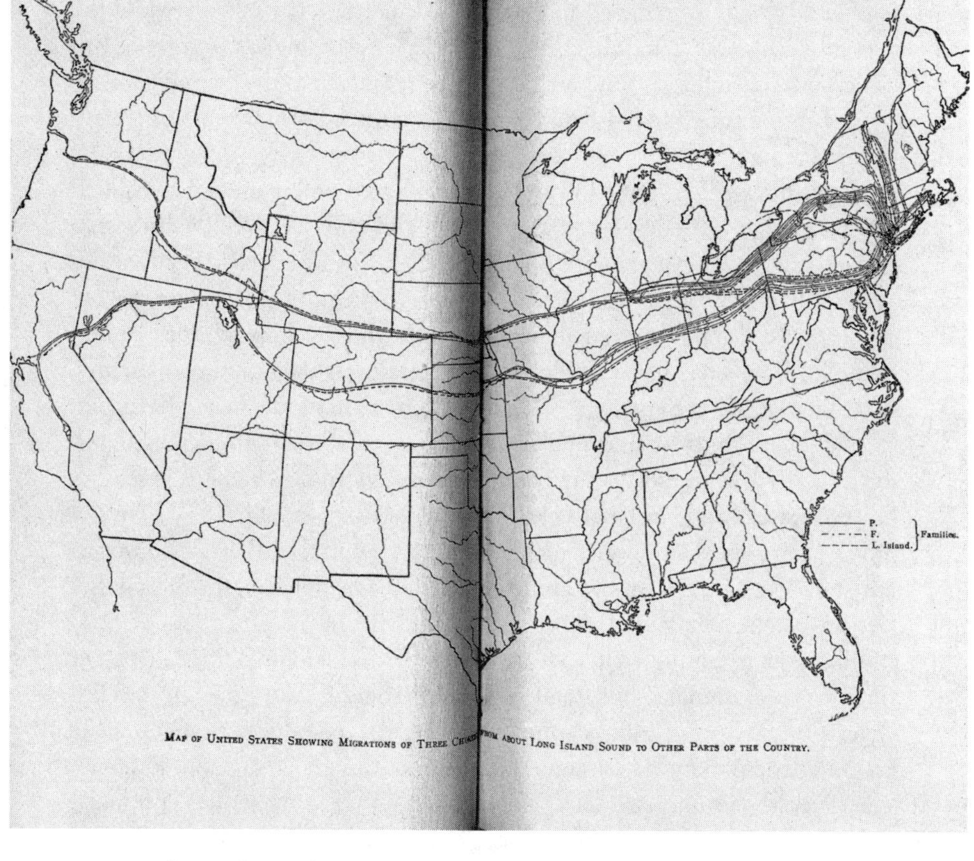

"Map of United States Showing Migrations of Three Choreics from about Long Island Sound to Other Parts of the Country." From the *American Journal of Insanity*, October 1916

families "were more prolific than normal families in the population at large." And Julia Bell reported in the 1930s that "individuals of both sexes have been noted to have very large families."[21]

The most egregious example of this line of thinking appeared in 1951 in the prestigious United States journal *Science*, in a paper titled "Social Fitness versus Reproductive Fitness." The authors, J. Daniel Palm, a graduate student at the University of Minnesota, and the medical geneticist Sheldon C. Reed, claimed to find enormously heightened fertility in men with Huntington's in relation to their unaffected siblings. Comparing the descendants of two nineteenth-century Minnesota brothers, Palm and Reed determined that the man with Huntington's had 787 descendants, while his brother without it had 186. The average number of children produced by the affected individuals was 6.07, while the average of their unaffected siblings was only 3.33. According to the authors, this result showed that the Huntington's chorea gene "increases the fecundity of the affected person compared with unaffected sibs," an effect that begins well before the onset of symptoms.[22]

These claims were eventually refuted by more responsible investigators, such as the Michigan geneticists T. Edward Reed and James V. Neel, writing in a 1959 issue of the *American Journal of Human Genetics,* who looked at all the offspring, both affected and unaffected, of parents with Huntington's in the state of Michigan. Reed and Neel argued that both those who developed the disease and those who did not had fewer children on average during their lifetime than men and women in the general (1940s Michigan) population. The fact of having an affected parent, in their study, led to a reduced, rather than an increased, fertility. The 1951 Minnesota study had generalized from one highly atypical instance. For Reed and Neel, not only was the disease not spreading out of control through heightened—or even average—fertility, but in fact, they found, recurrent mutation, a rare event, "seems to be the only way in which the present frequencies can be maintained."[23]

Still, warnings continued to appear. As the psychiatrist John Terry Maltsberger wrote in a sensationalist but frequently cited article, "Even unto the Twelfth Generation," in 1961, "If it is assumed that choreics reproduce as rapidly as the rest of the population, it should not take long for this malignant and dominant gene to replace its normal allele." Even as late as 1972, some writers continued to conjure up "the vast numbers of cases of Huntington's chorea in the United States," the "very large families" of affected persons, and "the apparently dysgenic fertility rates of potential victims of Huntington's chorea." Despite all the evidence to the contrary, the claim that Huntington's was rapidly increasing informed influential papers on the disease.[24]

STERILIZATION AND SURVEILLANCE

While Davenport and Muncey's 1916 paper emphasized the social problems posed by Huntington's chorea, it also proposed several ostensible solutions, helping to frame medical and political debate about the disease over the next several decades. The first was sterilization. "It would be a work of far-seeing philanthropy to sterilize all those in which chronic chorea has already developed," wrote Davenport, the actual author of the article.

> and to secure that such of their offspring as show prematurely its symptoms shall not reproduce. It is for the state to investigate every case of Huntington's chorea that appears and to concern itself with all of the progeny of such. That is the least the state can do to fulfill its duty toward the as yet unborn. A state that knows who are its choreics and knows that half of the children of every one of them will (on the average) become choreic and does not do the obvious thing to prevent the spread of this dire inheritable disease is impotent, stupid, and invites disaster. We think only of personal liberty and forget the rights and liberties of the unborn of whom the state is the sole protector. Unfortunate the nation when the state declines to fulfill this duty![25]

But Davenport understood well that sterilization of persons already known to be affected with Huntington's, even those in the earliest stages, would have little impact on the future prevalence of the disease, since most individuals developed symptoms only in their thirties or later, after they had had most of their children. It was the "progeny of such" that really concerned him. He considered Huntington's the one disorder for which prohibitions on marriage made sense, although he never went so far as to call for the sterilization of all those with an affected parent. In fact, he placed more emphasis on the "immense immigration of recent years" and on the need to exclude those destined to become choreic, his second proposed solution. "It requires little imagination to picture what the consequences of this new blood—these new centers of weakness—will mean to the population of this country three or four generations hence," he warned. Since Muncey's 962 "choreics" had supposedly descended from just half a dozen immigrant ancestors, exclusion, in his view, was an important strategy for control. For Davenport, Huntington's chorea was an especially compelling example of the urgent need for immigration restrictions. "Had it been known that one parent of the three brothers who came in the 17th century from England was choreic," he wrote, "and had they been excluded on that ground, we should have lost two leading educators, a surgeon or two, two state senators, two or three state assembly men and several ministers and 900 cases of one of the most dreadful diseases that man is liable to."[26]

Yet as Davenport acknowledged, this strategy too presented several quandaries. Only about half of those with an affected parent were destined to become ill themselves. Moreover, he agreed that even those who were affected later in life were often productive citizens before they became ill. Thus neither sterilization nor exclusion of middle-aged sufferers would have much impact on the number of those affected in the future.

Acknowledging this difficulty, Davenport proposed a third strategy. Although little noticed at the time, this proposal would prove the most influential. He called for developing a method of prediction that would indicate who, among the young offspring of an affected parent, was destined to develop this disease in the future. "Such a means of differential diagnosis would be of great eugenical importance," he noted in a 1913 talk at a meeting of the American Neurological Association, "and should be diligently sought after." Davenport insisted on the "great importance" of inquiring "whether there are any symptoms that will enable one to judge, 10 or 20 years before the usual age of incidence, which of a number of brothers and sisters are liable to be immune from the disease," and which are destined to become affected. Davenport himself proposed that within families where irritability preceded the onset of chorea, "the gradual or sudden appearance of this symptom some years before the usual age of onset should discourage marriage." The absence of irritability up to the age of thirty-six or forty meant that the individual should feel free to get married! As we shall see, Davenport's proposal would assume increasing importance in decades to come.[27]

EUGENICS, THERAPEUTICS, AND BIRTH CONTROL

Published in 1916, in the middle of the First World War, "Huntington's Chorea in Relation to Heredity and Eugenics" soon became a widely cited medical and scientific source. Especially as Davenport and other eugenicists came under criticism in the 1930s for their efforts to squeeze complex human behavioral traits into a narrow, single-gene, Mendelian frame, the Huntington's chorea study, as the historian Philip J. Reilly has noted, seemed to provide "convincing evidence of the wisdom of this enterprise."[28]

In addition, even if few clinicians were convinced by Davenport's analysis of "biotypes," the Davenport and Muncey paper helped shape a representation of Huntington's chorea as scientifically interesting and socially alarming, a public health emergency. The image of "962 choreics" descended from just half a dozen emigrant ancestors surfaced repeatedly in clinical and genetics papers as evidence of the proliferation of a dangerous and devastating disease that showed no signs of disappearing on its own.[29]

Ironically, the same year that the Davenport and Muncey paper was published, the young radical feminist Margaret Sanger opened the first birth control clinic in the United States, in New York City. And for families with Huntington's, accessible birth control and abortion could have offered options for family planning more effective and far more humane than legal prohibitions on marriage or recommendations for celibacy or sterilization. Indeed, by the 1920s many eugenicists themselves came to support birth control for eugenic ends, and some feminists such as Sanger used eugenic appeals in pressing for legalizing birth control. But neither Davenport nor Muncey raised the possibility of birth control. Although sterilization of those already affected, as Davenport acknowledged, did not really address the problem of Huntington's (since most people developed symptoms after they had had their children), it is important to note that his recommendation for sterilization emerged in a society in which sterilization programs in state institutions were already under way; his proposals were not mere abstract theorizing.[30]

By the 1920s, some clinicians also saw Huntington's chorea as an argument in favor of the legalization of birth control. More typically, however, physicians and social workers recommended abstinence or sterilization, whether voluntary or involuntary. As even the relatively progressive Estella Hughes wrote in 1925, "The main hope of prevention seems to lie through education of the public and the patients to a popular understanding of the disease, that they through their better knowledge of its causes and consequences, may promote its control, either through the avoidance of marriage, or through voluntary sterilization." For young people in families with Huntington's, such stark options in the age of Freud, flappers, and women's suffrage, with an emerging youth culture and growing freedom for women, must have seemed bitter indeed.[31]

HUNTINGTON'S IN PRINT

One might expect the Davenport and Muncey paper, and eugenics generally, to have increased medical and scientific interest in Huntington's chorea. Certainly the number of publications on Huntington's worldwide, and in the United States, had climbed steadily since the 1880s, as we have seen, and international publications continued to increase. Starting in the 1920s, however, the percentage of U.S. papers began to decline: from 1910 to 1919 about 42 such papers were published of a worldwide total of 170; from 1920 to 1929, the figure was 21, out of 187 worldwide; and from 1930 to 1939, with an international total of 231 publications, just 38 papers appeared in the U.S. medical press.[32]

The reasons for this situation are unclear. Davenport himself may have discouraged medical interest by promoting the view, in journals and at the medical meetings he frequently attended, that the solution to Huntington's lay in state control rather than medical or scientific research. On the other hand, medical publication on Huntington's continued in Germany even during the Nazi era: close to 50 percent of all medical and scientific papers on Huntington's worldwide were published in German-language journals in the 1920s, in the 1930s that figure was about 40 percent.[33]

But whatever the reasons, in the 1920s U.S. interest in Huntington's declined; therapeutics almost vanished from the literature, even the modest recommendations of earlier clinicians for such supportive strategies as enriched diets, assistance with eating, avoiding anxiety, exercising, and listening to music at mealtime. Discussions of prevention were limited mainly to sterilization and prohibitions on marriage, while researchers would not take up Davenport's suggestion to develop a method of "early diagnosis" until the 1940s. Therapeutics would not reappear as an important topic until after World War II.

"THE BAD CHARACTERS FROM BURES"

While Davenport and Muncey had laid out a compelling origin story about how Huntington's chorea in the United States had stemmed from just half a dozen respectable early English settlers, a Connecticut psychiatrist, Percy R. Vessie, turned this story on its head, making witchcraft and delinquency the linchpin of the tale. Whereas the earlier narrative told a story of decline and fall, Vessie told a story of "bad characters" from the beginning, and the passing down of a tainted inheritance that continued over twelve generations to the present. He based his account partly on Elizabeth Muncey's field work, partly on information from one of his own patients, and partly on his research in the Connecticut and Massachusetts archives, adding an additional set of images to the repertoire of historical representations of this disease.

In light of Vessie's role in shaping this narrative, it is useful to consider his unconventional path to psychiatry and neurology. Born in New York City in 1885 to a German father and Irish mother, Vessie earned his M.D. in 1909 from the Cleveland Homeopathic Medical College (later known as Cleveland-Pulte Medical College) in Ohio. Homeopathy, an alternative form of medicine developed in the early nineteenth century, was based on the idea that diseases could be cured by drugs—given in tiny amounts—that produced the same symptoms as the disease in a healthy person: the so-called "law of similars." Popular in the mid-nineteenth century, homeopaths struggled against efforts by "regular" physicians to marginalize them, finally gaining acceptance in the profession at the turn of the century. As they gained legitimacy, however, they lost popularity, especially as scientific medicine made significant advances in disease prevention and treatment. Gradually homeopaths merged with the "regulars" whom they had once bitterly opposed.[34]

VOL. 76 DECEMBER, 1932 No. 6

The Journal
OF
Nervous and Mental Disease
An American Journal of Neuropsychiatry, Founded in 1874

ORIGINAL ARTICLES

ON THE TRANSMISSION OF HUNTINGTON'S CHOREA FOR 300 YEARS—THE BURES FAMILY GROUP *

BY P. R. VESSIE, M.D.
GREENWICH, CONNECTICUT

Huntington's chorea[1] may be an ancient hereditary disease because of its wide distribution in the universe, still a definite record of this system of chorea and dementia did not appear in literature until the year 1816.[2] The grandfather of Huntington is reported to have positively identified the characteristics of this family disease in Long Island in the year 1797, yet there is no descriptive mention of this conspicuous malady for more than two hundred years of colonial life.

To establish a more remote continuity, we have focused our attention on the early colonial background and itinerary of a common ancestral group in New England, obtaining impressive information from public archives in the states of Massachusetts and Connecticut.[3] Most important of all, by following the ramifications in this mass of

* From the Clinical Service of the Blythewood Sanatorium; a study initiated by Dr. Frederick Peterson and Dr. Smith Ely Jelliffe.

[1] Huntington, George: On Chorea, Med. & Surg. Reporter, 26:317 (Apr. 13), 1872; Recollections of Huntington's Chorea, as I Saw It at East Hampton, Long Island, During My Boyhood, J. NERV. & MENT. DIS., 37:255 (Apr.), 1910.

[2] Jelliffe, S. E., and White, W. A.: Diseases of the Nervous System. Philadelphia: Lea & Febiger, 5th Ed., 1929, p. 669.

[3] Courts of Assistants, Particular Courts, General Courts, Crimes and Misdemeanors, New Haven Colonial, Fairfield and Stamford Records; Original Witchcraft Depositions, Cotton Mather's Magnalia Christi Americana, Taylor's Witchcraft Delusion in Colonial Connecticut, Ewen's Witch Hunting and Witch Trials, and Burr's Literature of Witchcraft; Life and Letters of John Winthrop, Hoadley's Records of the Colony and Jurisdiction of New Haven, Connecticut Historical Collections, and Encyc. Brit. Articles; Genealogies of Early Settlers by Bond, Savage, Pope, Stiles, and descendants of the Bures Family Group.

"On the Transmission of Huntington's Chorea for 300 Years—the Bures Family Group." From the *Journal of Nervous and Mental Disease*, December 1932

Vessie entered homeopathic medicine just as it was becoming assimilated into mainstream medicine. After completing his internship at the Cleveland City Hospital, he became an assistant physician at the upstate New York Gowanda State Hospital, a homeopathic institution at that time, where he remained for many years. In the late 1920s he secured a position at the elite Blythewood Sanitarium in Greenwich, Connecticut, a place with an atmosphere "rather like that of a delightfully luxurious country club," according to its advertisements. Soon he became medical director at Blythewood, a post he held during most of the 1920s, and again from 1938 to 1949. Despite his position, Vessie apparently felt somewhat insecure about his status, judging by his extreme deference to prominent practitioners with whom he corresponded, such as Smith Ely Jelliffe and Adolph Meyer at Johns Hopkins.[35]

Vessie came up with his origin theory when he traced the ancestry of one of his own Connecticut patients with Huntington's back to Elinor Knapp (whom he called "Ellin"), the seventeenth-century Connecticut women described by Elizabeth Muncey, and her husband Nicholas Knapp ("Nichols"), whom he identified as an emigrant from the village of Bures, in the southeastern English province of Suffolk, East Anglia. Borrowing Muncey's pedigree from Smith Ely Jelliffe, Vessie adopted Muncey's argument that since Elinor Knapp had descendants with Huntington's, and because she had (allegedly) been accused of witchcraft, she too probably suffered from the disease.[36]

Vessie also adopted Muncey's view that Elizabeth Knapp had suffered from Huntington's, citing as evidence "a detailed account in 1671 of the 'violent motions and agitations of her body'" in the witchcraft literature. He theorized that several other colonial Connecticut women accused of witchcraft—among them such well-known figures as Elizabeth Clawson, Mary Staples, Mercy Disborough—had also been afflicted with chorea. Ultimately, Vessie suspected all these women, but especially Elinor, "of being the lamentable means of transporting a family disease from England to the colonial states, which inheritance has spread throughout the United States." As he put it, "We believe the true story of this lesion to be revealed in the witchcraft trials of women in the Bures group."[37]

But Vessie did not stop with the women. He also portrayed Elinor's husband, Nicholas, his alleged brother William Knapp or Knopp ("Wilkie"), and another man, Jeffrey Ferris ("Jeffers"), as well as two men's wives, as possible cases of chorea. As evidence, Vessie emphasized the legal infractions of these men and women, citing such examples as Nicholas Knapp's selling quack medicine for scurvy, Jeffrey Ferris's harsh judgments as a juror and his "retaining a stolen calf,"

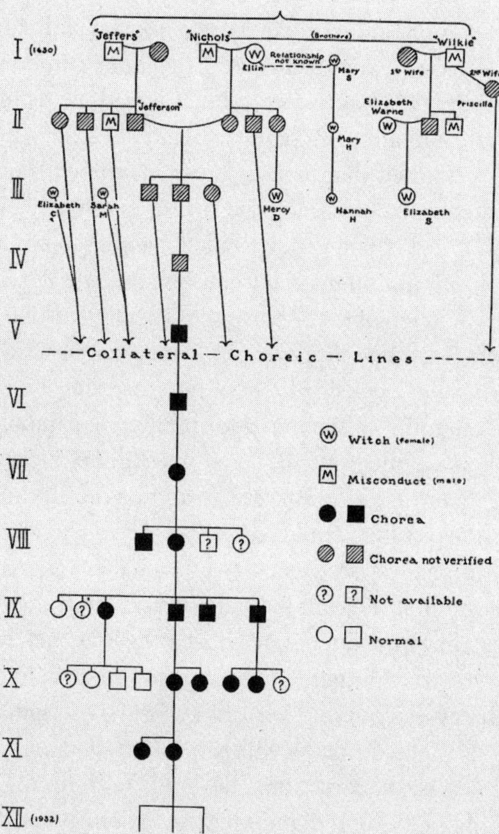

Pedigree chart of the Bures Family Group, showing members tried in colonial courts for witchcraft and misconduct, and the direct descent of Huntington's chorea in later generations.

We are indebted to Dr. Smith Ely Jelliffe for disclosing the collateral families, thus enabling us to trace this group and its background in early colonial archives. Approximately 1,000 cases in these branches were reported by the authors in footnotes 1, 6, 7, 8, 9, 10, 11, 12, 13, 15 and 17.

Pedigree chart alleging connections between witchcraft trials, "misconduct," and Huntington's chorea. From the *Journal of Nervous and Mental Disease,* December 1932 and William Knapp's public profanity, making speeches against the governor, and selling beer without a license. Vessie also noted that several of the second-generation males had charges against them while they were young, including "distemper" (drunkenness) and the serious charge of "bestialitie."[38]

For Vessie all this "misconduct" added up to a social pathology suggestive of Huntington's chorea. These mischief-making men and women were "notorious principals in unsavory colonial history" and "the bad characters from Bures." They were "illiterate and arrogant," and "none attained recognition or respectability." Vessie also claimed that their descendants shared their shortcomings. Within the first three generations, they began "to intermarry so freely and prolifically as to form a highly complex genealogy of consanguinity shot through with taint." Their insistence on marrying cousins and refusal to stop having children was, in his view, a sign of their "persistent stupidity," which "contributed to the dooming of many of their descendants." Their neighbors considered them "mean" and "despicable," accusing them of intermarrying "to keep their riches and property in the family." Suspicious and embittered, paranoid and resentful, these were neighbors no one wanted. "Their spitefulness, bickering, querulousness and blasphemy bring contempt, dislike and hatred to their doors," Vessie wrote; "therefore, the pity they would receive because of their bizarre and dance-like movements is in many cases prevented by their cantankerous behavior."[39]

Vessie emphasized that since all these individuals presumably suffered from an organic disease, they were not responsible for their bad behavior; as he put it, they constituted a "sorrowful march of victims to the scaffold, exile and social ostracism." He especially criticized what he called "these spiteful, furious, unyielding natures of witchcraft days," which he contrasted with "modern observations in the clinic." At the same time, his lurid descriptions of colonial Connecticut witches implied a kind of guilt by association. He portrayed the witch as a monster, with imps "hanging from the breasts and genitals" whom she dispatched to place curses on her enemies, make children die, kill hogs and cattle, and produce storms. "Caught in this web," Vessie wrote, "she is finally forced to submit to every conceivable temptation: stealing, murder and even suicide." In Vessie's portrait, it is difficult to decide whether these early settlers should be regarded as victims or villains.[40]

Here, then, was a cautionary tale about the "bad characters" who introduced Huntington's chorea to North America, an allegory of the dangers of bad heredity left uncontrolled. The implications for Vessie were clear. In 1932 he urged physicians to "warn all such choreics and their children against propagation." In 1939 he went much farther. The only solution to the problem of Huntington's chorea was "rigid sterilization."[41]

TRANSATLANTIC TRAFFICKING

Vessie's sensationalist thesis, published in two papers during the depths of the Great Depression and at the height of eugenic sterilization in the United States, Germany, and Scandinavia, stirred a lively interest on both sides of the North Atlantic. Abstracting the first paper in 1933, the prestigious British medical journal *The Lancet* boasted that Britons "may congratulate ourselves" on the loss of the three Bures couples to America, since they and their progeny were clearly "undesirable characters" who would nowadays be classed "as belonging to the social problem group." Reprinting the *Lancet* piece the following year, the popular U.S. magazine *Literary Digest* expressed sympathy for "the unfortunate victims of the witchcraft delusion," while referring to chorea as "the witchcraft disease."[42]

In 1934 an up-and-coming young English neurologist, MacDonald Critchley, published an elaboration of Vessie's thesis in the *British Journal of State Medicine*, claiming to identify the English mother of at least two of the three men from Bures, a woman he called "the wanton Mary Haste" and "the gay lady of Bures." Alluding to her "sinister charms," Critchley named her "the villainess of the piece and the probable source of the tainted germ-plasm." Going far beyond what even Vessie claimed, Critchley asserted that the descendants of Mary Haste, affected or unaffected with chorea, were "liable to bear the marks of a grossly psychopathic taint, and the story of feeblemindedness, insanity, suicide, criminality, alcoholism and drug addiction, becomes unfolded over and over again." Indeed, what one author wrote of Huntington's chorea might well describe the writings themselves: that "the tragic themes of this disease are repeated over and over again." Some later writers even claimed that Huntington's chorea had played a role in the famous Salem, Massachusetts, witchcraft trials of 1692, though Vessie had not made that claim.[43]

Despite Vessie's characterization of the women accused of witchcraft as victims of superstition, it is hard to miss the resonances between his and Critchley's Huntington's chorea narratives and the earlier eugenic family studies. The Bures family group was yet another version of the Jukes, the Kallikaks, the Hill folk, and all their allegedly "cacogenic" kin. Indeed, Vessie had made a sharp turn in narrating the history of Huntington's. Muncey, after all, had included many accomplished individuals in her pedigrees. Davenport had worried about "genius" in these families. They had both portrayed Huntington's across a wide swath of society. In their accounts, a "diabolical" disease had brought about the ruin of many capable, talented people who had contributed much to society before their illness became severe. The accounts of Vessie and Critchley (and those

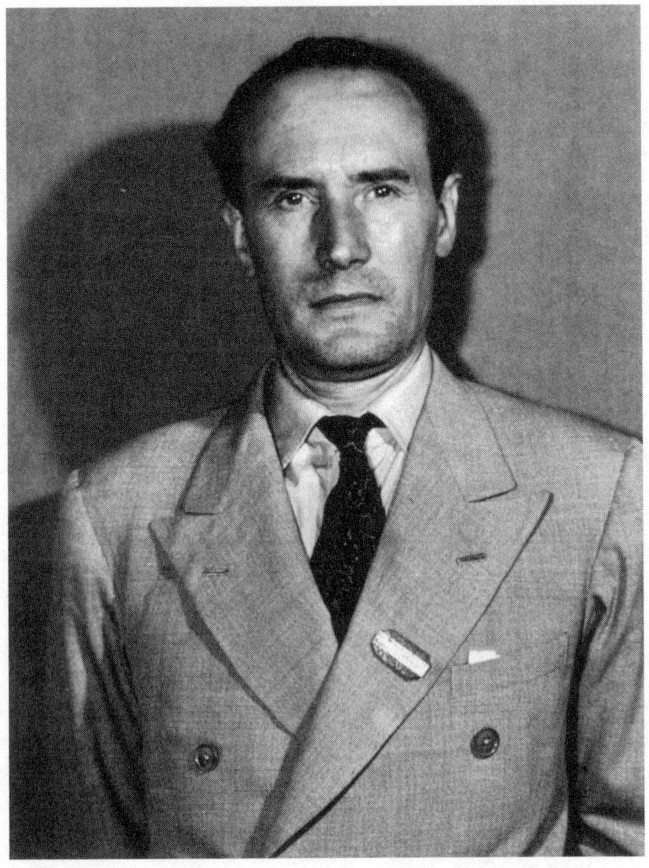

MacDonald Critchley (1900–1997), eminent British neurologist, at the Fourth International Neurological Congress, Paris, 1949. U.S. National Library of Medicine

who followed them) were entirely different. For them, the founding figures of the disease in America were already tainted. These lineages were spoiled from the beginning, their members inherently flawed. They had been "bad characters" from the start, passing down their ruined inheritance to their descendants.

The portrait Vessie and Critchley drew was so negative that the English geneticist Julia Bell wondered in 1934 whether the specific families they had studied just happened to be "uncommonly bad stock." Similarly, some geneticists in the United States, alluding to Vessie, compared those with the Huntington's chorea gene to carriers of a contagious disease, making an explicit equation between genes and germs. "Even the most hesitant of us to venture into the field of negative eugenics would probably agree upon the desirability of detection and exclusion of such immigrants," wrote James V. Neel in 1949, "on the same grounds that the United States Public Health Service now excludes those infected with certain contagious diseases."[44]

By this time, Huntington's chorea even surfaced on occasion in popular culture as an emblem of bad heredity, along with other more familiar disabilities targeted by the eugenics movement for elimination: when the California conservationist, environmentalist, and eugenicist Charles Goethe wanted to make claims, in 1949, about the benefits of a national park system, he proposed that parks would help create "a eugenically better nation" through the "gradual elimination of imbeciles, those insane through inheritance, carriers of congenital diseases, such as Huntington's chorea, haemophilia." Although he did not explain his reasoning, he nonetheless argued that eliminating such folk "would further reverse the tragic decline of the leadership type's birthrate."[45]

MISTAKEN IDENTITIES AND HISTORICAL FICTIONS

The narratives of Vessie and Critchley went unchallenged until 1969, when Mary Hans, a social worker, and Thomas Gilmore, a psychiatrist, at the Veterans Administration hospital in Albany, New York, used Vessie's pedigree to trace the ancestry of one of their own patients with Huntington's. To their surprise, they found numerous genealogical and historical errors, including the centerpiece of Vessie's pedigree claiming that Elinor Knapp had been executed as a witch. As Hans and Gilmore ascertained (from sources published before Vessie wrote his paper and therefore available to him), Elinor, the wife of Nicholas Knapp, had never been accused of witchcraft, much less been convicted and executed. Vessie (and Muncey) had apparently conflated her with a Goodwife Knapp, the wife of Roger Knapp. Goodwife Knapp had indeed been tried and executed as a witch in Fairfield, Connecticut, in 1653, while Elinor had lived in Stamford, where she died in 1658. Goodwife Knapp appeared to have no connection to the families with Huntington's chorea, while Elinor, who had no connection with witchcraft, did have descendants with the disease.[46]

Two other women whom Vessie surmised may have suffered from Huntington's—Elizabeth Knapp and Mercy Disborough—had been accused of either witchcraft or possession, but they had no known genealogical link either with Elinor or with Goodwife Knapp, nor did they have near descendants with symptoms evocative of Huntington's chorea. In 1671, the sixteen-year-old Elizabeth Knapp—the granddaughter not of Nicholas and Elinor but of William Knapp, as Vessie indicated—was the protagonist in a famous and well-documented episode of possession in Groton, Massachusetts, but she recovered, married a man named Scripture, and evidently went on to live a normal life.[47]

Critchley's argument also collapsed under close scrutiny. In the early 1970s two British researchers, Adrian Caro and Sheila Haines, demonstrated that his claims of a link between the Bures woman he called Mary Haste (whose name was actually Margaret, and of whom there is no evidence of chorea) and Vessie's emigrants to America were unfounded.[48]

More recent historical scholarship on early New England further undermines Vessie's thesis that witchcraft accusations might serve as a proxy for Huntington's chorea. As John Demos has written, while many writers have assumed that witches (or those accused) were "deranged, insane, or at least deeply eccentric, for New England the situation was largely otherwise." Historians today agree that seventeenth-century New England women accused of practicing witchcraft did not typically suffer from insanity or mental illness. New Englanders understood mental illness in a naturalistic way, as an illness of the body expressed through the mind, although they believed it could have supernatural causes as well. If women accused as witches were likely to be more assertive and independent than their neighbors, they did not, for the most part, appear to suffer from disorders such as St. Vitus's dance. And although the personality characteristics often attributed to early New England witches, such as irritability, melancholy, and bad temper, are sometimes found in persons with Huntington's, they are also found in many people without it. Moreover, many accused witches behaved in other ways entirely. As Demos has written, "What stands out about these people is their command of personal faculties, their ability to chart a given course of action, and to see it through." I have found no credible examples of an individual accused of witchcraft who behaved in ways evocative of this disease.[49]

More important, people suffering from chorea or other convulsive disorders in the seventeenth and eighteenth centuries were more likely to be seen as victims of witchcraft than as practicing witches, as many writers have noted. "Jerking helplessly like a marionette controlled by a careless puppeteer was to the popular mind a strong reason to suspect witchcraft," writes the historian Michael MacDonald, but "in spite of the contemporary readiness to believe that convulsive diseases were caused by supernatural powers, there was no single malady or cluster of symptoms that was popularly considered to be typical of witchcraft." William Buchan had put it bluntly. St. Vitus's dance, "wherein the patient is agitated with strange motions and gesticulations," was "by the common people . . . generally believed to be the effects of witchcraft." Witches might cause chorea in others. But they themselves were usually not affected.[50]

Vessie's portrait of "behavior problems" and "misconduct" in the men is similarly ahistorical. Most of the offenses he cited, such as selling beer without a license, drunkenness, and selling "quack" medicine (a judgment later rescinded), were minor infractions. Making speeches against the governor was a political act. Illiteracy was common among the early settlers and was evidence of class rather than chorea. The young man guilty of "bestialitie" went on to live a normal life. What Vessie called "disorderly conduct, theft, quackery, illicit sale of liquor, public prostitution, drunkenness, pauperism, religious dissension, family feuds and public denunciation of the Governor" were either trivial offenses or routine and typical acts for the litigious New Englanders of their time.[51]

NOT THE WITCHCRAFT DISEASE?

If neither witchcraft allegations nor conflicts with the law can be interpreted here as markers of Huntington's chorea, was there other evidence for Vessie's claims that some of these individuals may have been affected? With DNA analysis of their descendants, it may be possible to learn whether any of these seventeenth-century New England settlers carried the genetic mutation associated today with Huntington's. In fact, genealogy and genetics, not witchcraft accusations or legal misdemeanors, suggest a possible role in this story for the second generation of Vessie's characters: Joseph Ferris, a son of Jeffrey, and his wife, Ruth Knapp, a daughter of Elinor and Nicholas, were the common ancestors of several sets of early-twentieth-century sufferers, as shown in the pedigrees published by Vessie and by Hans and Gilmore. But contrary to Vessie's portrait of ostracism, scandal, and marginality, the lives of this couple, and certain of their close relatives, were marked more by social prominence than by social problems.[52]

The more important historical question, however, concerns the meaning of Vessie's interpretation in the twentieth century and its impact for affected families and for physicians. By portraying the supposed progenitors of Huntington's chorea in America as "bad characters" and their descendants as "mean" and "despicable," Vessie helped to legitimate a prejudicial and stigmatizing set of associations that surfaced in the medical literature on Huntington's for decades. Indeed, Vessie especially seemed to blame his female subjects for contributing "to the dooming of many of their descendants." In this regard his narrative is more revealing of the 1930s, when eugenics had wide legitimacy, than of the seventeenth-century era that it claimed to represent.[53]

Moreover, the fact that influential physicians such as Critchley, who served as president of the World Federation of Neurology in the 1970s, continued into the 1980s to cite Vessie's discredited thesis, conjuring up the "sociopathic traits and criminality" of the earliest alleged sufferers and their descendants, their "witchcraft, interbreeding, and crime," indicates just how uncontroversial this version of the history of Huntington's chorea had become. Critchley's claim that "the descendants of these three men were also undesirables and ne'er-do-wells" echoed as late as 2005 in the British novelist Ian McEwan's best-selling novel *Saturday*, where the thuggish, violent villain Baxter is a man whose every flaw the protagonist blames on Huntington's disease.[54]

And yet, many families with Huntington's have also embraced Vessie's witchcraft narrative, omitting his accusatory tone, his label of "misconduct," and his calls for sterilization, reinterpreting the story as an allegory of prejudice. For some, Vessie's "bad characters" became "outrageous nonconformists." The accused witches were simply persecuted women. Some readers and writers expanded his story, claiming that "practically all" of those affected by Huntington's on the east coast of the United States had descended from just two ancestors from Suffolk, England, and that some of the accused witches executed in the Salem witchcraft trials of 1692 also suffered from Huntington's, although, as we have seen, not even Vessie had made that claim.[55]

Despite its factual errors and eugenic associations, Vessie's thesis continues to exercise cultural power as a primal myth about the beginnings of Huntington's chorea in North America, a parable of modern medicine and science, and a story of injustice and unwarranted suffering. In this guise, it has a certain emotional truth, no matter how ungrounded in historical fact.

STERILIZATION AND SHAME

The 1920s through the 1940s constitute something of a nadir in the history not only of families with Huntington's chorea but also of people with other genetic disabilities and diseases. These were decades when hereditarian thought came to inform social agendas of all kinds, and the whole field of health reform "had been, in effect, 'eugenicized.'" Eugenics movements varied in different countries—eugenicists in Brazil and Mexico, for example, stressed kindergartens and prenatal care to improve the health of future generations, while those in Denmark, Sweden, and Norway embraced legislative regulation and sterilization. In Germany under the Nazi regime, the most extreme version of "racial hygiene" worldwide led first to the sterilization of those with mental and physical disabilities, between 1933 and 1939, and later to a policy of extermination.[56]

It is worth noting that Germany's 1933 Law for the Prevention of Progeny with Hereditary Defects (modeled partly on Indiana's 1907 sterilization law), which authorized the compulsory sterilization of those with mental disabilities, specifically named Huntington's chorea, along with such disorders as schizophrenia, manic depression, and severe alcoholism as grounds for compulsory sterilization. Historians have estimated that some 3,000–3,500 individuals affected with Huntington's may have been forcibly sterilized in Germany between 1933 and 1939 (out of a total of 350,000–400,000 people sterilized). With the start of World War II in 1939, sterilizations of the ill and disabled in Germany ceased and exterminations began, although I have found no specific figures for people with Huntington's who may have been killed during the war.[57]

In the United States during the 1920s, eugenic politics also became increasingly restrictive and exclusionist. As the Great Depression deepened during the 1930s, economic stringency intensified incentives to cut social welfare costs through exclusion of immigrants and compulsory sterilization. By this time many university-based geneticists had begun to criticize Davenport's efforts to tie complex behaviors to single genes; the Eugenics Record Office closed in 1939. But eugenic ideology continued to permeate educational materials and popular culture. As the historian of education Steven Selden has shown, eugenics "significantly penetrated" high school biology textbooks between 1914 and 1948, and informed mainstream American culture from the 1920s to the 1960s, popularized in magazines, films, books, lectures, exhibitions, and "fitter family contests." And practices of eugenic sterilization in the United States actually increased: whereas about 10,877 people had been sterilized by 1929, ten years later that number had tripled, to 33,035. Even after World War II, sterilizations continued: as Philip Reilly has shown, by the 1960s an estimated 60,000–66,000 persons, two-thirds of them women, had been involuntarily sterilized. Some sterilizations, even of children, were reportedly performed in the United States for Huntington's as well. Well into the 1960s eugenic notions of "better breeding" and "fitter families" continued to inform high school and college science texts.[58]

Even for critics of eugenics, Huntington's chorea stood out as one of the few conditions for which prohibitions against marriage and sterilization seemed an appropriate solution. The most telling statement of this position was the 1935 *Eugenical Sterilization: A Reorientation of the Problem*, "the definitive scientific critique of eugenic sterilization published in the United States." Written by a committee of the American Neurological Association under the leadership of Abraham Myerson, a professor of neurology at Tufts College Medical School in Boston, the Myerson report, as it was often called, sharply criticized practices of involuntary sterilization in state mental hospitals and asylums, and other strands of eugenics as well. It argued that many conditions for which sterilization was performed, such as "feeblemindedness" and "pauperism," were not actually hereditary, that mental illness was not increasing, and that the mentally ill and mentally disabled tended to have fewer children than average, not more. While isolated family reports might present instances of high fertility, "if the statistics as a whole are considered, a curious, not easily explainable, *complete contradiction* to the statements usually made in the eugenic literature appears." The report concluded that "the reputedly high fecundity of the mentally defective groups is a myth."[59]

At the same time the authors defended a policy of sterilization for Huntington's chorea (along with several other disorders) "with the consent of the patient or those responsible for him." They were certain that, in the case of Huntington's, "the indications for sterilization" would usually be "obvious to the physician and should be so to the patient." The report also called for widening the practice of sterilization in general, stating that sterilization laws "should be applicable not only to patients in State institutions but also to those in private institutions and those at large in the community." Even if there were "no new social or biological emergency," not only sterilization but restrictions on marriage "might well be strengthened by appropriate and early legislation." In this framework the meanings of "voluntary" were unclear.[60]

Well into the 1970s some clinicians worried that "there is probably no other disorder with such a strong argument against reproduction." If "reason alone and intellectual appreciation of future dangers" did not discourage reproduction, wrote John Pearson, a Kansas physician, in 1972, "what is left?"[61]

SILENCE INTO SPEECH

As we have seen, negative portraits of people with the magrums/St. Vitus's dance/Huntington's chorea did not begin with the era of eugenics. Nonetheless, the emergence of eugenics in the early twentieth century initiated a turn toward more hostile portrayals in medical writing and occasionally in popular media, raising questions about the social and emotional consequences of these representations for affected families. As the historian Nancy Leys Stepan has pointed out, "cultural codes have effects on how individuals live their lives and interact with one another." What impact, then, did this discourse have on the women and men living with Huntington's and on their families? To what extent did it influence the everyday practice of medical professionals dealing with them and with the disease?[62]

A window onto the attitudes and practices of family members and health professionals from about the 1940s through the 1970s is the testimony presented at a series of public hearings held in 1976 and 1977 by the Commission for the

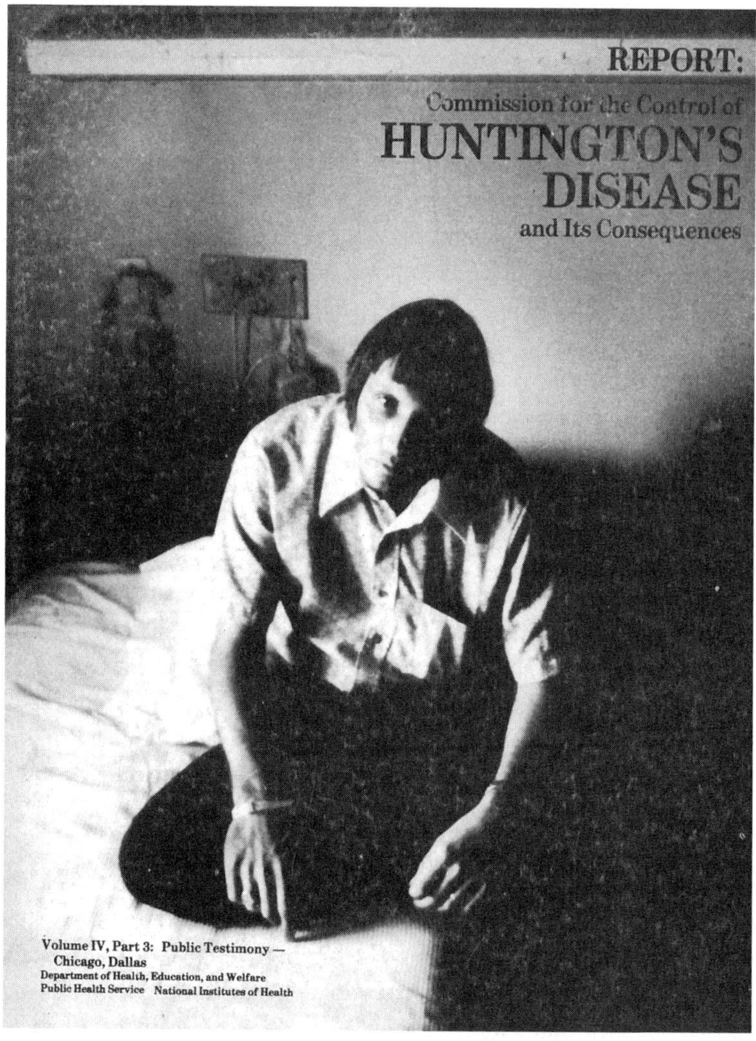

Report: Commission for the Control of Huntington's Disease and Its Consequences, 1977

Control of Huntington's Disease and Its Consequences, a panel mandated by the U.S. Congress in response to demands from affected families for an assessment of needs and recommendations for policy. Even before the commission, advocacy groups had begun to create spaces for these families to speak: groups such as the Committee to Combat Huntington's Disease (CCHD), organized in New York by Marjorie Guthrie, following the death from Huntington's of her husband, the songwriter and singer Woody Guthrie, in 1967; the California chapter of CCHD, in Los Angeles, headed by Milton Wexler, which in 1974 became the Hereditary Disease Foundation; and the Wills Foundation, started by Alice Pratt in Texas. In 1976 and 1977 the commission, led by Nancy Wexler, the executive director, and two cochairs, Marjorie Guthrie and Milton Wexler, held hearings around the country at which some two thousand people, family members (mostly unaffected individuals), caregivers, and health professionals—general practitioners, neurologists, nurses, and social workers among others—came to testify (or submit letters) about their experiences with the disease.[63]

One conclusion we can draw from this testimony is that from the 1940s through the mid-1970s, young people at risk for Huntington's sometimes received explicit warnings from physicians or counselors not to marry or not to have children, advice they found traumatic. "It's every girl's dream to have a baby and all of a sudden I was advised not to have a child," one young woman reported. "I really couldn't cope with a childless future." Another young woman reported that when she spoke with her pastor and school counselor about Huntington's, "they both advised me not to marry." A woman married to a husband with Huntington's testified that her adult children had repeatedly been told "not to plan on getting married, or having a family, or leading a normal life." A father whose wife was affected testified that his son was told at the National Institutes of Health that he should not have children since "the only way known to strike back at H.D. is to go childless." Clearly some physicians were offering direct eugenic advice to their patients well into the 1970s.[64]

And some family members agreed with this advice, but not for the reasons given by health professionals. More often they cited their own experience as the basis for their thinking. As a man who was one of the more extreme witnesses put it, "If potential victims have seen H.D. in their family, the way we did, getting sterilized would be a cause for rejoicing!" In his view, "it would be a good idea to try to track down every living H.D. patient. Give them the facts and encourage them to submit to sterilization, NOW!" But while most family members acknowledged the seriousness of childbearing decisions where a legacy of Huntington's was involved, they emphasized the importance of having a choice in the context of accurate information about the disease. As one woman married to a husband with Huntington's put it, "I love my daughters but I wish to God I had known about Huntington's disease years ago so I could have had the decision to make for myself." Others put their objections even more strongly. "One of the recommendations our first neurologist made was that we all ought to be sterilized," reported the wife of another man with Huntington's. "That was the first thing he said after he announced the diagnosis. That, I think, was not his place. That was something that we all had to come around to. It was like a slap in the face. . . . That's the way he dealt with us, and I think that was wrong. That was really the difficult thing we had to face in this."[65]

These responses point to a second theme woven through the commission testimony: that many individuals from affected families were unaware of Huntington's chorea in their ancestry until a relative close to them was diagnosed. As Marjorie Guthrie remarked ironically at one of the commission hearings, "because there are families who have not known their family background and history, eugenics will not work," although I would add that, in part because eugenics encouraged secrecy and silence, many families have not known their background and their history. Often a parent or grandparent had been misdiagnosed with something else—for instance "nervous breakdown," schizophrenia, Alzheimer's, Parkinson's, alcoholism, multiple sclerosis, even malingering. Sometimes physicians did not inform family members when they made a diagnosis of Huntington's. One woman reported that while her father had been at Pilgrim State Hospital on Long Island for six years, "never in all those 6 long years was H.D. ever mentioned by the hospital staff." Sometimes family members who knew did not inform their relatives, or did so only at a parent's death, usually years after those at risk had had their children. "It was at his death that my brothers, sister, and I were told about my father's hereditary disease," one woman reported, "and of course, warned not to have children." A man whose mother did not tell her children of their father's illness discovered it in medical school, when the news came as a tremendous shock. Indeed, some witnesses claimed that lack of knowledge caused them more difficulties than the disease itself. "It was the years wasted in not knowing what she had that really wrecked her," stated one woman of her sister. Once the sister had a correct diagnosis, "she knew now it was not her fault and she could accept it."[66]

Questions of knowledge emerged in commission testimony in yet another way, as both clinicians and many family members urged development of a predictive test. They did so, however, for sharply different reasons. Clinicians who spoke tended to support a test for eugenic purposes. If "it could be determined who could develop the disease," testified one representative New York neurologist, "taking appropriate measures after that might lead to a virtual absence of the disease," although just what these "appropriate measures" were he did not say. Even one of the commissioners proposed (in a minority position) that "if our attention is directed toward this early detection, accurate diagnosis, and genetic counseling, if we can combine this operation, then probably we [can] contribute more to the next generation than if we cure patients." Underlying this claim was the widely shared assumption that "rational" individuals would want to get tested and would "naturally" give up childbearing if they turned out to be gene carriers. Indeed some clinicians who testified compared Huntington's to Tay-Sachs, a recessive disorder that is fatal in early childhood, and whose implications differ considerably from a late-onset malady such as Huntington's. "Even though we do not have a cure for the disease," declared a pediatrician at UCLA, "we can now isolate those people who carry the [Tay-Sachs] gene, instruct them, and also ultimately prevent the birth of individuals who will become affected by the disease." He believed Tay-Sachs would cease to be significant in the near future, "and it is merely a matter of public health measures to prevent this disease from continuing." "What do we need," he asked, "to put Huntington's disease in this category?"[67]

Other physicians emphasized that a predictive test would "prevent discrimination against that half of the total population of at-risk individuals who are gene-free and who would otherwise be entitled to marriage, certain kinds of jobs, induction into the Armed Forces, and quite frequently the benefits of the Veterans Administration system," as if those who carried the gene were not entitled to marriage, jobs, or V.A. benefits. Many who testified shared the position expressed by the geneticist Ntinas Myrianthopoulos a few years earlier, that without a test, clinicians and counselors were faced with great difficulties. However compassionately they approached their clients, they had "nowhere to turn for help except to the sobering probability figure of one in two."[68]

Family members, on the other hand, often indicated that a test would be valuable for what they perceived was its subjective, psychological benefit to those at risk. If a test were to become available, some individuals said that they would take it to get rid of the anxiety their uncertain genetic status created. Without a test, as one woman put it, "it's like sitting in a courtroom for 40 years wondering if you're getting the electric chair or are going to be set free." Another woman compared being at risk to being 1-A for the draft during wartime. A predictive test would help them make important decisions about marriage, children, and career, although none indicated that a positive test would foreclose childbearing altogether. But other family members, including Marjorie Guthrie, worried about the long-term emotional impact of a test on those who received bad news. Do you really want to know, she asked, that you will die in twenty years of this disease?[69]

Some physicians shared their concern. These practitioners emphasized that a late-onset dominant disorder such as Huntington's differed from a recessive disease such as Tay-Sachs, where the parents themselves were not affected, and those affected died in early childhood. David L. Stevens, an English neurologist, worried that those found to carry the disease gene "will be plunged into despondency." He urged that a test be delayed until medicine had "something tangible" to offer. Other clinicians thought that although a test "would be welcomed" by many of those whom Stevens had characterized as "the unhappy frustrated people at risk," its accuracy had to be assured, and the question of whether the test itself could hasten onset of symptoms answered. Commission members themselves endorsed its development but stressed the need for great caution as well.[70]

Still, a predictive test was not the highest priority for most family members. They placed far more emphasis on the need for social services and affordable facilities for long-term care. As the commission summary put it, the basic message was everywhere the same: there was nowhere to go for help. People felt "almost totally deprived of support from any branch of society." Significantly, those few who reported positive experiences in caring for relatives were often from working-class families with good union pensions (the Teamsters, for example) or generous health insurance plans from their employers, or access to federal social welfare programs such as Social Security Disability, Aid to Dependent Children, and Medicaid. But many more, both working and middle class, had tremendous difficulties securing adequate insurance and financial coverage for care, and made greater social resources for caregiving a high priority for the future.[71]

Family members also advocated research toward treatments and a cure and demanded more informed and sympathetic health professionals who understood that incurable did not mean untreatable. Just getting an accurate diagnosis was often a challenge, as many physicians at the hearings acknowledged. "It's unbelievable how few doctors know about Huntington's Chorea," one neurologist exclaimed, "and even worse than that is the ones who know about it, but will drop the patient like a hotcake. They don't want to have anything to do with unpleasant, nasty diseases like that." Lay people agreed that the stigmatization of Huntington's extended to some health care workers, who were wary about the time needed to care for patients with this illness. As one woman testified, telephone calls to prospective nursing homes brought such responses as, "'Our doctor told us to stay as far away from you people as possible.' We're unpopular to our families, friends, and to society in general."[72]

No wonder, then, that many family members, men and women alike, emphasized the need to change this image of Huntington's, and to end the taboo against talking about it. "If I had one wish that this Commission could accomplish," said a young Ann Arbor woman, "it would be to take away the stigma of Huntington's disease and take it out of the closet." The burden of secrecy, within families as well as outside, resonated throughout the commission testimonies.

"Very little discussion about it takes place among us"; "I know in my own family I think it wasn't talked about"; "No one dared mention it"; "very hush-hush. No one wanted to talk about it"; and "Living with this Huntington's disease [in the family] is like the proverbial skeleton in the closet; everybody really slams the door in a hurry, and is intimidated by the fact that they have this peculiarity in the family that no one wants to talk about or to share or see." Everyone agreed that the silences within families were almost always damaging, inducing guilt and preventing relatives from sharing information and facing the illness in a realistic way.[73]

Talking about it outside the family, of course, was a complex matter, as witnesses' testimony regarding instances of discrimination illustrated the genuine risks of public disclosure. As one neurologist reported, "I have seen divorce, loss of employment, inability to get life insurance and rejection from the armed forces all revolve around the diagnosis of Huntington's disease in a family." Or as a plainspoken insurance man put it starkly to the commission: "Huntington's is considered in a class by itself. It is not grouped." If his company had information that someone's parent had it, or even that the applicant had been examined for it, that person could not be insured, at least not at the usual price. Huntington's was "the red flag."[74]

"A VAST COMMUNITY"

If the commission hearings highlighted the legacies of eugenics, it also illuminated possibilities and progress. By the 1970s the cultural landscape of Huntington's disease had changed, and indeed that of genetic disease and disability generally. The civil rights movements of the 1960s and 1970s, feminism, and the development of informed consent and patients' rights all challenged the bases of eugenic thought. The testimony of family members represented one strand in the larger repudiation of eugenics that was taking place during the 1970s, along with the legalization of abortion with *Roe v. Wade* in 1973, and the termination of the infamous Tuskegee experiments, in which southern black men with syphilis were followed from the 1930s to the 1970s without being given penicillin when it became available in the 1940s. With CCHD, the Hereditary Disease Foundation, and the commission, many members of families with Huntington's were stepping out of the closet. "Now at least, in my generation, those are no longer dirty, hush-hush, don't say them out loud words," acknowledged one young woman about the disease. People who had been isolated and secretive about the malady in their families began to form what the anthropologist Paul Rabinow has called a new biosocial community, centered around a shared identification with Huntington's. The Reverend Sidney Mink addressed this transformation at an October 1975 commission hearing in Boston: When Huntington's first struck his family in the 1940s, Mink recalled, it was "an esoteric disease and we thought very few people had it. Now we find that we're in a vast community of people involved all across the world."[75]

At the commission hearings some people at risk spoke of finding ways of living that had important values and rewards. "It is my objective to live each day to the fullest extent," affirmed one young man, "so that I would have nothing to regret if I am not around to live the next. In my opinion, living life with something hanging over my head is far superior to not living life at all." The wife of a man with Huntington's reported that her children say "quality, not quantity. In other words, their lives are going to be the best. We've been able to handle it that way." Some persons at risk spoke of their confrontation with Huntington's as a challenge and a quest, emphasizing that "it's made us appreciate life and do all the things we might have put off." Being at risk and knowing she might have a limited number of years to live encouraged one young woman "very strongly to want to make the best of those years, and I have made decisions that I might not otherwise have had the courage to make. Decisions that were good as to how to live my life." Rather than seeing her risk of Huntington's exclusively as a burden and source of dread, she took the possibility of the disease as a challenge to live her life as fully as she could.[76]

Only a few persons with Huntington's spoke at the commission hearings, an absence reflecting the difficulties of communication posed by the disease but also the unfamiliarity of a public forum for affected individuals, an unfamiliarity that would lessen as more persons with HD participated in meetings and conventions. At the hearings in the 1970s, others still did most of the speaking. After a diagnosis, stated Thomas Bird, a neurologist in Seattle, it's important "that the affected patient doesn't get the feeling that that's it, I've got to give up." As Bird emphasized, "people can have signs of the disease and continue on for many years with a very productive, useful, and interesting life; and we have to be sure that the individuals and the families know that, and that there isn't just a rejection of that individual." The commissioners stressed that lives with Huntington's disease had value, although affected individuals were often denied the chance to realize it. In a direct refutation of the ideology of eugenics, Marjorie Guthrie emphasized this point. "You know this, to me, is one of the most important parts of our testimony," she said at one of the commission hearings. "That people must not presume that because the doctor says you have

Huntington's, that your life is over. . . . You have certain capabilities and we must work then to use those to the utmost to give you an opportunity to live with what you've got."[77]

HUNTINGTON'S, DISABILITY, AND HISTORY

In many respects, the claims of Davenport, Vessie, Critchley, and others belonged to larger cultural narratives that informed much medical and popular discourse on disease and disability through much of the twentieth century. Ideas of neuropathic inheritance, of the "prolific" families of the "unfit"—especially the "unfit" woman—of associations between disability, criminality, and danger, were classic tropes of nineteenth- and early-twentieth-century eugenics that inflected the medical discourse on Huntington's as well. Indeed, the idea of the disabled figure as dangerous or evil has a long history in Western culture, represented in the many disabled villains of literature and film. Thus the portraits drawn by Vessie and Critchley built on a tradition of such stigmatizing images.[78]

This is not to say that all, or even most, health practitioners accepted these portrayals as realistic. Rather, many of the ideas that informed certain strands of medical and genetic thinking about Huntington's were not unique to this disease. Vessie's and Critchley's negative portrayals of people with Huntington's derived their credibility in part from their association with larger cultural myths. In this respect, Huntington's represents a useful case study in the two-way traffic between cultural expectations and medical knowledge: not only did cultural myths and stereotypes shape certain medical and scientific understandings of Huntington's, but medical and scientific narratives of Huntington's—for instance, the image of the woman with chorea as a witch—contributed to cultural associations between femaleness, illness, and evil. Understanding how these medical and historical narratives about Huntington's were constructed, then, can illuminate the relations between science and culture, suggesting ways that we can make new medical narratives less freighted with outworn stereotypes and clichés.

It is tempting to dismiss the older narratives as "bad science," or not science at all, merely the mythmaking of a few biased investigators speculating, outside their fields of expertise, about the historical origins of this disease. But the fact that these sources were published in mainstream, even prestigious medical and scientific journals, and repeatedly cited in the genetic and neurological literature, suggests that they cannot be so easily cast aside. Rather than simply dismiss them as outdated, we need to understand how they worked in the past in order to avoid falling into similar traps in the future.[79]

Indeed, this history calls into question the popular biomedical idea that substituting scientific "fact" for "superstition" necessarily lessens stigma and prejudice. As this history shows, "facts" about the Mendelian dominant inheritance of Huntington's chorea coexisted with arguments for eugenic sterilization just as easily, if not more so, than did allusions to hereditary curses and taints. Eugenics was a project of scientific modernity, and greater scientific knowledge about Huntington's, in the context of eugenics, did not lead to more enlightened treatment of those affected. As many scholars have noted, the sciences "are never 'simply scientific' but are complex constructions that always involve struggles over meaning and values." Constructing and employing biomedical knowledge in ways that benefit patients and families, women and men, children as well as adults, is also a question of politics and priorities.[80]

If viewing Huntington's disease through the lens of eugenics illuminates the secrecy that surrounded this illness throughout most of the twentieth century, viewing eugenics through the lens of Huntington's disease also extends the argument made by such scholars as Diane Paul, Alexandra Stern, Nancy Leys Stepan, and Wendy Kline, that "eugenics found its widest application" not in the 1910s and 1920s but in the 1930s and after. (As Stern put it, hereditarianism "did not perish after World War II; it was repackaged.") The example of Huntington's suggests, in fact, that the most intense impact of eugenic ideology on medical discourse in the United States may have been felt in the 1930s, 1940s, and 1950s, the years of the Great Depression, World War II, and the Cold War, haunted by McCarthyism, the Bomb, and anticommunism.[81]

In the 1960s and 1970s all this began to change, in response both to scientific advances and to social transformations. The civil rights movement challenged the racism of many strands of eugenics. Feminists reconfigured the choice to bear children as a private, not a public, concern. Indeed, feminism turned many women into health activists, demanding reproductive autonomy and legalized birth control and abortion. Within medicine, the development of L-dopa for treating Parkinson's disease led neurologists to organize a research group to pursue new treatments for Huntington's as well. The recombinant DNA revolution opened up powerful new methods for studying genes. And as persons from families with Huntington's began to organize and lobby for more research and services, they also rewrote the narratives surrounding the idea of a predictive test: instead of the eugenic strategy imagined by Charles Davenport, they defined it as one that must serve the interests of those who chose to obtain this information. They took the lead in writing guidelines for testing, after a genetic marker was identified in 1983, and again after the gene was found in 1993. They/we continue to lobby, organize, push for legislation against genetic discrimination, for better long-term health care, for more research.

Huntington's disease remains a reality. Members of the disability community remind us that "even when it involves pain and hardship, disability is not always a tragedy, hardship, or lack but in fact often provides much of value." Having a progressive fatal disease such as Huntington's is significantly different from living with a stable disability. Still, it does not preclude a worthwhile life, with the resources and support that can make this possible. Those of us at risk for this disease have learned to value our precarious relationship to the world, and the insights that it has given us. While we would prefer to gain this knowledge in other ways, nonetheless we have come to appreciate, not the disease, but the creativity and connections it has challenged us to pursue.

As we work toward a treatment that will make Huntington's a manageable disease, a curable illness, and possibly even a preventable one in those who carry the expanded gene, questions of values and priorities will become even more urgent. How to draw on our knowledge of the past to craft a wise and just future is the challenge before us.

Milwaukee. Huntington's Disease Society of America Annual Convention, June 2007.

See that willowy young woman in a bright red dress and matching lipstick who dances, already showing the slight twitches and grimaces of early Huntington's; the gray-haired woman jerking back and forth in her wheelchair, arms flying, head flopping; and that skinny young man in the backward baseball cap who shimmies and shakes out on the dance floor as if he didn't have a care in the world, who found out at the age of eighteen that he has the abnormal Huntington's disease gene and carries this knowledge with grace and strength. As we dance this dance of St. Vitus, this double dance of illness and of cure, the movements of chorea blend with those of hip hop, salsa, and rock and roll. Later, when I am no longer surrounded by people with Huntington's, I look at the still bodies near me and—just for an instant—I find something missing.

ABBREVIATIONS

AH	Abel Huntington
AJI	*American Journal of Insanity*
APS	American Philosophical Society, Philadelphia
CBD	Charles B. Davenport
CH	Cornelia Huntington
CHD	Elizabeth B. Muncey, "Classical Huntington's Disease (Huntington's Chorea) Families in the United States," ed. Sheldon C. Reed (1913; Minneapolis: Dight Institute for Human Genetics, University of Minnesota, 1964)
Davenport Papers	Charles B. Davenport Papers, American Philosophical Society, Philadelphia
EBM	Elizabeth B. Muncey
East Hampton History	Jeanette Edwards Rattray, *East Hampton History, Including Genealogies of Early Families* (Garden City, N.Y.: Country Life, 1953)
EHHS	East Hampton Historical Society
EHS	*East Hampton Star*
ERO	Eugenics Record Office Archives, ms. coll. 77, American Philosophical Library, Philadelphia
GH	George Huntington
GHS	Greenwich Historical Society, Greenwich, Connecticut
GLH	George Lee Huntington
HPH	Henry P. Hedges
JER	Jeanette Edwards Rattray
JNMD	*Journal of Nervous and Mental Disease*
Journal of Trustees	*Journal of the Trustees of the Freeholders and Commonalty of East Hampton Town*, 1725–1925, 7 vols. (East Hampton, N.Y., 1926)

LC	Library of Congress, Washington, D.C.
Main Street	Jeanette Edwards Rattray, *Up and Down Main Street: An Informal History of East Hampton and Its Old Houses* (East Hampton: *East Hampton Star,* 1968).
Osler Collection	Sir William Osler Collection, Osler Library of the History of Medicine, McGill University, Montreal
PLIC-EHL	Pennypacker Long Island Collection, East Hampton Library, East Hampton, N.Y.
Records of East Hampton	*Records of the Town of East Hampton, Long Island, Suffolk County, New York,* 5 vols. (Sag Harbor, N.Y.: J. H. Hunt, 1887–1905)
Refugees of 1776	Mather, Frederick Gregory, *The Refugees of 1776 from Long Island to Connecticut* (New York: J. B. Lyon, 1913)
SEJ	Smith Ely Jelliffe

NOTES

INTRODUCTION

1. See for example Gillian Bates, Peter S. Harper, and Lesley Jones, *Huntington's Disease*, 3rd. ed. (Oxford: Oxford University Press, 2002). In 1993, the mutant Huntington's disease gene was identified as a trinucleotide (CAG) expansion on the short arm of chromosome four, putting this malady into the category known as polyglutamine diseases, since CAG spells out instructions for the amino acid glutamine.
2. Robert A. Aronowitz, *Making Sense of Illness: Science, Society, and Disease* (Cambridge: Cambridge University Press, 1998), 11.
3. Medical works that include brief histories of the disease include Michael R. Hayden, *Huntington's Chorea* (New York: Springer-Verlag, 1981); Susan Folstein, *Huntington's Disease: A Disorder of Families* (Baltimore: Johns Hopkins University Press, 1989), and Peter S. Harper, ed., *Huntington's Disease* (London: W. B. Saunders, 1991; also Bates, Harper, and Jones, *Huntington's Disease*, 3rd ed.). On the dancing mania see H. C. Midelfort, *A History of Madness in Sixteenth-Century Germany* (Stanford: Stanford University Press, 1999), 25–79.
4. On the magrums see Alan Cobham, *A Glossary of Lancashire Words as Spoken in Mawdesley*, http://www.mawdesley-village.org.uk/dialect2.html; also George Wakeman, "Idioms," *The Galaxy: A Magazine of Entertaining Reading* 9 (February 1870), 271. Wakeman includes the "maggrums" or "megrims" among the "curious complaints" suffered by New Englanders.
5. Nora Ellen Groce, *Everyone Here Spoke Sign Language: Hereditary Deafness on Martha's Vineyard* (Cambridge: Harvard University Press, 1985). See also Sheila M. Rothman, *Living in the Shadow of Death: Tuberculosis and the Social Experience of Illness in American History* (Baltimore: Johns Hopkins University Press, 1994).
6. Percy R. Vessie, "On the Transmission of Huntington's Chorea for Three Hundred Years: The Bures Family Group," *JNMD* 76 (1932), 553–72; Vessie, "Hereditary Chorea: St. Anthony's Dance and Witchcraft in Colonial Connecticut," *Journal of the Connecticut State Medical Society* 3 (1939), 596–600.
7. Jeanette Edwards Rattray, local historian of East Hampton, signed her column "One of ours" in the *East Hampton Star* in the 1950s.

8. Averill Geus to author, April 28, 2001. See, for example, Emily K. Abel, *Hearts of Wisdom: American Women Caring for Kin, 1850–1940* (Cambridge: Harvard University Press, 2000); Sheila Rothman, *Living in the Shadow of Death: Tuberculosis and the Social Experience of Illness in American History* (Baltimore: Johns Hopkins University Press, 1994); Howard Kushner, *American Suicide* (New Brunswick: Rutgers University Press, 1991); Cornelia Dayton, "'A Burst Man': Joseph Gorham Presents the Puzzle of Autism to 18th-Century Cape Cod," paper presented to the Columbia Seminar on Early America, May 11, 1999.
9. The impact of eugenics on those deemed "unfit" is a topic that has intrigued and frustrated many scholars because of the elusiveness of evidence. Recent feminist scholars such as Nancy Gallagher, in *Breeding Better Vermonters: The Eugenics Project in the Green Mountain State* (Hanover, N.H.: University Press of New England, 1999), have speculated that well-intentioned eugenics workers may have contributed to the isolation and marginalization of so-called "degenerate" families in Vermont, including those with Huntington's chorea. As Gallagher writes, "the reproduction of evidence by eugenicists and well-intentioned social reformers and its propagation throughout the professional literature of diverse fields and the public domain were probably more toxic to children and families than real or imaginary genes" (90). Similarly, Wendy Kline, in *Building a Better Race: Gender, Sexuality, and Eugenics from the Turn of the Century to the Baby Boom* (Berkeley: University of California Press, 2001), has emphasized how eugenic ideology intensified anxieties and led some women especially to internalize beliefs about their unfitness for motherhood. "By arguing that only select bodies were fit to reproduce," writes Kline, "eugenicists added unprecedented pressure toward cultural uniformity and contributed to the increasing stigmatization of difference" (126). See also Nancy Leys Stepan, *"The Hour of Eugenics": Race, Gender, and Nation in Latin America* (Ithaca: Cornell University Press, 1991), 14.
10. See Staffan Müller-Wille and Hans-Jörg Rheinberger, "Heredity: The Production of an Epistemic Space," preprint 276 (Berlin: Max Planck Institute for the History of Science, 2004).
11. Marjorie Guthrie stated in hearings before the Congressional Commission of 1976 and 1977 that "until a certain year there was nothing in a textbook to find out." See *Report: Commission for the Control of Huntington's Disease and Its Consequences* vol. 4, part 5 (Washington D.C.: National Institutes of Health; Health, Education and Welfare, and Public Health Service, 1977), 496.

1. THE DEATH OF PHEBE HEDGES

1. Samuel Buell, *A Faithful Narrative of the Remarkable Revival of Religion, in the Congregation of East-Hampton, on Long Island* (Sag Harbor, N.Y.: Alden Spooner, 1808), 32–33.
2. Cited in Nancy Hayden Woodward, *East Hampton: A Town and its People, 1648–1994* (East Hampton: Fireplace, 1995), 91–92.
3. On the family of Phebe Mulford, see JER's informative but unreliable *East Hampton History*, 475–82, 585–87, and *Main Street*, n.p.; also *Records of East Hampton*, passim. See also William H. Pelletreau, comp., "Abstracts of Unrecorded Wills Prior to 1790 on File in the Surrogate's Office, City [i.e., County] of New York, 1665–1800," *Collections of the New-York Historical Society* 35 (1902), 380–81, 125–26, 290–91, 5–7. William H. Pelletreau, ed., *Early Long Island Wills of Suffolk County, 1691–1703* (New York: F. P. Harper, 1897), 123–27. Will of John Mulford, proved 1786, New York Surrogate Courts, liber 38, 421 (old number 374), Riverhead; will of John Mulford Jr.,

proved 1727, New York Surrogate Courts, liber 10, 408, New York City; will of John Stratton, New York Surrogate Courts, 1759, liber 25, 462, New York City; will of Thomas Chatfield, 1751, New York Surrogate Courts, liber 19, 11–14, New York City. See also "Ancient Burying Grounds of Long Island," *New York Genealogical and Biographical Register*, July 1900, 306–7; October 1900, 427–34; January 1901, 84–90; April 1900, 203–10; July 1901, 278; "South End Cemeteries," unpublished typescript, PLIC-EHL; on the "sweating sickness" see Lyman Beecher, "A Sermon Containing a General History of the Town of East-Hampton . . . January 1, 1806," *Journal of Trustees*, 1807–26), 179. See also East Hampton assessment rolls, passim, PLIC-EHL.

4. On Joseph and other Tillinghasts see Rose Tillinghast, *The Tillinghast Family, 1540–1971* (Rose Tillinghast, 1972), 179–86; JER erroneously identifies Phebe Mulford as Phebe Shaler in *East Hampton History*, 585–58, and *Main Street*, 15–16. I am grateful to Wayne G. Tillinghast for sharing his exhaustive fund of genealogical information on the Tillinghast family, especially on Joseph, who is described as a "mariner" in a 1759 Newport court case: Wayne Tillinghast to author, December 28, 1998. See also Tillinghast file, JER Papers, PLIC-EHL; Tillinghast family file, Suffolk County Historical Society, Riverhead. "Joseph Tillinghast of Rhode Island, distiller" appears on his marriage bond to Phebe Mulford, 1761; see *Marriage Bonds*, 4: 114, New York State Library, Albany; also *Marriage Licenses . . . of the Province of New York Previous to 1784* (Albany: Weed, Parsons, 1860), 275. George Huntington's report of the Rhode Island tradition is cited in *Neurographs* 1 (1908), 151–52. On the five families see *EHS*, January 18, 1973. In a letter to George Huntington written in 1908, Henry P. Hedges described what had been told to him "forty or fifty years ago" (in the 1850s or 1860s). His narrative seemed to identify Hannah Howell Pierson (1686–1726/7), daughter of Susannah Howell and Henry Pierson, as "the Howell woman from Southampton," pushing the story of the illness back to the late seventeenth century. Hannah Pierson married John Mulford Jr. (1683–1726/7), Phebe's grandfather, in 1707. Although she was only forty when she died, she was old enough to have been affected with St. Vitus's dance. Hedges's account is plausible, and he is certainly the earliest witness to give a genealogical account of the origins of St. Vitus's dance in East Hampton. (He heard this story from the great-great-grandson of Hannah Pierson, John T. Dayton, born in 1795 and died in 1874, who could have heard it from his own grandfather, Captain John Dayton, born in 1727. Captain Dayton had married a sister of Phebe Mulford, and he probably heard about Hannah from her or from his father-in-law, John Mulford. The latter was fifteen when his mother, Hannah, died, certainly old enough to remember her. But there are arguments against this interpretation as well. Hannah's father, Henry Pierson, was in the colonial legislature at the time of his death, at the age of forty-nine, and there is no direct evidence that either he or Susannah suffered from St. Vitus's dance. Hedges's account also implicates John Mulford as a sufferer from the disease. Mulford lived a long life, yet he had troubles toward the end. He suddenly dropped out of town governance at the age of fifty-two, around the time he was hit with several lawsuits for failure to pay his debts: events suggesting that something was amiss, although he lived for another twenty-one years. During the Revolution he spent three years in exile in Stonington, Connecticut, but was allowed to return to East Hampton in 1780, on grounds of being "very *infirm*." He was then sixty-six years old. He died in 1784 at the age of seventy-three.) Henry Hedges's letter is quoted in Charles S. Stevenson, "A Biography of George Huntington, M.D.," *Bulletin of the Institute of the History of Medicine* 22 (April 1934), 71. The original is at the ERO, ser. I-A: 3181, box 39, folder 3. On John Mulford see *Public Records of*

the State of Connecticut (Hartford: Press of the Case, Lockwood and Brainard, 1894), 332; Frederick Gregory Mather, *The Refugees of 1776 from Long Island to Connecticut* (Albany: J. B. Lyon, 1913), 875, 479. See also Suffolk County Court of Common Pleas, case file 22, March 30, 1763; case file 24, February 1764, July 16, 1764. Henry P. Hedges published *A History of the Town of East-Hampton* (Sag Harbor, N.Y.: John H. Hunt, 1897). See also George Roger Howell, *The Early History of Southampton, L.I., New York* (Albany: Weed, Parsons, 1887).

5. On East Hampton in the late eighteenth century see Buell, *A Faithful Narrative;* John Lyon Gardiner, "Notes and Observations on the Town of East Hampton, 1798," in E. B. O'Callaghan, ed., *The Documentary History of the State of New York* (Albany: Weed, Parsons, 1850–51), 674–86; Ilse O'Sullivan, *East Hampton and the American Revolution* (East Hampton: East Hampton Bicentennial Town Committee, 1976,) 55; David Gardiner, *Chronicles of the Town of Easthampton* (1840; New York: Bowne, 1871), rpt. as "Gardiner's East Hampton," in *New-York Historical Society Collections,* vol. 1 (New York: Printed for the Society, 1869); Woodward, *East Hampton;* Timothy Breen, *Imagining the Past: East Hampton Histories* (Athens: University of Georgia Press, 1996); *Records of East Hampton* and *Journal of Trustees;* "Census of Suffolk County 1776," in E. B. O'Callaghan, ed., *Calendar of Historical Manuscripts Relating to the War of the Revolution,* vol. 1 (Albany: Weed, Parsons, 1868), 400–404. See also East Hampton assessment rolls, passim, PLIC-EHL.

6. Gardiner, "Gardiner's East Hampton," 258; Woodward, *East Hampton,* 95; Timothy Dwight, *Travels in New England and New York,* vol. 1 (1811; rpt. Cambridge: Harvard University Press, 1969), 219; "Census of Suffolk County, 1776," in *Calendar of Historical Manuscripts,* 1: 400–404. On Lyman Beecher, see *Autobiography of Lyman Beecher,* ed. Barbara M. Cross, 2 vols. (1864; rpt. Cambridge: Harvard University Press, 1961); also Vincent Harding, *A Certain Magnificence: Lyman Beecher and the Transformation of American Protestantism,* 1775–1863 (Brooklyn: Carlson, 1991); Lyman Beecher letters, n.d., PLIC-EHL. On slavery in New York see Lynda R. Day, *Making a Way to Freedom: A History of African Americans on Long Island* (New York: Empire State Books, 1997), 19. On commerce see Breen, *Imagining the Past,* 147–84.

7. *Journal of Trustees,* 2: 1772–1807, 321; *Refugees of 1776,* 479, 597, 843, 914; Gaetano L. Vincitorio, "The Revolutionary War and Its Aftermath in Suffolk County, Long Island," *Long Island Historical Journal* 7 (Fall 1994), 68–85; Toby A. Appel, "Disease and Medicine in Connecticut around 1800," unpublished ms., 10; Henry Onderdonk, *Revolutionary Incidents of Suffolk and Kings Counties* (1848; rpt. New York: Kennikat, 1970), 321. On disease during the Revolution see Janice P. Cunningham and Elizabeth A. Warner, *Portrait of a River Town: The History and Architecture of Haddam, Connecticut* (Middletown, Conn.: Greater Middletown Preservation Trust, 1984), 22. For Phebe Tillinghast's allusion to the "peaceable Injoyment of our Liberties" see Connecticut State Archives, record group 1, "Public Records of the Colony of Connecticut," I series, vol. 20, 46, 47, rpt. in *Public Records of the State of Connecticut* (Hartford: Case, Lockwood and Brainard, 1894), 1: 77–78.

8. *Refugees of 1776,* 843, 913–14; with the military phase of the Revolution winding down and the fighting moving south, many women filed such petitions, one of the few ways in which they could express their relationship to a political enterprise, albeit in a "prepolitical" mode. See Linda Kerber, *Women of the Republic: Intellect and Ideology in Revolutionary America* (Chapel Hill: University of North Carolina Press, 1980), 80–87. For John Mulford's petition, see *Public Records of*

the *State of Connecticut*, 1: 1776–78, 332. Phebe Tillinghast's petition is in the Connecticut State Archives, record group 1, "Public Records of the Colony of Connecticut"; also *Refugees of 1776*, 913–14. While the petition states that she is from Southold and embarked from Southold, this petition is not in her handwriting, and because most refugees from East Hampton left from Sag Harbor, I infer that she did as well.

9. HPH, "Sag-Harbor in the Revolution," in Tom Twomey, ed. *Tracing the Past: Writings of Henry P. Hedges* (New York: Newmarket, 2000), 259; see "A List of Persons in Suffolk County on Long Island who took the following Oath of Allegiance and Peaceable behavior before Governor Tryon, 1778," P.R.O. Colonial Office, class 5, vol. 1109; photocopy in PLIC-EHL.
10. HPH, "Sag-Harbor in the Revolution," 259; HPH, "The Celebration of the Bi-Centennial Anniversary of East Hampton," in *Tracing the Past*, 27–28. See also Kenneth Scott, "Absentee Patriots from British-Occupied Suffolk County, L.I. 1778," *Long Island Source Records* (Baltimore: Genealogical Publishing, 1987), 600; Onderdonk, *Revolutionary Incidents*; Richard M. Bayles, *Historical and Descriptive Sketches of Suffolk County* (1874; rpt. Port Washington, N.Y.: Ira J. Friedman, 1962), 399–424; Vincitorio, "The Revolutionary War," 68–85. In 1800 about 68 slaves lived in thirty-three East Hampton households, while 119 free people of color also lived in the town. See U.S. federal census, 1800. There were still 26 slaves in East Hampton in 1810 and 17 in 1820, 12 of whom were women. See also Day, *African Americans on Long Island*, 24; Mary Esther Mulford Miller, *An East Hampton Childhood* (New York, 1938), 27.
11. See *East Hampton History*, 368–85; also *Records of East Hampton*, vols. 4–5; East Hampton assessment roll, 1806, PLIC-EHL. On the longevity of Hedges men see *Portrait and Biographical Record of Suffolk County* (New York: Chapman, 1896), 290: "The family was noted for its longevity, the average age [at death] being eighty-five years."
12. I base my claim for the residence of Phebe and David Hedges partly on the sessions records of the First Presbyterian Church of East Hampton, 1830–54, indicating that the families of two grandchildren, David A. and Stephen L. Hedges, both lived in the Hook. I am grateful to Barbara Borsack and the Reverend John Ames for permission to see records at the church on Main Street. The 1858 map of East Hampton village indicates a residence of D. Hedges (David A. Hedges) on a section of Pantigo Road called both "down Hook" and "down Pantigo." David A. Hedges's house on Pantigo was said to have been built in 1778, and I infer that Captain David and Phebe Hedges may also have lived there. See "D. Hedges" house on James Chace, "Map of Suffolk County, Long Island, New York" (Philadelphia: John Douglas, 1858). See also *Main Street*, 57–58; Thomas Edwards, "Reminiscences of Old East Hampton by the Sea," ms. (1929), 12–13, PLIC-EHL. For genealogy use with caution *East Hampton History*, 369–85; for births and deaths see also *Records of East Hampton*, vol. 5 passim; "Timothy Miller's Note Book," ms., PLIC-EHL.
13. On David Hedges's elected posts see *Records of East Hampton*, 4: passim; *Journal of Trustees*, passim; on "infidelity" see also "Records of the Clinton Academy," PLIC-EHL; Harding, *A Certain Magnificence*, 36–37; Cross, *Beecher*, 1: 68.
14. Quoted in Cross, *Beecher*, 1: 96–97.
15. GH, "Recollections," *JNMD* (1910), 37, 253; Anna Mulford, *A Sketch of Dr. John Smith Sage of Sag Harbor* (Sag Harbor, N.Y., 1897), PLIC-EHL; Richard M. Bayles, *The History of Suffolk County, 1683–1882* (New York: W. W. Munsell, 1882), 33; also "Early Physicians of Norwich," *Proceedings*, Annual Convention of the Connecticut Medical Association (Hartford, 1860), 167–81.

16. See, for example, Laurel Ulrich, *A Midwife's Tale: The Life of Martha Ballard Based on her Diary, 1785–1812* (New York: Vintage, 1990), especially 49–66; Paul Starr, *The Social Transformation of American Medicine* (New York: Basic, 1982), 30–54; Lester King, *The Medical World of the Eighteenth Century* (Chicago: University of Chicago Press, 1958); Lester King, *Medical Thinking: A Historical Preface* (Princeton: Princeton University Press, 1982); Charles E. Rosenberg, "Medical Text and Social Context: Explaining William Buchan's *Domestic Medicine*," *Bulletin of the History of Medicine* 57 (1983), 22–42. For changes in the early nineteenth century see John Harley Warner, *The Therapeutic Perspective: Medical Practice, Knowledge, and Identity in America, 1820–1885* (Princeton: Princeton University Press, 1997), 85–86.
17. See Paracelsus, *Selected Writings* (London: Routledge, 1951); Robert Burton, *The Anatomy of Melancholy* (Oxford: Lichfield and Short, 1621), 134–35; Thomas Sydenham, *Schedula Monitoria de Novae Febris Ingressae* (London: Walter Kettilby, 1686), 28; William Osler, "Historical Note on Hereditary Chorea," *Neurographs* 1 (1908), 5, 114–15. On the history of the medieval dancing mania see J. F. C. Hecker, *The Dancing Mania of the Middle Ages* (Philadelphia: Haswell, Barrington, and Haswell, 1837), and H. C. Erik Midelfort, *A History of Madness in Germany* (Stanford: Stanford University Press, 1999).
18. Ulrich, *A Midwife's Tale*, 11; for original spelling see Martha Ballard's diary, August 1, 1793. On the broad uses of *chorea* see Howard Kushner, *A Cursing Brain? The Histories of Tourette's Syndrome* (Cambridge: Harvard University Press, 1999), 33. William Buchan, *Domestic Medicine*, 2nd ed. (London: W. Strahan, 1772), 551–52. Buchan classified St. Vitus's dance under the heading of epilepsy, describing it as a "particular species of convulsion fits." In 1791 James Boswell diagnosed the tics and twitches of the great English author Samuel Johnson as "of the nature of that distemper called St. Vitus's dance," though scholars today consider Johnson's condition closer to the symptoms of modern-day Tourette syndrome. James Boswell, *The Life of Samuel Johnson* (1791; rpt. New York: Random House, 1952), 41.
19. "Hereditary" typically meant transmitted from earlier generation(s), but it could also mean that several siblings had the same condition even if their parents did not, or that children developed a condition at the same age as their parent(s) had when they were young. For testimony as to the early recognition of St. Vitus's dance in East Hampton see Edward Osborn to William Osler, January 28, 1898, Osler collection: "Every family in which chorea appears in East Hampton have had it since the earliest history two hundred years and more ago." George Huntington speculated that "with these earliest settlers, in all probability, came the disease"; also GH, "Recollections of Huntington's Chorea as I saw it at East Hampton, Long Island, During my Boyhood," *JNMD* 37 (April 1910), 255. On popular beliefs about the hereditary transmission of the magrums in other towns see Robley Dunglison, *The Practice of Medicine* (Philadelphia: Lea and Blanchard, 1842), 312–13, and Irving W. Lyon, "Chronic Hereditary Chorea," *American Medical Times*, December 19, 1863, 289. On widespread beliefs in the heredity of nervous disorders generally see Charles E. Rosenberg, "The Bitter Fruit: Heredity, Disease, and Social Thought in Nineteenth-Century America," in Donald Fleming and Bernard Bailyn, eds., *Perspectives in American History*, vol. 8 (Cambridge: Cambridge University Press, 1974), 203.
20. Nicolas Culpepper, *Culpepper's Works; or, The Complete Family* (1652; rpt. London: 1795), 1: 605; Cotton Mather, *The Angel of Bethesda* (1723; rpt. ed. Gordon W. Jones, Boston: American Antiquarian Society, 1972), 143. John C. Waller argues that a "binary opposition between heredity and curability persisted throughout the eighteenth century, and beyond." See Waller, "Poor Old

Ancestors: The Popularity of Medical Hereditarianism, 1770–1870," in "A Cultural History of Heredity II: 18th and 19th Centuries," preprint no. 247 (Berlin: Max Planck Institute for the History of Science, 2002), 132; also Waller, "'The Illusion of an Explanation': The Concept of Hereditary Disease," *Journal of the History of Medicine and Allied Sciences* 57(2002), 410–48; Rosenberg, "The Bitter Fruit," 203. On the other side of the debate see William Battie and John Monro in Battie, *A Treatise on Madness* (London: 1758), 24, 61; Buchan, *Domestic Medicine*, 9–10.

21. Waller, "'Illusion of an Explanation,'" 411; Rosenberg, "The Bitter Fruit," 198–99; Buchan, *Domestic Medicine*, 9–10; Benjamin Rush, *Medical Inquiries and Observations upon Diseases of the Mind* (Philadelphia: Kimber and Richardson, 1812), 51–52. According to Rush, the officer "was gratified in all his three wishes," since he was killed on the battlefield between his thirtieth and fortieth year of age, and though he was married, he left no children.
22. The literature on late eighteenth- and nineteenth-century concepts of heredity is vast. In addition to the abovementioned work of Charles Rosenberg and John C. Waller, I have found the following especially useful: Peter J. Bowler, *The Mendelian Revolution: The Emergence of Hereditarian Concepts in Modern Science and Society* (Baltimore: Johns Hopkins University Press, 1989); Ernst Mayr, *The Growth of Biological Thought: Diversity, Evolution, and Inheritance* (Cambridge: Harvard University Press, 1982); Rosenberg, "The Bitter Fruit"; Alan R. Rushton, *Genetics and Medicine in the United States, 1800–1922* (Baltimore: Johns Hopkins University Press, 1994); Staffan Müller-Wille and Hans-Jörg Rheinberger, "Heredity: The Production of an Epistemic Space," preprint no. 276 (Berlin: Max Planck Institute for the History of Science, 2004), and "Conference. A Cultural History of Heredity II, 18th and 19th Centuries," preprint no. 247 (Berlin: Max Planck Institute for the History of Science, 2002).
23. Rushton, *Genetics and Medicine*, 1–16.
24. Buchan, *Domestic Medicine*, 9–11; Rosenberg, "The Bitter Fruit," 207.
25. On Abel Huntington in East Hampton see Bayles, *Suffolk County*, 33; JER, "Looking Them Over," *EHS*, July 13, 1972; Mrs. Everett J. Edwards, "Early East Hampton Doctors," *EHS*, December 27, 1934; *East Hampton History*, 88–89; Richard L. Bushman, *From Puritan to Yankee: Character and the Social Order in Connecticut, 1690–1765* (New York: Norton, 1967), 123; AH Account Book, 1799–1809, PLIC-EHL; *East Hampton History*, 238. See also *Records of East Hampton*, vols. 3–5, passim, and *Journal of the Trustees*. Assessment rolls and Suffolk County censuses show Huntington's changing economic status. His political career can be followed in the pages of the *Corrector* and the *Express*. His daughter Cornelia mentions him occasionally in her Journal in the PLIC-EHL, which also contains several of his letters. The minister Lyman Beecher, who was "netops" ("cronies") with Abel Huntington, notes local gossip that he (Beecher) had "lowered his character twenty-five per cent. by going a hunting with Dr. H—, also a Deist.'" Beecher, *Autobiography*, 1, 69.
26. AH account book, May 20, 1802, September 9, 11, 12, 13, November 21, 1805; January 5, May 23, 27, June 7, November 21, 1806, PLIC-EHL.
27. See U.S. federal census of 1800 and East Hampton assessment roll of 1806; also, with caution, *Refugees of 1776* and the Tillinghast family file (PLIC-EHL); *East Hampton History*, 375, 478, 585–87, and *Main Street*, 15–16, 70–71. On widows' remarriage see Susan Grigg, "Toward a Theory of Remarriage: A Case Study of Newburyport at the Beginning of the Nineteenth Century," *Journal of Interdisciplinary History* 8 (Autumn 1977), 183–220.
28. *Main Street*, 70–71.

29. On Captain David Hedges's assets at this time see assessment roll, 1806, PLIC-EHL. On David Hedges's accident see the *Suffolk Gazette,* December 30, 1805.
30. HPH, *Tracing the Past,* 108; Beecher, "General History of the Town of East-Hampton," 155–89; Beecher, *Autobiography,* 2: 68, 90.
31. Beecher, "General History of the Town of East Hampton," 155–89.
32. On "so much of Hell & so much of Heaven" see Mary Dering to Elizabeth Dering Gardiner, 1792, Dering papers, PLIC-EHL. On "little unhappiness" see Martha Wickham [CH], *Sea-Spray: A Long Island Village* (New York: Derby and Jackson, 1857), 460. On the religious metaphors of melancholy see the diary of the Reverend Samuel Johnson describing an Amagansett woman convinced that "the Devil has her so completely in his power that she cannot be saved," that she will "haunt her family to death and then be cast with them into hell." September 21, 1852, PLIC-EHL. On nineteenth-century professional and vernacular understandings of illness among whites see Charles Rosenberg, *The Cholera Years: The United States in 1832, 1849, and 1866* (Chicago: University of Chicago Press, 1962), 40–54; Charles E. Rosenberg, *The Trial of the Assassin Guiteau: Psychiatry and the Law in the Gilded Age* (Chicago: University of Chicago Press, 1968); also Charles Rosenberg, "The Therapeutic Revolution: Medicine, Meaning, and Social Change in Nineteenth-Century America," in *Perspectives in Biology and Medicine* 20 (Summer 1977).
33. AH account book, May 27, 1806, PLIC-EHL. For nineteenth-century drugs see Robert Hooper, *The Physician's Vade-Medum* (Albany: E. F. Backus, 1809); John Redman Coxe, *The American Dispensatory* (Philadelphia: Carey and Lea, 1827), 479–83. George Huntington's 1872 paper also recommends some of these same drugs.
34. AH account books June 7, 1806, PLIC-EHL; see also *American Dispensatory,* 267–69.
35. See JER, *The Old Hook Mill* (New York: East Hampton Star, 1942); also "The Old Hook Mill," in *Discovering the Past: Writings of Jeannette Edwards Rattray, 1893–1974* (New York: Newmarket, 2001), 149–52, although these are unreliable. The account books of Nathaniel Dominy, who built the mill, show "Captain David Hedges and Co." involved in work related to this mill from April 29, 1806, through the summer of 1806. The most intensive phase appears to be from June 7 to July 3, when it was raised. See also Robert Hefner, "Hook Windmill," *Historic American Engineering Record,* HAER NY, 52-HAMTE 2, in "Historic American Engineering Record," American Memory: Library of Congress, http://www.memory.loc.gov.; *Suffolk Gazette,* June 30, 1806; AH account book, June 11, 1806; Timothy Miller, Notebook, June 10, 1806, ms., PLIC-EHL.
36. *Suffolk Gazette,* June 30, 1806. On St. Vitus see *Encyclopaedia Britannica* (Chicago: William Benton, 1958), 23: 226.
37. There is no record of an inquest, although the Suffolk County Court of Oyer and Terminer met on June 27, 1806, in Riverhead. A note in John Lyon Gardiner's account book for June 26, 1806, however, asking "what says the Attorney General" and alluding to a "petition," suggests that an inquest may have been considered. See John Lyon Gardiner, account book, Gardiner papers, PLIC-EHL; Lyman Beecher letter, n.d. [after 1811], Beecher papers, PLIC-EHL; see also Frances Huntting, journal, Huntting papers, PLIC-EHL; "Cousin Anna" to Frances Dering, February 12, 1824, Dering papers, PLIC-EHL; Samuel Buell, "A Sermon after the Funeral of Mrs. Jerusha Conkling," February 24, 1782, *Early American Imprints, First Series,* no. 17485.
38. Michael McDonald, "The Medicalization of Suicide," in Charles E. Rosenberg and Janet Golden, eds., *Framing Disease: Studies in Cultural History* (New Brunswick: Rutgers University Press,

1992), 86–100; Howard Kushner, *American Suicide* (New Brunswick: Rutgers University Press, 1991), 17. For a late determination of felo-de-se see the Court of Oyer and Terminer, July 4, 1810, Suffolk County Court, Riverhead.

39. *Suffolk Gazette,* January 19, 1807.

2. THE SOCIAL COURSE OF ST. VITUS'S DANCE

1. Arthur Kleinman, *Writing at the Margins: Discourse between Anthropology and Medicine* (Berkeley: University of California Press, 1995), 151.
2. Ibid.; Nora Groce, *Everyone Here Spoke Sign Language: Hereditary Deafness on Martha's Vineyard* (Cambridge: Harvard University Press, 1985), 108; In *Geographies of Disability* (London: Routledge, 1999), 95–98, Brendan Gleeson emphasizes the need for historians to investigate the particular social relations that surrounded impairment in specific settings, an approach I have tried to take here.
3. Timothy Dwight, *Travels in New England and New York* (1811; rpt. Cambridge: Harvard University Press, 1969), 1: 219, 222; Joyce Appleby, *Inheriting the Revolution: The First Generation of Americans* (Cambridge: Harvard University Press, 2000); Martha Wickham [CH], *Sea-Spray: A Long Island Village* (New York: Derby and Jackson, 1857), 10, 180. The Venezuelan revolutionary Francisco de Miranda, who visited East Hampton in 1784, was impressed by the "good character" of the inhabitants, whom he thought resembled "the people of Connecticut," and by the large number of books in the public library, albeit mostly on theological subjects. See Ettie Hedges Pennypacker, *Francisco de Miranda's Visit to Long Island in 1784* (East Hampton: privately printed, 1937). See also John Demos, "Old Age in Early New England," *American Journal of Sociology* 84 (1978), S249.
4. Prentice Mulford, "P. Mulford Takes Notes on the East End," *Corrector,* February 6, 1875; Wickham, *Sea-Spray,* 10, 180.
5. On Betsy Hedges and her husband, Squires Miller, see *East Hampton History,* 457, 459; also East Hampton tax assessment roll, 1815, PLIC-EHL. The Dominy account book for November 22, 1821, shows a bill to Captain David Hedges "To Coffin for your Daughter," Dominy papers, PLIC-EHL. Their son Squires H. Miller is listed as the ship's carpenter on the whaleman's shipping list, August 24, 1843, Cold Spring Harbor Whaling Museum. Either Squires or his son joined the Presbyterian church in Bridgehampton in 1848. See sessions records, First Presbyterian Church, East Hampton, 1830–54, September 27, 1848.
6. On November 12, 1808, Stafford married the stepdaughter of Lieutenant Thomas Baker, a man of modest assets, descended from one of the town founders, with property in 1806 valued at about one-fifth that of David Hedges. See *Suffolk Gazette,* November 12 [21], 1808; *East Hampton History,* 209; tax assessment rolls, PLIC-EHL; HPH to GH, July 9, 1908, in ERO, ser. I-A: 3181, box 39, folder 3, quoted in Charles S. Stevenson, "A Biography of George Huntington, M.D.," *Bulletin of the Institute of the History of Medicine* 2 (April 1934), 71–77; see Stafford Hedges in the *Records of East Hampton,* 4: 377, 383, 401, 414; tax assessment rolls especially 1820, 1831 and 1832 ("Stafford Hedges heirs" after 1833); the account book of Abel Huntington for June 3, 1809, shows that Stafford's first child was born on that day. See also June 4, 1809. In 1832 Stafford Hedges had 33 acres assessed at $280, plus $50 in personal assets; his father, Captain David Hedges, had 381

acres worth $4,830. See East Hampton assessment roll of 1832. Stafford's white marble gravestone lies in the North End cemetery.

7. On Hiram B. Hedges see JER, "Looking Them Over," *EHS*, January 30, 1941; December 2, 1954; *East Hampton Records*, 4: 508; Hiram B. Hedges logbook from the *Monmouth*, 1839–45, Kendall Whaling Museum, Sharon, Massachusetts. Hiram Hedges is mentioned in Frederick P. Schmitt, *Mark Well the Whale! Long Island Ships to Distant Seas* (Cold Spring Harbor, N.Y.: Whaling Museum Society, 1971). Letters, bills of sale, and whaleman's shipping lists from Hedges's voyages are at the Cold Spring Harbor Whaling Museum, Cold Spring Harbor, New York. Joseph Redfield's logbook from the *Josephine*, 1846–49, Hiram Hedges captain, is at the PLIC-EHL. The gravestone of Abby Dwight, wife of Hiram B. Hedges, died May 9, 1848, age twenty-two, is at the Riverside Cemetery, Plattsburgh, New York. Hiram Hedges's whaling voyages to the South Pacific suggests the possibility of a genetic link between East Hampton families with chorea and families in Papua New Guinea and New Britain. See Euan M. Scrimgeour, "Possible Introduction of Huntington's Chorea into Pacific Islands by New England Whalemen," *American Journal of Medical Genetics* 14 (1983), 607–13; also Scrimgeour, "Huntington's Disease in Two New Britain Families," *American Journal of Medical Genetics* 17 (1980), 197–202.
8. J. Madison Huntting, diary, August 1849, PLIC-EHL; Carleton Kelsey, *Amagansett: Lore and Legend* (Amagansett, N.Y.: Amagansett Village Improvement Society, 1996), 46; S. S. Smith *Travels in Siberia* (London: Longman, 1854), 2: 394–95; "Reminiscences of H. H. Frary," typescript, New Bedford Whaling Museum, New Bedford, Massachusetts.
9. Fred Lockley, "Impressions and Observations of the Journal Man," *Oregon Daily Journal* (Portland), June 19, 1933, contains a brief mention of Hiram Hedges by his son Clarence Hedges, as does *The History of Oregon*, vol. 3, *Biographical* (Chicago: Pioneer Historical Publishing Company, 1922), 354. On David A. Hedges see above sources; also *Records of East Hampton*, 4: 499, 509, 522, 524, 548, 572; 5: 21, 29, 30, 32; J. Madison Huntting, diary, January 24, 28, 1845, PLIC-EHL. Hiram Hedges is listed as a farmer in the U.S. census, Multnomah County, Oregon, 1860. After the death of Mary Nicolson Hedges, around 1863, David A. Hedges became the guardian for Hiram's seven-year-old son Clarence, who soon ran away; neighbors brought charges of ill-treatment and neglect, and the court appointed another guardian. See Clarence Hedges, guardianship case no. 35, Clackamas County Court, Oregon City, Oregon. Clarence Hedges became a highly successful newspaper publisher in The Dalles, Oregon. An obituary for "Mr. D. H. Hedges" appeared in the *Daily Oregonian* on October 18, 1880, presumably referring to D. A. Hedges: his gravestone in East Hampton indicates that he died in Portland, Oregon, 1880. The will of Jerusha Hedges, widow of David A. Hedges, indicated that she wished "to be buried in the North End cemetery [in East Hampton] as near to the grave of my deceased infant child (which died many years since) as is practicable." Jerusha Hedges, July 10, 1884. PLIC-EHL.
10. See Lockley, "Impressions and Observations," also *History of Oregon*, 3: 354.
11. EBM, "Huntington's Disease," B-3; JER, "Looking Them Over," *EHS*, December 2, 1954; GLH, account book, May 2, 1870: "DA Hedges returned from Oregon." The 1870 census for East Hampton shows that David had brought Hiram's ten-year-old daughter Minnie Hedges with him from Oregon to East Hampton, and both were staying with his younger sister Margaret. Thus Hiram's niece could have heard the story directly from her uncle.
12. On Schuyler Conkling see *East Hampton History*, 255; *Journal of Trustees, 1725–1845*, for the years

1835–40 passim; *East Hampton Records*, 4: 482, 507, 534, 536, 539, 548, 561, 564, 568–69; 5: 3; JER, "Looking Them Over," *EHS*, April 10, 1952; see also U.S. census, Suffolk County, Town of East Hampton, Village of Amagansett, 1850, 1860.

13. On Conkling's difficulties see logbook of the bark *Monmouth*, 1843–45, Kendall Whaling Museum: on December 21, 1844, near the Marianas, all hands were called on deck while a crewman was "put in the Brigging and flogged with a cat [-o'-nine-tails] by the Capt. in presence of the whole crew for abusing the second mate!" Also February 1, 1845, "The captain and 2 mate (who was sick) onshore." The second mate got better but then worse again, and continued sick for some time. Conkling is listed as second mate on the whaleman's shipping list, August 1843, CSHWM. On Conkling's "continued neglect of church ordinance," see sessions records, First Presbyterian Church, East Hampton, February 3, March 1, June 3, September 27, December 5, 1848; January 5, 1849. The report of the committee appointed to "visit" him was accepted October 6, 1849, with no further mention of "visits," suggesting either that he was too ill to attend, that he convinced the elders to excuse him for other reasons, or that he resumed attendance, which seems unlikely.
14. Everett J. Edwards and Jeanette Edwards Rattray, *Whale Off: The Story of an American Whaler* (New York: Frederick A. Stokes, 1932), 41. On Phebe Conkling and chorea see Edward Osborn to William Osler, June 15, 1888; GH to Osler, June 9, 1888, Osler collection. See also The *Sag Harbor Express*, January 23, 1868; Juliet Hand, journal, 1867–69, January 17, 1868: "Schuyler Conklin's widow died last night," PLIC-EHL.
15. See obituary of Margaret Hedges Cartwright in *EHS*, January 26, 1917. The diary of J. Madison Huntting, July 23, 1843, mentions the marriage of Margaret Hedges and Frederick Cartwright, PLIC-EHL; George Lee Huntington mentions her in his account book, January 7, 1869, "Mrs. Cartwright here sewing," and May 5, 1875, PLIC-EHL. Mary Hoogland Huntington complains about being pressured to pay off the widow Cartwright's mortgage while other people's bills remain outstanding; see her diary, March 19, 1860. I am grateful to Jean Lominska for a copy of this diary.
16. For Stephen Hedges's participation in town governance, see *East Hampton Records*, 4: 1812, 1816, 1817–19, 1821, 1822–23, 1825, 1827, 1829, 1831, 1833, 1841; *Journal of Trustees*, vols. 3–6. See also the sessions records of the First Presbyterian Church, 1830–54, 1854–88, passim.
17. See *Portrait and Biographical Record*, 290; account book of the First Presbyterian Church, East Hampton; Frances S. Huntting, journal, August 12, 1866, PLIC-EHL; quoted in JER, "Looking Them Over," *EHS*, January 31, 1952; Mary Esther Mulford Miller, *An East Hampton Childhood* (East Hampton, N.Y.: Star Press, 1938), 20.
18. F. Huntting, journal, January 6, 1874; quoted in JER, "Looking Them Over," *EHS*, June 4, 1952; also in account book of GLH, January 7, 1874; I am grateful to Cornelia Dayton for pointing out the resonance between the searches for Phebe and Stephen Hedges. See Edward Osborn's account of S.H. in his letter to William Osler, June 28, 1898, Osler collection. George Huntington's biographer cites his 1909 reference to "Stephen C.," whom Huntington said he had known as a boy, when Stephen was "an old man, insane, and a terror to the boys." I am certain this is a reference to Stephen Hedges, however, since there is no other Stephen in the town who fits the description, and who would have been related to the two women ("near relatives of his of the same name") young George had seen on the road. See Charles S. Stevenson, "A Biography of George Huntington, M.D.," *Bulletin of the Institute of the History of Medicine* 2 (April 1934), 72. See also

will of Stephen Hedges, filed March 13, 1872, proved August 28, 1875, file 7794, liber 12, 135, Suffolk County Surrogate Courts, Riverhead.

19. On Stephen Lewis Hedges see *Portrait and Biographical Record of Suffolk County* (New York: Chapman, 1896), 290–91; *East Hampton History*, 162–63, 382–83; *Journal of Trustees*, 5: 1845–70, passim; *Records of East Hampton*, 4: 525–79, passim; 5: 5–390, passim; Woodward, *East Hampton*, 160–61; GLH account book, 1859–62, 1863–73; tax assessment rolls; obituary in scrapbook 2; PLIC-EHL. Will of Stephen L. Hedges, filed March 1, 1897, proved February 21, 1891, is in the Suffolk County Surrogate Courts, file 13717, liber 33, 22, Riverhead.
20. On East Hampton's sympathy for the South see Miller, *East Hampton Childhood*, 24, 27; CH, diary, April 16, 1861: "There is glaring wrong on both sides"; also Thomas Edwards, "Reminiscences of Old East Hampton by the Sea," ms. (1929), 26, PLIC-EHL. On meetings to find army substitutes see GLH day book, October 23, 1862: "Town Meeting—Agree to raise $4000 and send the Supervisor to NY to procure 40 substitutes to fill the Quota of East Hampton and prevent the draft"; September 18, 1863, "Town meeting to keep men from the war," PLIC-EHL.
21. *Portrait and Biographical Record*, 290–91; also CHD, B-7.
22. On Betsy Hedges and Edward Dayton see *East Hampton History*, 273; 379–82; *Portrait and Biographical Record*, 989–90; R. G. Dun credit reports, 586 (January 18, 1892), 162, Baker Library, Harvard University Graduate School of Business, Cambridge; J. M. Huntting, diary, August 6, 1863, PLIC-EHL. On Mary Hedges and Jeremiah Mulford see Miller, *East Hampton Childhood*. For references to William H. Hedges and Nathan M. Hedges see the U.S. census, California, Sonoma County, Petaluma, 1870, 1880.
23. CHD, B-7, B-8. While familial objections to a potential spouse appear occasionally in nineteenth-century East Hampton letters and diaries, none that I have found allude to any of these families or to issues of inherited illness; rather, they concern the age, wealth, race, religion, and current health of the intended. For instance, see Julia Parson to John S. Sherrill, March 23, 1870, Julia Parson papers, PLIC-EHL: "His parents have forbidden his coming to see Ella Osborne anymore. . . . She is older than he is and I suppose they want him to do better, that is *more money*." See also JER, "Looking Them Over," *EHS*, April 10, 1952, referring to the mid-nineteenth century: "The parents objected to their marriage (presumably because of her delicate health)." See also CH, diary, 1821, n.d.: "I saw my handsome Jew beau in the street today twice . . . but alas he's a Jew—and I can't change *my religion*!!! so farewell my beautiful Jew—." March 1826: "I hope she will not fall in love with the interesting Tuscarora invalid. I don't know why either, for I see no reason why the 'tincturing' of the skin should form so powerful an objection to that unfortunate people. But prejudice is everything and no matter what may be the beauty of the person or the endowments of the mind—no matter how brilliant his talents and how fervent his piety—he is an Indian—and though deemed worthy of an admittance into heaven he is excluded from all intimacy of intercourse upon earth." I am grateful to Jean Lominska for providing me with a typescript of parts of this diary. PLIC-EHL.
24. See David Hedges, will of November 17, 1841, proved January 2, 1847, file 3638, liber 4, 438–41, Suffolk County Surrogates Court, Riverhead, directing his grandson David A. Hedges to support Margaret until she married, or, or if she failed to marry, for the rest of her life. On the other hand, David Hedges left nothing to the son of his deceased daughter Betsy but $250 and "all of the personal property that shall be in my house at my decease that belonged to his mother." To his daughter Phebe Conkling he left a mere $60. He left most of his property to his son Stephen, and

two grandsons, Hiram and David. Of the seven offspring of Joseph Tillinghast and Phebe Mulford, five survived to adulthood, all of whom married and had children. Two left East Hampton: Joseph Tillinghast Jr. married a Southold woman and became a farmer in that town, where he lived to the age of seventy-three; Mary Tillinghast married an East Hampton "yeoman" from a middling family, William King, and moved with him to Huntington, Long Island. See Rose Tillinghast, *The Tillinghast Family, 1540–1971* (Rose Tillinghast, 1972), 179–86; also Tillinghast family file, Suffolk County Historical Society, Riverhead.

25. While Captain David Hedges in 1801 possessed assets worth some $3,543, putting him among the wealthiest men in the town, Elisha Payne had assets worth $30. In 1806 Hedges paid taxes on property worth $3,730, while Payne paid taxes on $60. See East Hampton tax assessment rolls, 1801, 1806. PLIC-EHL.

26. On premarital pregnancy and marital choice in the late eighteenth century see Mary Beth Norton, *Liberty's Daughters: The Revolutionary Experience of American Women, 1750–1800* (Ithaca: Cornell University Press, 1980), 55–56; also Estelle Freedman and John d'Emilio, *Intimate Matters: A History of Sexuality in America* (New York: Harper and Row, 1988), 43.

27. Interview with Carleton Kelsey, May 17, 2001, Amagansett. See also *East Hampton History*, 528–32; Edwards, "Reminiscences," 343. See references to Elisha Payne in the account books of John Lyon Gardiner, Nathaniel Dominy, and Nathaniel Hand; also in East Hampton tax assessment rolls, PLIC-EHL. See Payne's letter of administration, April 1, 1834, no. 2616, liber F, 95, at the Suffolk County Surrogate Courts, Riverhead. For George Huntington's diagnosis of Nancy's son Elias see GH, "Excerpts from a Paper Read at a Regular Meeting of the New York Neurological Society Dec. 7, 1909." I am grateful to Charles Gardiner Huntington 3rd for granting me access and permission to quote from this manuscript.

28. Elisha's children are listed in his 1834 letter of administration. Sylvanus Payne (born 1795) moved to Southampton, became a shoemaker, married at the age of twenty-two, and had several children. Stafford T. Payne (1809–65) and Ezra Payne (1799–1855) became farmers and also married and had children. A fifth son, Nathaniel, received aid from the town in 1837 and again in 1858, and may have been the N. G. Payne who died April 13, 1862, at the Brattleborough (Vermont) Asylum "with a severe attack of Epilepsi." *Sag Harbor Express*, April 17, 1862. I cannot trace the two daughters, Maria and Clarissa, though both were alive in 1830.

29. On the pension record of Albert M. Payne in Company H, 48th New York Regiment, see soldier's certificate 196385, can no. 3769, bundle no. 40, U.S. National Archives; that of Elias R. Payne in Company K, 127th New York Regiment, is soldier's certificate 153170, can no. 2883, bundle no. 35, U.S. National Archives. On East Hampton in the Civil War see Harrison Hunt, "East Hampton and the Civil War," in Tom Twomey, ed., *Awakening the Past: The East Hampton 350th Anniversary Lecture Series, 1998* (New York: Newmarket, 1999), 323–31; Miller, *East Hampton Childhood*, 23–26; Edwards, "Reminiscences," 18, 26, 41.

30. On Albert M.'s postwar difficulties see his soldier's certificate 196385, especially the "General Affidavit, 1881"; for Elias R. see his soldier's certificate 153170; also U.S. census, 1870, 1880; *Records of East Hampton*, 5: 301, 305; "Thomas Rose, Old Fisherman, Dies," *EHS*, July 3, 1928; also GH, "Excerpts from a Paper."

31. On Nancy Payne Rose see CHD, B-12; "Thomas Rose," *EHS*, July 3, 1928; East Hampton death records 358, December 28, 1890.

32. *East Hampton History*, 588, describes Edmund as an orphan from Southold, the story evidently

passed down in the family. However, a variety of evidence persuades me that Edmund was the son of Lydia Bennett: first, U.S. censuses show that Lydia Bennett, born in Connecticut ca. 1777, lived with Edmund Tillinghast and his family at least from 1850 until she died in 1870. The New York state census of 1865 specifies that "Lydia Bennett," eighty-eight, living with him, was his mother. Second, GLH's account book indicates numerous visits to Edmund Tillinghast "to vstg mother"; see account book, November 22, 1860; October 31, November 1, 1865; April 19, December 10, 1869; March 17, 1870, PLIC-EHL. Third, Edmund Tillinghast, his wife, Mary, and Lydia Bennett are buried side by side in the South End Cemetery. The Southold story may have arisen because Lydia's brother Joseph Tillinghast had married into a Southold family and settled there in the early 1800s; there were many Tillinghasts in that town. See Tillinghast family file, SCHS. For Edmund Tillinghast's economic status see East Hampton tax assessment rolls and U.S. census, 1860, 1870, 1880. For his town offices see *Records of East Hampton*, vols. 4–5 passim. Use with caution *East Hampton History*, 586–89; Tillinghast, *Tillinghast Family*, 183–84; *Main Street*, 15–16. On William Bennett see Timothy Miller notebook, July 13, 1809, PLIC-EHL; Nathaniel Dominy also notes William Bennett's death in his account book, July 14, 1809, "To Coffin for his Corps"; Dominy account book, PLIC-EHL. On William A. Bennett see *EHS*, March 2, 1950. William A. lived in the house once owned by the elder Phebe Tillinghast. See *Main Street*, 15; also *East Hampton History*, 229, 587 (although JER on 229 mistakenly identifies William A. as the son of Gamaliel Bennett, rather than of Lydia and William Bennett).

33. See *Records of East Hampton*, 5: 642. On remarriage rates see Susan Grigg, "Toward a Theory of Remarriage: A Case Study of Newburyport at the Beginning of the Nineteenth Century," *Journal of Interdisciplinary History* 8 (Autumn 1977), 183–220. I am grateful to Cornelia Dayton for this reference. On changing ideals of marriage in the late eighteenth century see Helena M. Wall, *Fierce Communion: Family and Community in Early America* (Cambridge: Harvard University Press, 1990), 133–34. Neither of Abel Huntington's two daughters, Cornelia and Abby, ever married. Nor did the widely admired John Wallace, founder of the local Episcopal Church and a boarder with the Huntington family, ever marry, nor many members of families with no relation to St. Vitus's dance: "bachelor lords" and maiden aunts were a familiar part of the social landscape. Single status did not necessarily indicate social exclusion; however, marriage did suggest integration into the community, and all the children and grandchildren of Phebe Hedges and her sisters married at least once.

34. See sessions records, First Presbyterian Church, East Hampton; register of inmates in the Suffolk County Alms House, 1878–79; also case book of the Suffolk County Asylum, Westhampton Records Center, Westhampton, New York. Diagnostic entries clearly distinguished between "St. Vitus's dance" (in adults) and other maladies such as "lunacy," "epilepsy," "deranged," "palsy," and "feeble mind." Moreover, when one forty-one-year-old woman diagnosed with St. Vitus's dance died, the "Remarks" stated, "died of Chorea." See register, 1881, 143.

35. See, for example, Mary Huntington, diary, January 6, 9, 1860, PLIC-EHL; GLH, account book, January 6, 9, 1860, PLIC-EHL; Mary E. Miller, *East Hampton Childhood*, 34–36.

36. See GH, "On Chorea," *Medical and Surgical Reporter* 26 (April 13, 1872), 320; *East Hampton History*, [211].

37. GH, "On Chorea," 320–21; also GH, "Excerpts," 1909.

38. For accidents see GLH account book, July 11, 1856; July 30, 1869; Dec. 3, 1870; Jan. 2, March

22, 1872, PLIC-EHL. See also *Sag Harbor Express*, November 27, 1862; May 21, 1874; CH, diary, July 4, 1826, PLIC-EHL; H. Dering to F. Dering, February 12, 1812; October 30, 1814, Dering papers, PLIC-EHL; *Sag Harbor Express*, March 14, 1861; on consumption, CH, diary, June 13, 1824, PLIC-EHL. On consumption as a hereditary disease see Sheila M. Rothman, *Living in the Shadow of Death: Tuberculosis and the Social History of Illness in American History* (Baltimore: Johns Hopkins University Press, 1994), 14, 24. John Waller argues that long-standing links between the idea of incurable disease and a relatively unchanging constitution helped forge the idea of "hereditary disease." See John C. Waller, "'The Illusion of an Explanation': The Concept of Hereditary Disease, 1770–1870," *Journal of the History of Medicine and Allied Sciences* 57 (2002), 411.

39. F. Huntting, journal, August 21, 1855, December 15, 1856, PLIC-EHL; CH, diary, 1867, n.d., PLIC-EHL. Writing to John Dominy in 1814, the teenaged Jeremiah Mulford observed that a mutual friend "has lately executed himself with a gun, the means of this fatal event was caused by his father talking to him and opposing his going to see Caroline," a young woman to whom he had been engaged. See Jeremiah Mulford to John Dominy, August 1, 1814, Dominy papers, PLIC-EHL. J. Madison Huntting noted crisply in his diary entry for March 28, 1841, that "Mulford Parsons hung himself this afternoon." On early American and English perceptions and practices toward mental illness see Gerald Grob, *Mental Institutions in America: Social Policy toward the Mentally Ill* (New York: Free Press, 1973); Grob, *The Mad among Us: A History of the Care of America's Mentally Ill* (New York: Free Press, 1994); Ellen Dwyer, *Homes for the Mad: Life inside Two Nineteeth-Century Asylums* (New Brunswick: Rutgers University Press, 1987); Norman Dain, *Concepts of Insanity in the United States, 1789–1865* (New Brunswick: Rutgers University Press, 1964); Roy Porter, *Mind-Forge'd Manacles: A History of Madness in England from the Restoration to the Regency* (Cambridge: Harvard University Press, 1987); Charles E. Rosenberg, *The Trial of the Assassin Guiteau: Psychiatry and the Law in the Gilded Age* (Chicago: University of Chicago Press, 1968); Benjamin Rush, *Medical Inquiries and Observations upon the Diseases of the Mind* (Philadelphia: Kimber and Richardson, 1812); Michael MacDonald, *Mystical Bedlam: Madness, Anxiety, and Healing in Seventeenth Century England* (Cambridge: Cambridge University Press, 1981).

40. Frances Sage to Frances Dering, 1815, n.d., Dering papers, PLIC-EHL; HPH to GH, July 9, 1908; Edward Osborn to SEJ, February 25, 1905, ERO, ser. 1, box 39, folder 3, A:3181S, 3; also CHD, B-1, B-3, B-10, B-12.

41. Frances Sage to Frances Dering, 1815, n.d., Dering Papers, PLIC-EHL. Some mentions of St. Vitus's dance may have been oblique, for instance Cornelia Huntington's remark in her diary that one of her neighbors was "quite unwell and I think not a little fidgety," April 28, 1861, PLIC-EHL.

42. Clarence King, "A Third Case of Hereditary Chorea," *Medical News* 55 (July 13, 1889), 40.

43. Transcript, Martha Kalser and Elizabeth Davis, October 23, 1998. I am grateful to Martha Kalser for this transcript. Personal communication, Elizabeth Davis, May 17, 2001, East Hampton.

44. See GH, "On Chorea," 320; also CHD, A-13, B-17, B-10, B-12.

45. Although alcoholism in the late nineteenth century was increasingly considered an illness rather than a vice, it was still viewed with disapproval, as a moral flaw and sign of weakness, yet it did not carry the taboo on speech that surrounded St. Vitus's dance, possibly because it was not generally

seen as hereditary. See W. J. Rorabaugh, *The Alcoholic Republic: An American Tradition* (New York: Oxford University Press, 1979). Muncey said drinking was a common strategy for men with chorea; see CHD, B-91, B-12–13. Hattie reported in 1909 that heavy drinking was so prevalent among the affected families in one Nova Scotia community that local lay people believed the disease resulted from alcoholism, even though numerous sufferers with chorea were not alcoholics. See W. H. Hattie, "Huntington's Chorea," *AJI* 66 (July 1909), 125. But Estella Hughes, in 1925, reported few instances of heavy drinking among people with Huntington's in her Michigan study, and "in no instance does it appear that they drank for mental relief." See Hughes, "Social Significance of Huntington's Chorea," *American Journal of Psychiatry* 4 (January 1925), 550.

46. GH, "Recollections," *JNMD* 1910, 255–56. Gamaliel was a first-century Jewish leader and one of the greatest teachers of ancient Judaism; George Huntington's comment is a tribute to his father's wisdom.

47. I am using Lennard Davis's definition of disability as "a disruption in the visual, auditory, or perceptual field as it relates to the power of the gaze," a definition well suited to the visual drama of chorea. Lennard Davis, *Enforcing Normalcy* (New York: Verso, 1995), 140–42.

48. See William Osler, "On the General Etiology and Symptoms of Chorea," *Medical News* 51 (October 15, 1887), 437–41, and (October 22, 1887), 470.

49. Charles E. Rosenberg, "The Bitter Fruit: Heredity, Disease, and Social Thought in Nineteenth-Century America," in Donald Fleming and Bernard Bailyn, eds., *Perspectives in American History,* vol. 8 (Cambridge: Cambridge University Press, 1974), 203, 223; John Higham, *Strangers in the Land: Patterns of American Nativism 1860–1925* (New York: Atheneum, 1965), 95; Gail Bederman, *Manliness and Civilization* (Chicago: University of Chicago Press, 1995).

50. Daniel Pick, *Faces of Degeneration: A European Disorder, c. 1848–1919* (Cambridge: Cambridge University Press, 1989), 59. Gianna Pomata has emphasized the importance of class to European physicians' conceptions of heredity. "When dealing with aristocratic diseases," she writes, "physicians had taken an optimistic view of hereditary stock as improvable over the generations, but in dealing with the disease of the urban poor, in contrast, they adopted a much more negative attitude, one that emphasized the social need to prevent the reproduction of people from tainted stock." See Gianna Pomata, "Comments," in "A Cultural History of Heredity III: 19th and Early 20th Centuries," preprint 247 (Berlin: Max Planck Institute for the History of Science, 2005), 151.

51. Pick, *Faces of Degeneration,* 59; on Francis Galton see Peter J. Bowler, *The Mendelian Revolution: The Emergence of Hereditarian Concepts in Modern Science and Society* (Baltimore: Johns Hopkins University Press, 1989), 64–73; Diane B. Paul, *Controlling Human Heredity, 1865 to the Present* (Amherst, N.Y.: Humanity Books, 1998), 30–36; see also Rosenberg, "The Bitter Fruit," 223. According to Rosenberg, Americans "now explained phenomena as varied as class identity, criminality, and 'pauperism' in terms increasingly hereditarian and deterministic." While drawing on the earlier concepts of predisposition and diathesis, the idea of neuropathic constitution or neuropathic inheritance placed more emphasis on the inheritance of antisocial behavior, and on the cumulative effects of inherited disorders. See also Garland Allen, *Life Sciences in the Twentieth Century* (New York: John Wiley, 1975), 20–40; Rosenberg, *Trial of the Assassin Guiteau,* 244.

52. GH to William Osler, July 25, 1887, Osler collection.

53. On Edward Osborn, see *Portrait and Biographical Record,* 1896, 400–401; *History of East Hampton,* 89–90.

54. Osborn to Osler, July 7, 1887, Osler collection; Osler to Jelliffe, February 16, 1905, ERO, series 1,

3182S, box 39, folder 3; also William Osler, "Historical Note on Hereditary Chorea," *Neurographs* 1 (1908), 113–16.

55. GH to Osler, June 9, 1888, Osler collection. It is unclear whether Mrs. Stratton's unmarried sister with chorea was regarded as a member of the family or treated rather as a domestic servant, as the census taker described her when he came to the house in 1880.

56. Osborn to Osler, June 15, 1888, Osler collection.

57. See William Osler, "Remarks on the Varieties of Chronic Chorea," *JNMD* 18 (February 1893), 97–111; William Osler, *On Chorea and Choreiform Affections* (Philadelphia: Blakiston and Son, 1894); Osborn to Osler, January 28, 1898, Osler collection.

58. It is possible, of course, that Osborn was unusually reticent or timid—George Huntington expressed no similar qualms about discussing the subject with the family in question. But then he had been away from East Hampton for twelve years and, as he himself acknowledged in a subsequent letter, was no longer abreast of current developments. Osborn was closer to the families, and more aware of their sensitivities. The families may have feared a situation such as that described by the anthropologist Mary Douglas, who detailed instances of mentally ill persons whose peculiar behavior was tolerated as merely eccentric so long as they stayed in the community. Once they were formally classified as abnormal, the same behavior was counted as intolerable. See Mary Douglas, *Purity and Danger: An Analysis of the Concepts of Pollution and Taboo* (1966; rpt. London: Routledge, 1996), 98.

59. See Landon Carter Gray, *A Treatise on Nervous and Mental Diseases* (Philadelphia: Lea Brothers, 1895), 348, 351. William C. Porter in 1918 concurred, stating that he had obtained "much contradictory information" partly because of "the natural reticence of members of the family in discussing what is well known to them to be the curse of their family. They have been more apt than not to deny the presence of chorea." See Porter, "Huntington's Chorea," *State Hospital Quarterly* 4 (1918–19), 65–66. But C. R. McKinniss stated in 1914 that "it is comparatively easy to trace the genealogy of a family which has such conspicuous landmarks to guide us and only occasionally have we seen attempts to conceal the facts." See McKinniss, "The Value of Eugenics in Huntington's Chorea," *Medical Record* 86 (1914), 105.

60. Henry P. Hedges, *A History of the Town of East-Hampton* (Sag Harbor: John H. Hunt, 1897); GH to SEJ, July 13, 1908, ERO, series 1, A:3181, box 39, folder 3; HPH to GH, July 9, 1908, ibid. Huntington's term *magrums* was common to Dutchess County, where he was living.

61. See JER, *East Hampton History*, 172; Henry Maudsley is cited in Vida Skultans, *Madness and Morals: Ideas on Insanity in the Nineteenth Century* (London: Routledge, 1975), 65. See also "P. Mulford Takes Notes on the East End"; Breen, *Imagining the Past*, 138.

62. See Irving P. Lyon to SEJ, February 25, 1905, ERO. On Bedford and Pound Ridge, see Alvah P. French, ed., *History of Westchester County, New York* (New York: Lewish Historical Publishing, 1925), 2: 645–793.

63. Irving W. Lyon, "Chronic Hereditary Chorea," *American Medical Times* 7 (December 19, 1863), 289–90. Fifty years later, Elizabeth Muncey too noted that "the public sentiment that has existed for years against marriage into the affected families," although whether she was citing Lyon's claim or arguing from her own data is unclear; CHD, 1–2. However, her field notes from Greenwich, Stamford, Bedford, and Pound Ridge mentioned only a few cases of overt ostracism: one family was "so badly affected with chorea that no one would allow his children to marry them" (four of the six children of this couple who survived to adulthood remained unmarried); CHD, A-55.

In another case, "there was much opposition" to a marriage "on account of heredity of chorea," although in this case the marriage did take place; CHD, B-118. Given these negative perceptions, were members of these families socially ostracized? Were they less likely to marry than those in the unaffected clans? The available genealogical evidence for Bedford and Pound Ridge suggests that family members did get married, although it is unclear whether they married into families of similar social rank or into other kinships perceived as "migrims" families. In the largest such family in Pound Ridge and Bedford, nearly all the individuals whom we can trace, both men and women, were married. These were the descendants of Jesse Bouton, a large landowner in Pound Ridge, and Rachel Ferris (1751–1806). She had been "highly respected as a young woman," according to a published Bouton family genealogy. But later in life she "was afflicted with that terrible nervous disease then known as 'magrums' (inherited as has been said from the English ancestry and has appeared in the descendants of the Ferris family here and there to the present day [1890]." All of Rachel's eleven surviving children married, and of her approximately sixty surviving grandchildren, all except three males also married: figures suggesting that negative perceptions surrounding the magrums in this region during the first half of the nineteenth century may have coexisted with an everyday practice that was more accepting. For marriages in this family see *Bouton-Boughton Family* (Albany: Joel Munsell Sons, 1890), 472–93; also Bouton family bible (typescript), the journal of Judge Ezra Lockwood, typescript, and notes from church records in the Alice Thatcher Tomlinson papers, all at the Pound Ridge Historical Society, Pound Ridge. I have also drawn on *Town of Bedford: Bedford Historical Records*, vols. 5, 9 (Bedford Hills: Town of Bedford, 1976, 1978); Bedford assessment rolls, U.S. census records for Westchester County, and records of the Westchester County Almshouse, Westchester County Archives, White Plains. See also Irving P. Lyon to SEJ, February 25, 1905, ERO, series I, A:3181, box 39, folder 3; Irving P. Lyon to SEJ, March 12, 1912, ibid. Also see "Ferris Family Notes," GHS. One great-grandson of Rachel's became a patient of the Philadelphia neurologist Wharton Sinkler, who wrote up his case and in 1889 published his family tree. See Wharton Sinkler, "Two Additional Cases of Hereditary Chorea," *JNMD* 14 (February 1889), 82–84.

64. P. R. Vessie, "On the Transmission of Huntington's Chorea for Three Hundred Years: The Bures Family Group," *JNMD* 76 (1932), 565.
65. See Belle Ferris to Mrs. Henry, December 17, 1931, Ferris family papers, GHS. See also "Lady Ann Millington," Hendrie genealogy notebook 3, GHS. The Ann Millington story circulated widely in the Ferris family, in connection more often with class consciousness than with chorea. According to a descendant, Isabella (Belle) Ferris, "her title made the messiest mess that ever landed on the old Greenwich shore." See Belle Ferris to Mrs. Henry, December 17, 1931, Ferris family papers, GHS. See also "Lady Ann Millington," Hendrie genealogy notebook 3, GHS. According to another descendant, E. A. Ferris, "the early Ferrises and Lockwoods had a sense of 'our kind' deriving from the Millington ancestry. European history suggests, however, that superior offspring have not always resulted from consanguinous marriages in royalty." E. A. Ferris reported also that "Aunt Belle blamed both physical and emotional problems on consanguinity," explaining "the breeders' practice of inbreeding, then outbreeding." These "problems" alluded to may have included Huntington's, particularly since this narrator refers to "original sin and its expiation," noting that "it came up recurrently" in the family. See E. A. Ferris, "Family Story," unpublished ms. (1972), 16–17, 98, 89, Connecticut Historical Society, Hartford. In this version, Lady Ann "pursued her lover, a British army officer, from England to the New World," supporting herself as a teacher.

"Not finding the one she loved, she loved the one who was near." This narrator notes that Lady Anne's descendants "worshipped her memory—and tried to crowd her genes into future generations"; ibid., 89. While not referring explicitly to Huntington's, Ruth Moxcey Martin's paper on "Intermarriage of Blood Relatives in Three Old New England Communities," published in 1923, also reports stories about "pride, miserable pride," and intermarriage similar to those reported by Ann Millington's Greenwich descendant. "'I've heard my great grandfather say it and other old people and folk in the family on down, that no families along this coast were anywhere near of so fine blood as we,'" reported Martin's informant. According to this narrator, young people married "'to keep property here'" (probably Stamford), and because they believed no one outside of their own relatives were good enough to marry. The result was a trail of suicides, so that the town itself was called "suicide town." See *Genetics, Eugenics, and the Family*, vol. 1, International Congress of Eugenics (New York: American Museum of Natural History, 1923), 278–79.

66. Belle Ferris to Mrs. Henry, December 17, 1931, Ferris family papers, GHS.

67. Ibid.

68. Jerome M. Sundin, "Huntington's Chorea in Lake Lillian: The Destruction and Stigmatization of a Founding Family," honors thesis, Hamline University, 1999, 23, 27, 14. I am grateful to Jerome Sundin for permission to cite this manuscript.

69. Social practices in two other communities merit comparison: Euan M. Scrimgeour, a clinician who practiced in Papua New Guinea in the 1970s, reported that relatives of individuals affected with Huntington's on the Gazelle Peninsula of East New Britain were "very sensitive and ashamed that the condition is in their lineage and one senses that the families involved tend to be ostracized." However, he added that the "affliction, while feared, is accepted stoically enough, at least on the surface, by patients and their families once it has become established. There is little or no rejection." According to Scrimgeour, families cared for their affected members in the village, and there were no known cases of suicide. See Euan M. Scrimgeour, "Huntington's Disease in Two New Britain Families," *Journal of Medical Genetics* 17 (1980), 197–202. In contrast, Americo Negrette described two impoverished communities on the shores of Lake Maracaibo, Venezuela, in the 1960s, where husbands and wives abandoned their spouses when they developed Huntington's chorea, and the entire community was stigmatized on account of its association with the disease. Negrette claimed that those who became affected accepted their destiny with a fatalistic resignation born of the realization that salvation was impossible. Yet their individual narratives also suggest protest and, often, a determination to keep on living as best they can. See Americo Negrette, *Corea de Huntington* (Maracaibo: Universidad de Maracaibo, 1963), 213, 205.

70. Paul Longmore, "The League of the Physically Handicapped and the Great Depression: A Case Study in the New Disability History," *Journal of American History* (December 2000), 892; Helen Rattray, "Dr. Huntington's Disease Still with Us," *East Hampton Star*, January 18, 1973; Helen Rattray, "A Village at Odds with Its Glamour"; "Research Hits Home," *East Hampton Star*, April 8, 1993.

3. INVENTING HEREDITARY CHOREA

1. See Andre Barbeau, Thomas N. Chase, and George W. Paulson, eds., *Advances in Neurology*, vol. 1, *Huntington's Chorea, 1872–1972* (New York: Raven, 1973); William Osler, "Remarks on the Varieties of Chronic Chorea," *JNMD* 18 (February 1893), 97–98.

2. On earlier assessments see David L. Stevens, "The History of Huntington's Chorea," *Journal of the Royal College of Physicians* 6 (April 1972), 272–76; also George W. Bruyn, "Huntington's Chorea: Historical, Clinical, and Laboratory Synopsis," in P. J. Vinken and G. W. Bruyn, eds., *Handbook of Clinical Neurology*, vol. 6 (Amsterdam: North Holland Publishing, 1968), 298–378.
3. Peter English, "Emergence of Rheumatic Fever in the Nineteenth Century," in Charles E. Rosenberg and Janet Golden, eds., *Framing Disease: Studies in Cultural History* (New Brunswick: Rutgers University Press, 1992), 22; Howard Kushner, *A Cursing Brain? The Histories of Tourette's Syndrome* (Cambridge: Harvard University Press, 1999), 33–34.
4. See Stevens, "History of Huntington's Chorea," 273; Thomas Jeffreys, "On Chorea, with Two Cases to Illustrate the Nature and Treatment of That Disease," *Edinburgh Medical and Surgical Journal* 23 (1825), 273–86; *Western Medical Gazette of Cincinnati, Ohio* 4 (1832), 58. See also Russell N. de Jong, "George Huntington and His Relationship to the Earlier Descriptions of Chronic Hereditary Chorea," *Annals of Medical History* 9 (May 1937), 201–10.
5. John Elliotson, "St. Vitus's Dance," *Lancet* 1 (November 3, 1832–33), 163; Stevens, "History of Huntington's Chorea," 272–74.
6. Robley Dunglison, *The Practice of Medicine* (Philadelphia: Lea and Blanchard, 1842), 2: 312–13.
7. Ibid.
8. When Dunglison published his *Medical Lexicon: A Dictionary of Medical Science* (Philadelphia: Lea and Blanchard, 1848), he defined the magrums as "a singular convulsive affection which resembles chorea," and made no reference to heredity at all (520). See William Browning, "Charles Rollin Gorman," *Neurographs* 1 (1908), 144–47.
9. Eight years later Lund published a second report noting that "the disease still keeps to the same families." Johan Christian Lund, "Chorea Sancti Viti i Saetesdalen," and "Om Saetesdalen," *Beretning om Sundhedstilstanden og medicinal forholdene i Norge* (Oslo, 1856–72), 137, 163; see Alf L. Orbeck, "An Early Description of Huntington's Chorea," *Medical History* 3 (April 1959), 165–68.
10. See Orbeck, "Early Description," 168; August Hirsch, *Handbuch der historisch-geographischen Pathologie* (Erlangen: F. Enke, 1859–64), 2: 572; see also English translation by the New Sydenham Society, 1883–86; Irving W. Lyon, "Chronic Hereditary Chorea," *American Medical Times* 7 (December 19, 1863), 289–90.
11. Lyon, "Chronic Hereditary Chorea," 289–90. Peter Harper argues that Lyon's cases were of benign chorea, not Huntington's. See Peter S. Harper, "Huntington's Disease: A Historical Background," in Gillian Bates, Peter S. Harper, and Lesley Jones, eds., *Huntington's Disease*, 3rd. ed. (Oxford: Oxford University Press, 2002), 10–11. Because Lyon's cases were not his patients but people he evidently recalled from his youth—according to his son, Lyon had observed these cases of the magrums in and around his home town of Bedford—he may have misremembered certain elements or reported uncritically what the neighbors told him. See Irving P. Lyon to SEJ, February 25, 1905; Irving P. Lyon to H. H. Laughlin, March 12, 1912, ERO, ser. I-A:3181, folder 3; Wharton Sinkler, "Two Additional Cases of Hereditary Chorea," *JNMD* 14 (February 1889), 82–85. See also Peter S. Harper, "Introduction: A Historical Background," in Bates, Harper, and Jones, *Huntington's Disease*, 11–12; for biographical sketches of Lyon see William Browning, "Irving Whitall Lyon, M.D.," *Neurographs* 1 (1908), 147–49; Horace S. Fuller, "Irving Whitall Lyon, M.D., of Hartford," Proceedings 104th Convention of the Connecticut State Medical Society (Bridgeport, 1896), 327–31.
12. Stevens, "History of Huntington's Chorea," 273.

13. On demography in New England and England see John Demos, "Old Age in Early New England," *American Journal of Sociology* 84 (1978), S248–87.
14. Maris A. Vinovkis, "Mortality Rates and Trends in Massachusetts Before 1860," *Journal of Economic History* 32 (March 1972), 184–213; Richard Archer, "New England Mosaic: A Demographic Analysis for the Seventeenth Century," *William and Mary Quarterly* 47 (October 1990), 477–502; E. A. Wrigley and R. S. Schofield, *The Population History of England, 1541–1871* (Cambridge: Cambridge University Press, 1981), 299–320; Peter Laslett, "Necessary Knowledge: Age and Aging in the Societies of the Past," in David I. Kertzer and Peter Laslett, eds., *Aging in the Past: Demography, Society, and Old Age* (Berkeley: University of California Press, 1995), 4–77; E. A. Wrigley et al., *English Population History from Family Reconstitution, 1580–1837* (Cambridge: Cambridge University Press, 1997); Daniel Scott Smith, "The Demographic History of Colonial New England," *Journal of Economic History* 32 (March 1972), 165–83; Joyce Appleby, *Inheriting the Revolution: The First Generation of Americans* (Cambridge: Harvard University Press, 2000), 189.
15. Demos, "Old Age in Early New England," S256, 259.
16. Staffan Müller-Wille and Hans-Jörg Rheinberger, "Heredity: The Production of an Epistemic Space," preprint 276 (Berlin: Max Planck Institute for the History of Science, 2004), 10: "Breeding new varieties for specific marketable characteristics, the exchange of specimens among botanical and zoological gardens, experiments in fertilization and hybridization of geographically separated plants and animals, the dislocation of Europeans and Africans that accompanied colonialism, and the appearance of new social strata in the context of industrialisation and urbanisation, all these processes interlocked in relaxing and severing cultural and natural ties and thus provided the material substrate for the emerging discourse of heredity." See also Peter Bowler, *The Mendelian Revolution: The Emergence of Hereditarian Concepts in Modern Science and Society* (Baltimore: Johns Hopkins University Press, 1989), 162; Roger J. Wood and Vítězslav Orel, *Genetic Prehistory in Selective Breeding: A Prelude to Mendel* (Oxford: Oxford University Press, 2001).
17. Bowler, *Mendelian Revolution*, 162.
18. Carlos López Beltrán, "Heredity Old and New: French Physicians and *L'heredite naturelle* in the Early Nineteenth Century," in *A Cultural History of Heredity II: 18th and 19th Centuries*, preprint 247 (Berlin: Max Planck Institute for the History of Science, 2003), 10; Charles E. Rosenberg, "Framing Disease: Illness, Society, and History," in Rosenberg and Golden, *Framing Disease*, 202–3; Gianna Pomata, "Comments," in "A Cultural History of Heredity II," 145–47.
19. For patients with magrums see Bloomingdale Asylum minutes, March 4, 1848; July 5, 1849, in vol. 9, December 31, 1847–December 30, 1854; also medical register, vol. 1844–1866, archives, Weill Cornell Medical Center–New York Presbyterian Hospital; see also William Logie Russell, *The New York Hospital: A History of the Psychiatric Service, 1771–1936* (New York: Columbia University Press, 1945), 219.
20. See Armand Trousseau, *Lectures on Clinical Medicine*, trans. P. Victor Bazire (1868; London: The New Sydenham Society, 1882), 393; Charles E. Rosenberg, "The Bitter Fruit: Heredity, Disease, and Social Thought in Nineteenth-Century America," in Donald Fleming and Bernard Bailyn, eds., *Perspectives in American History*, vol. 8 (Cambridge: Cambridge University Press, 1974), 198; Jean-Martin Charcot, "Original Lectures," *Medical Times and Gazette* 1 (March 9, 1878), 245–46; also Jean-Martin Charcot, *Charcot the Clinician: The Tuesday Lessons, Excerpts from Nine Case Presentations on General Neurology Delivered at the Salpêtrière Hospital in 1887–88*, trans. with commentary by Christopher G. Goetz (New York: Raven, 1987), 71–101. See also

Ellen Dwyer, *Homes for the Mad: Life Inside Two Nineteenth Century Asylums* (New Brunswick: Rutgers University Press, 1987), 103. Dwyer notes that asylum superintendents felt that while heredity might predispose a person to madness, it was not a sole cause.

21. On the domestic setting of American medical practice see Starr, *Social Transformation*, 60–72; also Judith Walzer Leavitt, "'A Worrying Profession': The Domestic Environment of Medical Practice in Mid-19th-Century America," *Bulletin of the History of Medicine* 69 (1995), 10–29. See Susan Lindee, *Moments of Truth in Genetic Medicine* (Baltimore: Johns Hopkins University Press, 2005), 6. For biographical sketches of Waters, Gorman, and Lyon see essays by William Browning in *Neurographs* 1 (1908), 137–49. I cannot help wondering whether the so-called "refinement of America" in the 1830s and 1840s helped make the odd movements and sometimes difficult behavior of adults suffering from St. Vitus's dance and magrums more visible both to observers and to sufferers themselves by the mid-nineteenth century—more evidently a disease than a mere eccentricity. The emergence of modern posture standards that were part of the redefinition of middle-class etiquette taking shape from the 1750s onward made some Americans in the early Republic more conscious of stance and physical carriage as a sign of class and of character. "Here was an important means of distinguishing oneself not only from an earlier, effete upper class but also from bent workers and lounging frontiersmen. . . . Proper posture constituted a demonstration of good character." Popular advice books such as Lord Chesterfield's best-selling *Letters to his Son,* first published in 1775 and widely circulated in the mid-nineteenth-century United States (the East Hampton Library had a copy), railed against "vulgar, low expressions, awkward motions and address" that "vilify as they imply either a very low turn of mind, or low education and low company." Presenting oneself with "a constant smirk upon the face, and a whiffling activity of the body" gave strong indications of "futility," as did "an awkward address and ungraceful attitudes and actions." In a cultural climate of growing attention to issues of bodily control, the involuntary movements of chorea may have seemed more salient to observers and more embarrassing and shameful to the sufferers. See David Yosifon and Peter N. Stearns, "The Rise and Fall of American Postures," *American Historical Review* 103 (October 1998), 1059; Richard Bushman, *The Refinement of America: Persons, Houses, Cities* (New York: Random House, 1993), passim; Olivia H. Leigh, ed., *Letters to His Son by the Earl of Chesterfield* (New York: Tudor, 1937), 199, 218.

22. On medical regionalism see Warner, *Therapeutic Revolution*, 72–75. New medical journals included the *Boston Medical and Surgical Journal*, precursor to the *New England Journal of Medicine*, started in 1828, the *Medical and Surgical Reporter* in 1856, the *American Medical Times* in 1860, the *New York Medical Journal* in 1865, and the *Medical Record* in 1866.

23. Lyon, "Chronic Hereditary Chorea," 289–90.

24. GH, "On Chorea," *Medical and Surgical Reporter* 26 (April 13, 1872), 320.

25. On the Huntington family see "Abel Huntington," in Richard Bayles, *History of Suffolk County, 1683–1882* (1882; rpt. Smithtown, N.Y.: Suffolk County Tercentenary Commission, 1983), 33; James Macfarlane Winfield, "A Biographical Sketch of George Huntington, M.D.," *Neurographs* 1 (1908), 89–95; Katherine Huntington, "Extracts from the Childhood of the Huntington Family," November 27, 1933, unpublished ms.; Charles S. Stevenson, "A Biography of George Huntington, M.D.," *Bulletin of the Institute of the History of Medicine* 2 (April 1934), 53–76; JER, "Looking Them Over," *East Hampton Star,* July 13, 1972; Russel N. de Jong, "George Huntington and His Relationship to the Earlier Descriptions of Chronic Hereditary Chorea," *Annals of Medical*

History 9 (May 1937), 201–10; Nadia Durbach and Michael R. Hayden, "George Huntington: The Man behind the Eponym," *Journal of Medical Genetics* 30 (1993), 406–9; Douglas Lanska, "George Huntington and Hereditary Chorea," *Journal of Child Neurology*, 10 (January 1995), 46–48; Douglas Lanska, "George Huntington (1850–1916) and Hereditary Chorea," *Journal of the History of the Neurosciences* 9 (2000), 76–89; Mrs. Everett J. Edwards, "Early East Hampton Physicians," *EHS*, December 27, 1934. George Lee reported his son George's exploits in his account book, PLIC-EHL.

26. See JER, "Looking Them Over," *East Hampton Star*, July 13, 1972; also Joseph Osborne, "Autobiography of Joseph Osborne," typescript, 10–11; Edwards, "Early East Hampton Physicians."
27. Osborne, "Autobiography," 11; on Mary Hoogland Huntington's ideas of parenting see her diary, 1859–60, unpublished ms., courtesy of Jean K. Lominska.
28. In 1860 George Lee Huntington reported assets of $4,700, well above the average of free white adult males at that time, which was $2,580, but below the average wealth of urban physicians in the North, which was $8,063. Over the years George Lee became more established. Compared with the truly wealthy East Hampton families, however, the Huntingtons were relatively modest: in 1857, while the two Huntington physicians Abel and George Lee had combined assets of $2,200, Deacon Stephen Hedges and his sons Stephen L. and George had assets (mostly land) of $6,750. See U.S. census, 1850, 1860, 1870; also East Hampton tax assessment rolls for 1857, PLIC-EHL; also E. Brooks Holifield, "The Wealth of Nineteenth-Century Physicians," *BHM* 64 (1990), 9–85; George Lee Huntington, account book, October 6, 1855; December 1, 1862; September 29, October 20, 1865, PLIC-EHL.
29. Martha Wickham [CH], *Sea-Spray: A Long Island Village* (New York: Derby and Jackson, 1857), 5, 179, 350; CH, diary, "April Sunday," 1826–27, PLIC-EHL; also "Journals of Cornelia Huntington, 1821–1827, 1863–1867," typescript, courtesy of Jean Lominska; Sherrill Foster, "By Choice or By Chance: Single Women's Lives in Nineteenth Century Suffolk County, N.Y.," in *Awakening the Past: The East Hampton 350th Anniversary Lecture Series, 1998* (New York: Newmarket, 1999), 227–33.
30. Wickham, *Sea-Spray*, 179.
31. There is no good biographical portrait of John Wallace. However, the Huntington papers at the PLIC-EHL contain many items referring to him, including references in GLH's account books; a letter from GLH to Wallace's friends and relatives after his death, n.d.; Wallace's will; and a number of letters alluding to the mysterious circumstances under which he had abruptly left Scotland in 1840, including one from Henry P. Hedges to O. B. Ackerly, November 16, 1894; from James Spaulding dated October 26, 1930; from Robert MacKenzie to "My Dear Keyes," November 23, 1878, concerning Wallace's origins in Scotland; and from Captain Wolfe Murray of the Tweedale Shooting Club in Peebles, Scotland, of which Wood had been a member. The local history section of the Rogers Memorial Library in Southampton, New York, also contains two letters pertaining to Wallace: W. S. Pelletreau, a local historian, to "Friend Howell," August 31, 1885, and J. H. Foster to "Dear Cousin," September 1, 1888, in an untitled scrapbook, 183–85. According to Cornelia, the Huntington family believed that Wallace had been exiled on account of a political crime. However, Foster claimed that the "crime" of which Wallace was accused was sodomy, a charge that would better explain the secrecy surrounding his flight from Scotland. See also "Talk Given by Charles G. Huntington in His Later Years," n.p., courtesy of Jean Lominska; Huntington, "Huntington Family," [8–9]; A. A. Hayes, "Mystery of Easthampton," in *Harper's*, August

1885. L. Clarkson, *The Shadow of John Wallace* (New York: White, Stokes and Allen, 1884), is a romantic fictionalization of Wallace's life.

32. On physicians as "intimate travelers," see Starr, *Social Transformation*, 76; on the domestic practice of nineteenth-century physicians see Starr, *Social Transformation*, 60–72; Judith Walzer Leavitt, "'A Worrying Profession': The Domestic Environment of Medical Practice in Mid-19th-Century America," *Bulletin of the History of Medicine* 69 (1995), 6, 10–29. See also Susan Lindee, *Moments of Truth in Genetic Medicine* (Baltimore: Johns Hopkins University Press, 2005), 6.

33. GLH, account books, September 28, 1868; March 3, April 27, September 20, 1869, PLIC-EHL; also GH, "Notes on the Lectures of Drs. Parker and Markoe; Session of '69–'70"; "Notes on October 5, 18, 1869, Dr. Parker." I am indebted to Charles Gardiner Huntington 3rd, Simsbury, Connecticut, for allowing me to see these notes. See also Warner, *Therapeutic Revolution*, 24, 75; Kenneth Ludmerer, *Learning to Heal: The Development of American Medical Education* (New York: Basic, 1985), 26; Charles A. Flood, "P and S: The College of Physicians and Surgeons of Columbia University," ms., 1989; Charles E. Rosenberg, "The Practice of Medicine in New York a Century Ago," *Bulletin of the History of Medicine* 41 (1967), 223–53; Benjamin Rush, *Medical Inquiries and Observations upon the Diseases of the Mind* (Philadelphia: Kimber and Richardson, 1812). Medicine was not the preferred career choice of George Huntington—he later told his children that, had he had the resources, he would have preferred to become an artist. However, a traumatic boyhood incident may have influenced his decision. On August 7, 1863, while swimming at the beach, the thirteen-year-old George found himself trying to rescue a fellow swimmer, a boy about the same age who was the nephew of the local minister. "Georgie held him above water until his own strength was exhausted, when to save his own life he was forced to let go his hold & by the mercy of God was permitted to reach shore," his father wrote in his account book. "Every effort has been made to recover the body but without success." In her diary Cornelia Huntington also noted how the search for the body went on the following day, and that after this day, "Georgie has been told that he must give it up, for he is wearing himself out with labor and exposure in this terrible stifling heat; but he begs so hard, and is so anxious to aid in the searching, that it is hard to deny him; he saw him last in life, and he feels as if *he must find him.*" We know no more about the impact of this traumatic event on young George Huntington's life, for he himself did not write about it. But it is tempting to speculate that perhaps he sought to save others as he could not save his childhood friend. See account book, August 7, 1863; CH, diary, August 7, 1863, PLIC-EHL.

34. Asthma dominated Huntington's life so much so that one of his daughters later referred to him as a "semi-invalid," indicating that "our lives were overshadowed by Father's poor health—his attacks of asthma, his hay fever had always to be reckoned with"; Huntington, "Huntington Family," 38. See also GH, "An Inaugural Thesis on Opium Submitted to the Examination of the Trustees and Faculty of Medicine of the College of Physicians and Surgeons, Medical Department of Columbia College. For the degree of Doctor in Medicine, March 4th, 1871"; courtesy of Charles G. Huntington 3rd. On the family's use of opium see the diary of Mary Hoogland Huntington, April 14 [1860]: "been sick all day—have taken an opiate, put my feet into hot water and now will go to bed—"; April 16 [1860], "taken opium and under its influence am going to bed"; courtesy of Jean Lominska; GLH, account book, May 16, September 23, 1871, PLIC-EHL. See also Bonnie Ellen Blustein, "New York Neurologists and the Specialization of American Medicine," *Bulletin of the History of Medicine* 53 (1979), 170–83.

35. GLH, "Account Book," February 28, March 4, 1871, and passim, PLIC-EHL.

36. James Macfarlane Winfield, "A Biographical Sketch of George Huntington, M.D.," *Neurographs* 1 (1908), 93. No family trees made by George Huntington or his father have come to light, and possibly the two physicians did not make any of the families with chorea in East Hampton, though George Huntington later referred to "figures." See GH, "Chronic Progressive Hereditary or Huntington's Chorea," *Transactions of the Fifth Annual Session, Tri-State Medical Association of the Carolina's and Virginia* (Raleigh: Edwards and Broughton, 1903), 183.
37. GH, "Excerpts," December 7, 1909, ms., courtesy of Charles G. Huntington 3rd.
38. Jeanette Edwards Rattray, herself a distant descendant of Phebe Hedges, mentions "a David or Daniel Hedges" who had allegedly jumped to his death from the window of the house on North Main Street that once belonged to David A. Hedges, Phebe Hedges's grandson. But as we have seen, although David A. Hedges returned to East Hampton from Oregon in 1870, he was evidently back in Oregon in 1880, and reportedly died there in late 1880, after falling off a horse. See *Main Street*, 34. Two others with the initials D.H., both named David Hedges, died in East Hampton when George Huntington was a boy: the silversmith known as Colonel David Hedges died in 1857 at age seventy-eight, and another with the same name died at the age of sixty-four in 1870. See *East Hampton History*, 377. However, I have found no evidence of suicide for either of these men. Thomas Edwards mentions a man who hanged himself in an old barn, but gives no name. See "Reminiscences of Old East Hampton by the Sea," ms. (1929), 63–64, PLIC-EHL. Diaries, letters, coroners' reports, and the newspapers recorded occasional suicides in East Hampton, none of which was specifically attributed to St. Vitus's dance; for instance, in 1797, the forty-year-old Daniel Dayton Jr., "Not being in His Right Mind," climbed into the garret of his father's house, and hanged himself with a rope. See "An Inquisition taken on the body of Daniel Dayton Junior," June 26, 1799; also Suffolk County Oyer and Terminer, minutes, June 5, 1799, Suffolk County Court Center, Historical Documents Division, Riverhead. In 1815 young Hedges Parsons shot himself with a gun because his father refused to allow him to see his fiancé and forced him to break off his engagement. See Jeremiah Mulford to John Dominy, August 1, 1814, Dominy papers, PLIC-EHL. Mulford Parsons hanged himself in 1841, and in 1858 Roswell Bushnell, "being in a State of Mental Aberration, left the house of Aaron Fithian & voluntarily threw himself into the sea." See diary of J. Madison Huntting, March 28, 1841, PLIC-EHL; coroner's report, November 11, 1852, FB3–12, Suffolk County Court Center, Riverhead. In 1846 fifty-seven-year-old Isaac S. Van Scoy hanged himself, while in 1854 his cousin Abraham Van Scoy cut his throat. See Sag Harbor *Corrector*, December 26, 1846; *East Hampton Records*, vol. 5, 633. Jonathon Parsons in 1856 survived a second attempt to cut his throat. See Fanny Huntting, journal, December 15, 1856, PLIC-EHL. I have not discerned a link between any of these individuals and St. Vitus's dance, although fear of the disease may have motivated some who in fact were not vulnerable. When they noted a motive, witnesses almost always attributed the suicides to mental illness or severe mental distress.
39. See Huntington, "Huntington Family," [10]; also Stevenson, "George Huntington," 58.
40. GLH, account book, November 6, 1871, PLIC-EHL; Huntington, "Huntington Family," [10].
41. GH, "A Letter from Pomeroy," *Sag Harbor Express*, April 4, 1872.
42. GH account books, December 1871–March 1872 passim, courtesy of Charles G. Huntington 3rd; GLH, account book, February 18, 1871, February 25, March 3, 1872, PLIC-EHL; J. Q. A. Hudson, "Letter," *Medical and Surgical Reporter* 26 (February 10, 1872), 114. GH, "On Chorea." All quotations are from this paper.

43. GH, "On Chorea," 320. These included the London physician Thomas Watson (1792–1882), author of *Lectures on the Principles and Practices of Physic,* first published in the United States in 1844; the Scotsman James Copland (1791–1870), author of an enormous *Dictionary of Practical Medicine,* first published in its entirety in 1860; the American David Francis Condie (1796–1875), whose book on childhood diseases Huntington cited; the Philadelphia physician George Bacon Wood (1797–1879), whose case of incurable adult chorea George Huntington specifically referenced in his paper; the German Heinrich Moritz Romberg (1795–1873), author of a *Manual on the Nervous Diseases of Man,* translated into English in 1853; and the Frenchman Armand Trousseau (1801–67), author of the influential *Lectures on Clinical Medicine,* published in English in 1866. Many of these authors noted occasional adult cases of chorea, and also generally mentioned heredity as a predisposing factor in childhood chorea. But they were usually more concerned with exciting or precipitating causes, such as fright, worms and other digestive upsets, and especially rheumatic fever (the latter sometimes considered as a predisposing cause), all of which Huntington also mentioned. The passage from Ezekiel 21:27 reads "I will overturn, overturn, overturn, it: and it shall be no more, until he come whose right it is; and I will give it him."
44. GH, "On Chorea"; William Osler, "Historical Note on Hereditary Chorea," *Neurographs* 1 (1908), 113–16.
45. GH, "On Chorea"; GH, "Recollections," *JNMD* (1910), 255; GH, "Excerpts," December 7, 1909.
46. GH, "On Chorea," 317–21.
47. Ennalls Martin, "Hereditary Blindness," *Baltimore Medical and Surgical Recorder* 1 (January 1809), 277–79.
48. Bowler, *Mendelian Revolution,* 95–96; Conway Zirkle, "Gregor Mendel and His Precursors," *Isis* 42 (1951), 97–104; Ernst Mayr, *The Growth of Biological Thought: Diversity, Evolution, and Inheritance* (Cambridge: Harvard University Press, 1982), 649–52. Lyman Beecher, a great friend of Abel Huntington's, had planted an experimental orchard soon after his arrival in East Hampton in 1799, and years later he recalled that "people had had the impression that fruit would not do well so near the salt water, and laughed when they saw me setting out trees." If Beecher was familiar with horticulturalists such as Knight—a remote but interesting possibility—then others in East Hampton might have read this work as well. See *Autobiography of Lyman Beecher,* ed. Barbara M. Cross, 2 vols. (1864; rpt. Cambridge: Harvard University Press, 1961), 1: 90. References to books appear often in the daybooks of GLH, although just what books we do not know: "Geo at Sag Harbor, gets his books," writes his father on September 6, 1870; "Geo's box of Books . . . all right," on July 30, 1872; "Pack and Send off George's box of Books," on June 19, 1873; and so forth. GLH refers to sending papers such as the *New York Times* and also the *Boston Journal of Chemistry* to his son. See GLH account book, February 2, 1872, PLIC-EHL.
49. Edward Osborn to William Osler, June 28, 1898, Osler collection.
50. Ibid.
51. GH, "Recollections," 255; see also Nadia Durbach and Michael R. Hayden, "George Huntington: The Man Behind the Eponym," *Journal of Medical Genetics* 30 (1993), 406–9. Sally Gregory Kohlstedt has emphasized the role of domestic interactions in the development of modern science. See her "Parlors, Primers, and Public Schooling: Education for Science in Nineteenth-Century America," *Isis* 81 (September 1990), 424–45. While I cannot trace the specific contributions of women in the family to George Huntington's portrayal of chorea, I am drawing here on

Kohlstedt's insights, as well as on diaries, memoirs, the testimonies of neighbors such as Thomas Edwards in his "Reminiscences," and Cornelia Huntington's novel *Sea-Spray.*

52. Huntington, "Huntington Family," [33–34].
53. See Elizabeth Gasking, "Why Was Mendel's Work Ignored?" *Journal of the History of Ideas* 20 (January 1959), 60, 78–79; also N. Russell, *Like Engend'ring Like: Heredity and Animal Breeding in Early Modern Europe* (Cambridge: Cambridge University Press, 1986); Charles Darwin, *The Variation of Animals and Plants under Domestication* (New York: Appleton, 1900), 1: 461. While nineteenth-century naturalists tended to think holistically, in terms of species, farmers and animal and plant breeders tended to focus on discrete isolated characteristics, hoping to "fix" desirable features that could be reproduced reliably generation after generation. Conversely, they hoped to avoid undesirable features that might suddenly reappear after several generations of absence. See Roger J. Wood and Vítězslav Orel, *Genetic Prehistory in Selective Breeding: A Prelude to Mendel* (Oxford: Oxford University Press, 2001), 272–74.
54. On George Huntington's visit to the Suffolk County Agricultural Fair see GLH, account book, June 22, 1870; Robert Stewart, *The American Farmer's Horse Book* (Cincinnati: C. F. Vent, 1867), 435. On earmarks see *East Hampton Records*, passim; J. L. Gardiner, "Gardiner's East Hampton, 1798," in *Collections of the New York Historical Society* (New York: NYHS, 1868), 256; T. H. Breen, *Imagining the Past: East Hampton Histories* (Athens: University of Georgia Press, 1996), 90–91. On the agriculture and animal husbandry of Long Island see Roger Wunderlich, "Go East, Young Man: Nineteenth-Century Farm Life on the South Fork of Long Island," *Long Island Historical Journal* (Fall 2000), 1–10; Richard King, "The Nineteenth-Century Agricultural Transition in an Eastern Long Island Community," *Agricultural History* 55 (January 1981), 50–63. On the breeding and agricultural activities of the Gardiner family see *East Hampton History*, 451–55; also, John Lyon Gardiner, "Farmbook," PLIC-EHL.
55. See SEJ note, ERO, A31812S, box 40; GH, "Excerpts," December 7, 1909, ms., courtesy of Charles G. Huntington 3rd; Stevenson, "George Huntington," 72–73. See also William Bateson, *Mendel's Principles of Heredity* (Cambridge: Cambridge University Press, 1909), 229–30: "The one essential point in such collections [pedigrees] is that the *normal* members of families should be recorded with as much care as the abnormals. In all cases, where possible, inquiry should be made respecting the children of the normals."
56. James Finch, Tillinghast notes, Papers of JER, PLIC-EHL; *Suffolk Gazette*, June 30, 1806; Edward Osborn to William Osler, June 15, 1888, Osler papers. For Henry P. Hedges's construction of the genealogy of the disease in East Hampton see Stevenson, "George Huntington," 71–72.
57. For the Tillinghast genealogy see Chapter 1, note 4.
58. GH, "On Chorea," 321.
59. GH, "From Our Correspondents," *Sag-Harbor Express*, March 7, 1872; G.H., "A Letter from Pomeroy," *Sag Harbor Express*, April 4, 1872.
60. Stevenson, "George Huntington," 72.
61. Rudolf Virchow and August Hirsch, *Jahresbericht über die Leistungen und Fortschritte in der Gesammten Medicin für 1872* (Berlin: Verlag von August Hirschwald, 1873), 32. Camillo Golgi, "Sulle alterazioni degli organi centrali nervosi in un caso di corea gesticolatoria associata ad alienazione mentale," in *Camillo Golgi: Opera Omnia* (Milan: Ulrico Hoepli, 1903), 3: 868–99; see also Paolo Mazzarello, *The Hidden Structure: A Scientific Biography of Camillo Golgi*, trans. and ed. Henry A. Buchtel and Aldo Badiani (Oxford: Oxford University Press, 1999), 85–86.

62. Those who wrote about adult cases of chorea in the 1870s usually mentioned the affected relatives of their patients without comment. In 1873 Louis Landouzy, a medical professor in Paris, reported the case of a thirty-seven-year-old housepainter from Belgium who had suffered from choreic movements for seven years without any improvement. The patient indicated that his father had died, at about forty years of age, "of symptoms absolutely similar to those which led him today to the hospital," and that one sister had died of the same disease while another sister was hospitalized for similar symptoms. But what made the illness interesting to Landouzy was "the age of the patient, the long duration of his illness, and its localization almost exclusively in the pelvis [aux membres pelviens]." Similarly, James MacFaren, an assistant physician at the Royal Edinburgh Asylum, reported in 1874 on his patient J.C., a forty-six-year-old sawyer who had been arrested on charges of being drunk. When the symptoms did not abate after a couple of days in jail, he was "certified insane and sent to the asylum." Although MacFaren suspected a "neurosis" in the family—the man's older brother had reportedly suffered from "brain fever"—he too was more interested in the advanced age of the patient, the duration of the symptoms—which had begun six years earlier and showed no signs of abatement—and the apparent absence of predisposing or exciting causes. See Landouzy, "Société de Biologie," *Gazette Medicale de Paris* 48 (1873), 329–30; James MacFaren, "A Case of Chorea," *Journal of Mental Science* 29 (April 1874), 98; Allan McLane Hamilton, *Nervous Diseases* (Philadelphia: Henry C. Lea, 1978), 404; R. T. Wright, "Subcutaneous Injection of Curara for Chorea," *Lancet* 2 (August 24, 1878), 23; Charcot, "Original Lectures"; see also *Charcot the Clinician*, 85–92; P. Berdinel, "Chorée des Adultes," *Gazette Medicale de Paris* 49 (1878), 336–37.
63. GH, "Letter from Pomeroy," *Sag Harbor Express*, April 4, 1872; GH, account book, 1872–73, passim.
64. *Sag Harbor Express*, August 15, 1872.
65. GLH, account book, passim; *Sag Harbor Express*, December 18, 1873.
66. GLH, account book, January 20, 1874.
67. GH, "Huntington's Chorea," *Brooklyn Medical Journal* 9 (1895), 173–74; GH, "Chronic Progressive Hereditary or Huntington's Chorea," *Transactions of the Tri-State Medical Association* (Raleigh, Va.), 1903: 180–85; GH, "Recollections of Huntington's Chorea as I Saw It at East Hampton, Long Island, During My Boyhood," *JNMD* 37 (1910), 255–57. On the late-nineteenth-century transition from a manhood defined in terms of self-restraint and self-mastery to a masculinity centered on assertiveness and dominance see Gail Bederman, *Manliness and Civilization: A Cultural History of Gender and Race in the United States, 1880–1917* (Chicago: University of Chicago Press, 1995).
68. GLH, account book, March 20, 1874. PLIC-EHL.

4. CHOREA AND THE CLINICAL GAZE

1. A. Harbinson, "Sclerosis of the Nervous Centres Mainly Cerebral," *Medical Press and Circular* 1 (February 18, 1880), 123–25.
2. For British examples see G. MacKenzie Bacon, "Chorea at an Advanced Age of Life," *Journal of Mental Science* 26 (1880–81), 253–54; T. W. McDowall, "Chorea in an Aged Person," *Journal of Mental Science* 27 (July 1881), 201–3; M. D. MacLeod, "Cases of Choreic Convulsions

in Persons of Advanced Age," *Journal of Mental Science* 27 (1882), 194–200; W. P. Herringham, "Chorea in the Adult, and in the Old," *Brain* 11 (October 1888), 134–39. On early accounts of juvenile chorea in families with adult hereditary chorea see G. W. Bruyn, "Huntington's Chorea: Historical, Clinical, and Laboratory Synopsis," P. J. Vinken and G. W. Bruyn, eds., *Handbook of Clinical Neurology*, vol. 6 (Amsterdam: North Holland Publishing, 1968), 316–29; also G. W. Bruyn, F. Baro, and N. C. Myrianthopoulos, *A Centennial Bibliography of Huntington's Chorea, 1872–1972* (Louvain: Leuven University Press, 1973). Clarence King, born in 1861 in Machias, New York, had a strong appreciation for the seriousness of the illness, which "seemed to demand a more thorough and extended study of its pathology and mode of treatment than it has yet received." See Clarence King, "Hereditary Chorea," *New York Medical Journal* 41 (April 25, 1885), 468–70; Clarence King, "Another Case of Hereditary Chorea," *Medical Press of Western New York* 1 (1885–86), 674–77; also Clarence King, "A Third Case of Huntington's Chorea," *Medical News* 55 (July 13, 1889), 41. On his father, T. J. King, see William Adams, ed., *Historical Gazetteer and Biographical Memoir of Cattaraugus County, N.Y.* (Syracuse: Lyman, Horton, 1893), 146–47. On Huber's contribution to the nomenclature see A. Huber, "Chorea hereditaria der Erwachsenen (Huntington'sche Chorea)," *[Virchows] Archiv für pathologische Anatomie und Physiologie und für klinische Medicin* 108 (1887), 267–85. On children with hereditary chorea see J. Hoffman, "Über Chorea chronica progressiva (Huntington'sche Chorea, Chorea hereditaria)," *[Virchows] Archiv für pathologische Anatomie und Physiologie und für klinische Medicin* 111 (1888), 513–48; L. C. Stephens, "Hereditary Chorea," *Transactions of the South Carolina Medical Association* (April 1892), 99–100; William Osler, "Remarks on the Varieties of Chronic Chorea," *JNMD* 18 (February 1893), 98; W. F. Menzies, "Cases of Hereditary Chorea (Huntington's Disease)," *Journal of Mental Science* 38 (October 1892), 560.

3. L. C. Stephens, "Hereditary Chorea," *Transactions of the South Carolina Medical Association* (April 1892), 99–100; William Osler, "Remarks on the Varieties of Chronic Chorea," *JNMD* 18 (February 1893), 98; W. F. Menzies, "Cases of Hereditary Chorea (Huntington's Disease)," *Journal of Mental Science* 38 (October 1892), 560.
4. Harbinson, "Sclerosis of the Nervous Centres," 123–25; U.S. Bureau of Census, *Historical Statistics of the United States from Colonial Times to 1970* (White Plains, N.Y.: Kraus International, 1989), B 37–91.
5. See Bonnie Ellen Blustein, "New York Neurologists and the Specialization of American Medicine," *Bulletin of the History of Medicine* 53 (1979), 170–83; Charles E. Rosenberg, *The Trial of the Assassin Guiteau: Psychiatry and the Law in the Gilded Age* (Chicago: University of Chicago Press, 1968); SEJ, "Fifty Years of American Neurology: Fragments of an Historical Retrospect," *Semi-Centennial Anniversary Volume of the American Neurological Association, 1875–1924* (New York: American Neurological Association, 1924); F. G. Gosling, *Before Freud: Neurasthenia and the American Community, 1870–1910* (Urbana: University of Illinois Press, 1987).
6. Blustein, "New York Neurologists," 170–83; Howard I. Kushner, *A Cursing Brain? The Histories of Tourette Syndrome* (Cambridge: Harvard University Press, 1999); Bonnie Ellen Blustein, *Preserve Your Love for Science: Life of William A. Hammond, American Neurologist* (Cambridge: Harvard University Press, 1999). See also Elizabeth Lunbeck, *The Psychiatric Persuasion: Knowledge, Gender, and Power in Modern America* (Princeton: Princeton University Press, 1994), 336–37.
7. Charles E. Rosenberg, "The Bitter Fruit: Heredity, Disease, and Social Thought in Nineteenth-

Century America," in Donald Fleming and Bernard Bailyn, eds., *Perspectives in American History*, vol. 8 (Cambridge: Cambridge University Press, 1974), 223; see also Ian R. Dowbiggin, *Inheriting Madness: Professionalization and Psychiatric Knowledge in Nineteenth-Century France* (Berkeley: University of California Press, 1991).

8. Gerald Grob, *The Mad among Us: A History of the Care of America's Mentally Ill* (New York: Free Press, 1994); Rosenberg, *Trial of the Assassin Guiteau*, passim; Abraham Myerson et al., *Eugenical Sterilization: A Reorientation of the Problem* (New York: Macmillan, 1936), 24.

9. On the theories of Weissman see Ernst Mayr, *The Growth of Biological Thought: Diversity, Evolution, and Inheritance* (Cambridge: Harvard University Press, 1982), 698–707; Peter J. Bowler, *The Mendelian Revolution: The Emergence of Hereditarian Concepts in Modern Science and Society* (Baltimore: Johns Hopkins University Press, 1989), 83–92.

10. On the hostility toward Weissman's theory of "hard heredity" see Mayr, *Biological Thought*, 701; also Alan R. Rushton, *Genetics and Medicine in the United States, 1800–1922* (Baltimore: Johns Hopkins University Press, 1994), 48; Kenneth M. Ludmerer, *Genetics and American Society: A Historical Appraisal* (Baltimore: Johns Hopkins University Press, 1972), 63–73; Leila Zenderland, *Measuring Minds: Henry Herbert Goddard and the Origins of American Intelligence Testing* (New York: Cambridge University Press, 1998), 150. One of the earliest positive references to Weissman in the literature on Huntington's is by James J. Putnam, who emphasized that acquired traits were not passed on, and that germ cells were not affected by the bad habits or diseases of the parents. See "A Case of Huntington's Chorea: Its Social Aspects," *Boston Medical and Surgical Journal* 150 (April 1904), 399–401.

11. See Jean-Paul Gaudilliere and Ilana Lowy, eds., *Heredity and Infection: The History of Disease Transformation* (New York: Routledge, 2001); Paul Starr, *The Social Transformation of American Medicine* (New York: Basic Books, 1982), 189–97; see also Daniel Pick, *Faces of Degeneration: A European Disorder, c. 1848–c. 1918* (Cambridge: Cambridge University Press, 1989), 59, and Rosenberg, *Trial of the Assassin Guiteau*, 251.

12. See Paolo Mazzarello, *The Hidden Structure: A Scientific Biography of Camillo Golgi*, trans. and ed. by Henry A. Buchtel and Aldo Badiani (Oxford: Oxford University Press: 1999), 86–88; see also *Fifth Annual Report*, Board of Trustees of the General Hospital for the Insane of the State of Connecticut (Hartford: General Hospital for the Insane, 1871), 32–33.

13. Golgi's patient, a man with a "hysterical" mother, "had been devoted to Bacchus and Venus from early life," and had suffered for ten years from choreic movements, along with personality changes and loss of intellectual acuity, suggesting a diagnosis of hereditary chorea. See Mazzarello, *Hidden Structure*, 86–88. For other early autopsy reports see H. von Ziemssen, *Cyclopedia of the Practice of Medicine* (New York: William Wood, 1877), 14: 445–60. "All authorities agree": Harbinson, "Sclerosis of the Nervous Centres," 124–25; MacLeod, "Cases of Choreic Convulsions," 194–200; Herringham, "Chorea," 415–18.

14. Mazzarello, *Hidden Structure*, 87; on early neuropathological studies see Bruyn, "Huntington's Chorea," 329–30; also Peter Harper and Michael Morris, "Introduction: A Historical Background," in Peter S. Harper, ed., *Huntington's Disease* (London: W. B. Saunders, 1991), 18.

15. Mazzarello, *Hidden Structure*, 87. Bruyn emphasizes the role of P. Anglade in 1906, G. Jelgersma in 1908, and Alois Alzheimer in 1911 in the acceptance of the degenerative thesis after about 1911; Harper argues that this acceptance did not come until the 1920s. Wharton Sinkler, "On Heredi-

tary Chorea, with a Report of Three Additional Cases and Details of an Autopsy," *Medical Record* 41 (March 12, 1892), 285. See also Osler, "Chronic Chorea," 107; Osler, *Principles and Practice of Medicine* (New York: Appleton, 1899), 1091; von Zeimssen, *Practice of Medicine*, 453. A few writers mention W. R. Gowers's theory of "abiotrophy," defined as "a degeneration or decay in consequence of a defect of vital endurance" in his paper "Abiotrophy," *Lancet* 2 (April 12, 1892), 1003. However, Gowers himself does not include hereditary chorea in his account of abiotrophy. On efforts to link abiotrophy to Huntington's chorea see Malcolm MacKay, "Hereditary Chorea in Eighteen Members of a Family, with a Report of Three Cases," *Medical News* 85 (September 10, 1904), 498.

16. Clarence King, "Hereditary Chorea," *New York Medical Journal* 41 (April 25, 1885), 468.
17. See Theodore Diller, "Some Observations on the Hereditary Form of Chorea," *American Journal of Medical Science* 98 (December 1889), 592; Osler, "Chronic Chorea," 111; GH to Osler, June 9, 1888, Osler collection; also L. C. Stephens, "Hereditary Chorea," 99–111. W. R. Gowers also alluded to this association in *A Manual of Diseases of the Nervous System* (London: J. and A. Churchill, 1893), 2: 624. On David Barkley's theory of an inherited retrovirus see Alice Wexler, *Mapping Fate: A Memoir of Family, Risk, and Genetic Research* (Berkeley: University of California Press, 1995), 128–29, 132–33. For George Huntington's reference to tetanus on eastern Long Island see GH to William Osler, June 9, 1888, Osler collection.
18. Charles L. Dana, "The Pathology of Hereditary Chorea," *JNMD* 20 (September 1895), 581–82. See also Joseph Collins, "The Pathology and Morbid Anatomy of Huntington's Chorea," *JNMD* 25 (January 1898), 57–61; Clarence A. Good, "A Review of Chronic Progressive Chorea (Huntington's) with Report of a Case," *AJI* (July 1900), 33. Good emphasizes the atrophy of the brain and degenerative change throughout the cortex.
19. Dana, "The Pathology of Hereditary Chorea"; on the use of such analogies see Nancy Leys Stepan, "Race and Gender: The Role of Analogy in Science," in Sandra Harding, ed., *The "Racial" Economy of Science* (Bloomington: Indiana University Press, 1993), 359–76; see also Douglas C. Baynton, "Disability and the Justification of Inequality in American History," in Lauri Umansky and Paul K. Longmore, eds., *The New Disability History: American Perspectives* (New York: New York University Press, 2001), 33–57.
20. See William Francis Drewry, "Chronic Progressive Chorea," *Charlotte Medical Journal* 7 (September 1895), 318–23. Drewry claimed that he had "never known of but one or two cases. I do not recall the record of a single authentic case of Huntington's chorea in the African." Yet he apparently believed that his patient did in fact suffer from this disease. Drewry also thought "the Negro" exempt from locomotor ataxia, paralysis agitans, or delirium tremens; of five thousand patients at the Freedman's Hospital in Washington, D.C., he had encountered only one or two cases of delirium tremens. On the other hand, epilepsy and hysteria were "quite common among Negroes," a frequency he attributed to race rather than to the demographics of institutionalization. Other early cases of African descent include that described by J. L. Bower, "Notes on Some Cases of Chorea and Tremor, Including a case in a Negro," *JNMD* 15 (1890), 131–42; also that reported by Arthur Conklin Brush in "Huntington's Chorea," *New York Medical Journal* 61 (March 9, 1895), 305.
21. Clarence King, "Hereditary Chorea," *Medical Record* 70 (November 17, 1906), 765. A few prominent twentieth-century clinicians, including MacDonald Critchley and George Bruyn, consid-

ered that "the Jewish race appears to show conspicuous indemnity from the disease." However, Ntinos Myrianthopoulos, a geneticist at the U.S. National Institutes of Health, noted in 1966 that it was his impression, from counseling many Jewish families with Huntington's, that "the proportion of Jewish cases is, if anything, higher than that of non-Jewish cases." See Ntinos Myrianthopoulos, "Huntington's Chorea," *Journal of Medical Genetics* 3 (1966), 300; Bruyn, "Huntington's Chorea," 303; MacDonald Critchley, "The History of Huntington's Chorea," *Psychological Medicine* 14 (1984), 726.

22. On early neuropathological studies see Bruyn, "Huntington's Chorea," 329–30; also Harper and Morris, "Introduction," 18. See also Frank K. Hallock, "A Case of Huntington's Chorea, with Remarks upon the Propriety of Naming the Disease 'Dementia Choreica,'" *JNMD* 24 (1898), 852; James J. Putnam, "A Case of Huntington's Chorea," *Boston Medical and Surgical Journal* 101 (April 14, 1904), 399; Pick, *Faces of Degeneration*, 8–9.
23. As the historian Daniel Pick has written, "degeneration slides over from a description of a disease or degradation as such, to become a kind of self-reproducing pathological process—a causal agent in the blood, the body and the race—which engendered a cycle of historical and social decline perhaps finally beyond determination"; *Faces of Degeneration*, 22. On families with Huntington's dying out, see Henry F. Perkins, *The First Annual Report of the Eugenical Survey of Vermont* (Burlington: University of Vermont, 1927), 9.
24. On the medieval association of "uncontrolled bodily motion, thrashing about, and convulsions" with madness and pain, see Esther Cohen, "The Animated Pain of the Body," *American Historical Review* (February 2000), 58–59, 63–68, and Barbara Newman, "Possessed by the Spirit: Devout Women, Demoniacs, and the Apostolic Life in the Thirteenth Century," *Speculum* 73 (1998), 733–70. See also James Boswell, *The Life of Samuel Johnson* (1791; rpt. New York: Random House, 1952), 42–43; Thomas Jeffreys, "On Chorea, with Two Cases to Illustrate the Nature and Treatment of That Disease," *Edinburgh Medical and Surgical Journal* 23 (1825), 285. On the term *insanity* see SEJ to CBD, December 26, 1910, APS-ERO. Hereditary insanity was a staple of such gothic fictions as Edgar Allen Poe's "Fall of the House of Usher" (1839) and Louisa May Alcott's "A Nurses's Story" (1865) and "The Skeleton in the Closet" (1867). On chorea as a "mania of the motor centres" see Ernest S. Reynolds, "Hereditary or Huntington's Chorea," *Medical Chronicle* 16 (1892), 128.
25. Ellen Dwyer, *Homes for the Mad: Life inside Two Nineteenth-Century Asylums* (New Brunswick: Rutgers University Press, 1987), 158.
26. Hallock, "A Case of Huntington's Chorea," 858; Theodore Diller, "Chorea in the Adult as Seen among the Insane," *American Journal of the Medical Sciences* 99 (April 1890), 340. Clarence King found that "the patient, recognizing the character of his disease and the future doom that surely awaits him, is generally sad and downcast, and, in consequence, seeks seclusion." It was "during this stage that the patient may attempt the destruction of his own life." He was personally familiar with a lady who twice "through shame and mortification, attempted suicide" in this early stage of the disease. See King, "Hereditary Chorea" (1885), 469. For Jelliffe's critique of the term *insanity* as a single "entity," see SEJ to Davenport, December 26, 1910, Davenport papers.
27. Arthur S. Hamilton, "A Report of Twenty-Seven Cases of Chronic Progressive Chorea," *AJI* 64 (January 1908), 469–70; Allan Diefendorf, "Mental Symptoms of Huntington's Chorea," *Neurographs* 1 (1908), 128–36.

28. King, "Hereditary Chorea" (1885), 469; Clarence King, "Another Case of Hereditary Chorea," *Medical Press of Western New York* 1 (1885–86), 676; King, "Third Case," 41; King, "Hereditary Chorea" (1906), 767; Clarence King, "Hereditary Chorea," *New York Medical Journal* 1040 (August 12, 1916), 306–8.
29. The English geneticist William Bateson, for instance, referred to "the peculiar form of insanity known as Hereditary Chorea" in his influential 1909 text *Mendel's Principles of Heredity* (Cambridge: Cambridge University Press, 1909). The Vermont eugenicist Henry F. Perkins also referred to "the dreadful form of insanity known as Huntington's Chorea" in his 1927 *Eugenical Survey of Vermont.*
30. On Huntington's chorea as an "interesting" disease see C. M. Hay, "Hereditary Chorea, with a Contribution of Eight Additional Cases of the Disease," *University Medical Magazine* 2 (June 1890), 465. See also Wharton Sinkler, "Chorea," in William Pepper, ed., *A System of Practical Medicine,* vol. 5, *Diseases of the Nervous System* (Philadelphia: Lea Brothers, 1886), 439–56; Wharton Sinkler, "Hereditary Chorea," *Boston Medical and Surgical Journal,* 119 (October 11, 1888), 368; Wharton Sinkler, "Two Additional Cases of Hereditary Chorea," *JNMD* 14 (February 1889), 69–91; Wharton Sinkler, "Hereditary Chorea, with a Report of Three Additional Cases and Details of an Autopsy," *Medical Record* 41 (March 12, 1892), 281–85; Wharton Sinkler, "Family Diseases," *Journal of the American Medical Association* 34 (February 10, 1900), 331–35. Others who wrote on Huntington's in the 1880s and 1890s, such as Theodore Diller, Frank K. Hallock, Charles Eugene Riggs, Eugene D. Bondurant, George J. Preston, and Edward N. Brush, were active in medical societies at the state and local level.
31. Rushton describes Huntington's chorea in the late nineteenth century as "the preeminent 'hereditary' neurologic disease." See Rushton, *Genetics and Medicine,* 99–100.
32. See W. F. Menzies, "Cases of Hereditary Chorea (Huntington's Disease)," *Journal of Mental Science* 164 (January 1893), 53; E. M. Phelps, "A New Consideration of Hereditary Chorea," *JNMD* 18 (October 1892), 775; William Osler *The Principles and Practice of Medicine* (New York: Appleton, 1892), 944; William Osler, *On Chorea and Choreiform Affections* (Philadelphia: Blakiston, 1894), 108. See Sinkler, "Two Additional Cases," 88. On the differences between similar or direct and dissimilar or transformational heredity see Jean-Martin Charcot, *Charcot the Clinician: The Tuesday Lessons, Excerpts from Nine Case Presentations on General Neurology Delivered at the Salpêtrière Hospital in 1887–88,* trans. with commentary by Christopher G. Goetz (New York: Raven, 1987), 87. On the development of pedigrees see Yoshio Nukaga and Alberto Cambrosio, "Medical Pedigrees and the visual production of family disease in Canadian and Japanese genetic counselling practice," in Mary Ann Elston, ed., *The Sociology of Medical Science and Technology* (Oxford: Blackwell, 1997); also Yoshio Nukaga, "Between Tradition and Innovation in New Genetics: The Continuity of Medical Pedigrees and the Development of Combination Work in the Case of Huntington's Disease," *New Genetics and Society* 21 (2002), 39–64, and Yoshio Nukaga, "Inscribing Heredity: The Development and Use of Family Trees in the Case of Hereditary Chorea," unpublished ms.
33. See, for instance, Diller, "Some Observations," 585–93; Diller, "Chorea in the Adult," 329–49; Stephens, "Hereditary Chorea," 99–100; Hallock, "A Case of Huntington's Chorea," 862.
34. See, for instance, Charcot, *Charcot the Clinician,* 86; Osler, "Historical Note on Hereditary Chorea," *Neurographs* 1 (1908), 115; R. M. Phelps, "A New Consideration of Hereditary Chorea,"

JNMD (October 1892), 772; Hay, "Hereditary Chorea," 463–72; Osler, "Chronic Chorea," 97–98.

35. GH, "On Chorea," *Medical and Surgical Reporter* 26 (April 13, 1872), 320; Landon Carter Gray, A *Treatise on Nervous and Mental Diseases* (Philadelphia: Lea Brothers, 1895), 344; King, "Hereditary Chorea" (1906), 766; Hamilton, "Twenty-Seven Cases," 460. Clarence Good also thought that it was transmitted "probably more frequently through the female." See Good, "A Review of Chronic Progressive Chorea (Huntington's), with Report of a Case," *AJI* 57 (July 1900), 27–28; Julia Bell, "Huntington's Chorea," *The Treasury of Human Inheritance* (Cambridge: Cambridge University Press, 1948), 4: 22.
36. On the allegedly heightened fertility of women who later became choreic see Sinkler, "Two Additional Cases," 89; also Good, "Chronic Progressive Chorea (Huntington's)," *AJI* (1900), 27–28.
37. On warnings against marriage see William Buchan, *Domestic Medicine,* 2nd ed. (London: W. Strahan, 1772), 10; also King, "Hereditary Chorea" (1906), 767. On the fertility of the feebleminded woman see James W. Trent Jr., *Inventing the Feeble Mind: A History of Mental Retardation in the United States* (Berkeley: University of California Press, 1994), 164–65, and Wendy Kline, *Building a Better Race: Gender, Sexuality, and Eugenics from the Turn of the Century to the Baby Boom* (Berkeley: University of California Press, 2001), 16, 24–26, 46–48.
38. See Janet Farrell Brodie, *Contraception and Abortion in Nineteenth-Century America* (Ithaca: Cornell University Press, 1994), 2, 253–58; Linda Gordon, *Woman's Body, Woman's Right: A Social History of Birth Control in America* (New York: Penguin, 1974), 159–245.
39. Arthur Hamilton in 1908 complained that members of affected families lacked an understanding of the "impropriety" of marriage; "Twenty-Seven Cases," 470. McKinniss noted that "we cannot emphasize the danger too much, and should advise always against marriage of these individuals"; C. R. McKinniss, "The Value of Eugenics in Huntington's Chorea," *Medical Record* 86 (July 18, 1914), 106. Sherman See wrote in 1923: "The crime of it, which can be laid at the door of no one, is the freedom with which these people multiply and, by multiplying, intensify the curse of chorea"; "Huntington's Chorea in Montgomery County," *Kentucky Medical Journal* 21 (May 1923), 228. I also draw here on my mother's experience in the 1920s and 1930s.
40. Horace Marion, "A Many-Phased Case of Chorea," *Boston Medical and Surgical Journal* 150 (April 14, 1904), 397–99, and J. J. Putnam, "A Case of Huntington's Chorea: Its Social Aspects," *Boston Medical and Surgical Journal* 150 (April 14, 1904), 399–401.
41. Putnam, "A Case of Huntington's Chorea"; Marion, "A Many-Phased Case of Chorea." On the criminalization of abortion see Brodie, *Contraception and Abortion,* 253–88.
42. Putnam, "A Case of Huntington's Chorea"; Marion, "A Many-Phased Case of Chorea."
43. See King, "Hereditary Chorea" (1906), 767; Osler, *On Chorea,* 108, 111; Sinkler, "Two Additional Cases." As Osler put it, diagnosis was easy in the familial form but exceedingly difficult in cases without it.
44. For Waters see Robley Dunglison, *Diseases of the Nervous System* (Philadelphia: Lea and Blanchard, 1848), 217–18; also James MacFaren, "A Case of Chorea," *Journal of Mental Science* 89 (April 1874), 97. King, "Hereditary Chorea" (1885), 470; Osler, *On Chorea* (1894), 112; L. C. Gray, A *Treatise on Nervous and Mental Diseases,* 2nd ed. (Philadelphia: Lea Brothers, 1895), 569; Dana, "Hereditary Chorea" (1895), 569; Bondurant, "Chronic Adult Chorea" (1896), 682.

45. Sinkler, "Two Additional Cases," 90; Hay, "Hereditary Chorea" (1890), 472; Stephens, "Hereditary Chorea" (1892), 106–7; King, "Hereditary Chorea" (1906), 767.
46. Nicholas Dynan, "The Physical and Mental States in Chronic Chorea," *AJI* 7 (January 1914), 627; King, "Hereditary Chorea" (1916), 307.
47. Sinkler, "Two Additional Cases," 90–91; Putnam, "Huntington's Chorea" (1904), 399–401; Hamilton, "Twenty-Seven Cases," 473–74; McKinniss, "Value of Eugenics," 106; William C. Porter, "Huntington's Chorea," *State Hospital Quarterly* 4 (1918–19), 74.
48. I am relying here on entries in Bruyn, Baro, and Myrianthopoulos, *Centennial Bibliography.*
49. William Browning, "Editorial," *Neurographs* 1 (1908), 85–88.
50. *Neurographs* 1 (1908).
51. See John C. Burnham, *Jelliffe: American Psychoanalyst and Physician* (Chicago: University of Chicago Press, 1983); *Semi-Centennial Volume of the American Neurological Association* (1924), 191–93.
52. See Burnham, *Jelliffe*, 6; SEJ, "A Contribution to the History of Huntington's Chorea: A Preliminary Report," *Neurographs* 1 (1908), 116–24; Edward Osborn to SEJ, May 24, 1905, ERO, ser. 1-A:31812 S, box 39, folder 4.
53. SEJ, "Contribution to the History."
54. On Davenport see Garland Allen, "The Eugenics Record Office at Cold Spring Harbor, 1910–1940," *Osiris*, 2nd ser. (1986), 225–64; Daniel J. Kevles, *In the Name of Eugenics: Genetics and the Uses of Human Heredity* (Berkeley: University of California Press, 1985), 41–56; Mark A. Largent, "'Zoology of the Twentieth Century': Charles Davenport's Prediction for Biology," http://www.amphilsoc.org/library/bulletin/2002/davenport.htm; Charles E. Rosenberg, "Charles Benedict Davenport and the Beginning of American Genetics," *Bulletin of the History of Medicine* 35 (1961), 266–76; CBD, *Heredity in Relation to Eugenics* (New York: Henry Holt, 1911), 259.
55. See Barbara A. Kimmelman, "The American Breeders' Association: Genetics and Eugenics in an Agricultural Context, 1903–13," *Social Studies of Science*, 3 (May 1983), 163–204, especially 183–89; Rushton, *Genetics and Medicine*, 116, 125; Kenneth M. Ludmerer, *Genetics and American Society: A Historical Appraisal* (Baltimore: Johns Hopkins University Press, 1972), 50–51; CBD to SEJ, March 21, 1911, Davenport papers; Steven Selden, *Inheriting Shame: The Story of Eugenics and Racism in America* (New York: Teachers College Press, 1999), 6, 53–54, 69; CBD, *Heredity in Relation to Eugenics*, 259–60, 224.
56. See H. H. Laughlin, "Report on the Organization and the First Eight Months' Work of the Eugenics Record Office," *American Breeders Magazine* 2 (1911), 107–12; SEJ to MacDonald Critchley, January 13, 1936, SEJ papers, Library of Congress, Washington, D.C.; CBD to SEJ, March 21, 1911, Davenport papers.
57. Browning, "Editorial," 85; C. Eugene Riggs, "Three Cases of Huntington's Chorea," *JNMD* 38 (September 1901), 519.

5. THE EYES OF ELIZABETH B. MUNCEY, M.D.

1. See, for example, Susan Sontag, *Illness as Metaphor and AIDS and Its Metaphors* (New York: Doubleday, 1989); Jesse F. Ballenger, *Self, Senility, and Alzheimer's Disease in Modern America: A History* (Baltimore: Johns Hopkins University Press, 2006); Rosemarie Garland Thomson, *Ex-*

traordinary Bodies: Figuring Physical Disability in American Culture and Literature (New York: Columbia University Press, 1997); Sander L. Gilman, *Disease and Representation: Images of Illness from Madness to AIDS* (Ithaca: Cornell University Press, 1988).

2. Paul K. Longmore and Lauri Umansky, eds., *The New Disability History: American Perspectives* (New York: New York University Press, 2001), 22.
3. Diane B. Paul, *Controlling Human Heredity, 1865 to the Present* (Amherst, N.Y.: Humanity Books, 1998), 19–21, 50–96; Nancy Leys Stepan, *"The Hour of Eugenics": Race, Gender, and Nation in Latin America* (Ithaca: Cornell University Press, 1991).
4. On marriage restrictions see CBD, *Bulletin No. 9: State Laws Limiting Marriage Selection* (Cold Spring Harbor, N.Y.: Eugenics Record Office, June 1913). On the social contexts of eugenics see Alexandra Minna Stern, *Eugenic Nation: Faults and Frontiers of Better Breeding in Modern America* (Berkeley: University of California Press, 2005); Wendy Kline, *Building a Better Race: Gender, Sexuality, and Eugenics from the Turn of the Century to the Baby Boom* (Berkeley: University of California, 2001); Daniel J. Kevles, *In the Name of Eugenics* (Berkeley: University of California Press, 1985), 84–112; Philip R. Reilly, *The Surgical Solution: A History of Involuntary Sterilization in the United States* (Baltimore: Johns Hopkins University Press, 1991), 41–56; Martin S. Pernick, *The Black Stork: Eugenics and the Death of "Defective" Babies in American Medicine and Motion Pictures since 1915* (New York: Oxford University Press, 1996). Although Huntington's chorea was not listed among those conditions rendering a person excludable from the United States, the 1903 *Book of Instructions for the Medical Inspection of Immigrants* (Washington, D.C.: Government Printing Office, 1903), 12, specified locomotor ataxia, spastic paraplegia, "and other incurable nervous diseases" as liable to render a person unable to work and therefore subject to exclusion. Immigration regulations of 1917 specified "spastic gaits, caused by disorders of the nervous system," as reasons for proscription, and included "chorea," although not specifically Huntington's chorea. See Treasury Department, U.S. Public Health Service, *Regulations Governing the Medical Inspection of Aliens* (Washington, D.C.: Government Printing Office, 1917), 19. See also Stepan, *Hour of Eugenics,* 133. *Buck vs. Bell* was a Supreme Court case designed to test the constitutionality of the state of Virginia's compulsory sterilization law. It involved the sterilization of a young, allegedly feebleminded woman who had been institutionalized by her adoptive mother. See Reilly, *Surgical Solution,* 67–68.
5. On eugenic family studies see Nicole Hahn Rafter, ed., *White Trash: The Eugenic Family Studies, 1877–1919* (Boston: Northeastern University Press, 1988), and Leila Zenderland, *Measuring Minds: Henry Herbert Goddard and the Origins of American Intelligence Testing* (New York: Cambridge University Press, 1998), 150. See also Florence H. Danielson and Charles B. Davenport, *The Hill Folk: Report on a Rural Community of Hereditary Defectives* (Cold Spring Harbor, N.Y.: Eugenics Record Office, 1912); Henry Herbert Goddard, *The Kallikak Family: A Study in the Heredity of Feeblemindedness* (New York: McMillan, 1912).
6. The literature on Mendel is vast. For placing Mendel within a historical context I have found especially useful Garland Allen, *Life Sciences in the Twentieth Century* (New York: John Wiley, 1975); Ernst Mayr, *The Growth of Biological Thought: Diversity, Evolution, and Inheritance* (Cambridge: Harvard University Press, 1982), 710–26; Robert C. Olby, "Mendel, Mendelism, and Genetics," 1997, www.mendelweb.org/MWolby.intro.html; Roger J. Wood and Vítězslav Orel, *Genetic Prehistory in Selective Breeding: A Prelude to Mendel* (Oxford: Oxford University Press, 2001); Peter J.

Bowler, *The Mendelian Revolution: The Emergence of Hereditarian Concepts in Modern Science and Society* (Baltimore: Johns Hopkins University Press, 1989). Bowler suggests that "eugenics created a demand for theories which stressed the role of heredity over environment in the shaping of human character" (165–66).

7. Mayr, *Growth of Biological Thought*, 710–26.
8. On the neglect of Mendel for forty years see Bowler, *Mendelian Revolution*, 1–20, 105–11; Mayr argues, however, that most of Mendel's methodology came from physics. See Mayr, *Growth of Biological Thought*, 722–24; Elizabeth Gasking, "Why Was Mendel's Work Ignored?" *Journal of the History of Ideas* 20 (January 1959), 60, 78–79. See also Vítězslav Orel, "Heredity before Mendel," 1996, www.mendelweb.org/MWorel.html.
9. See Mayr, *Growth of Biological Thought*, 710–26; Bowler, *Mendelian Revolution*, 93–109; Gasking, "Why Was Mendel's Work Ignored?" 78–79.
10. William Bateson, "An Address on Mendelian Heredity and Its Application to Man," *Brain*, part 2 (June 1906), 155; see also Bowler, *Mendelian Revolution* 116–27; Mayr, *Growth of Biological Thought*, 544–45, 733–34.
11. Bateson to Nettleship, February 1, April 13, October 13, 1906; January 7, 1907, Braugham papers, special collections, University College London (hereafter UCL). See also Bateson, "An Address on Mendelian Heredity," 176. On the relationship between Bateson and Nettleship see Alan R. Rushton, "Nettleship, Pearson, and Bateson: The Biometric-Mendelian Debate in a Medical Context," *Journal of the History of Medicine* 55 (2000), 134–57.
12. Reginald C. Punnett, "Mendelism in Relation to Disease," *Proceedings, Royal Society of Medicine* 1 (March 1908), 144; SEJ, "A Contribution to the History of Huntington's Chorea: A Preliminary Report," *Neurographs* 1 (1908), 124. Jelliffe wrote that his own figures concerning the pattern of inheritance "seem to show a very close approximation to the results of Mendelian crossing." However, without more data he was "unwilling to present any conclusions."
13. William S. Church, William S. Gowers, Arthur Latham, and E. F. Bashford, *The Influence of Heredity on Disease* (London: Longmans, 1909), 27–28; William Bateson, *Mendel's Principles of Heredity* (Cambridge: Cambridge University Press, 1909), 229.
14. CBD, "Heredity and Mendel's Law," *Proceedings of the Washington Academy of Sciences* 9 (July 31, 1907), 179–87; CBD, "Determination of Dominance in Mendelian Inheritance," *Proceedings of the American Philosophical Society* 46 (January–April 1908), 59–63; CBD, *Heredity in Relation to Eugenics* (New York: Henry Holt, 1911), 102–3 (Davenport cites *Mendel's Principles of Heredity* in his bibliography but does not credit Bateson in the text). See also Bateson to CBD, November 8, 1908; CBD to Bateson, November 20, 1908, CBD diary, May 1909, Davenport papers.
15. CBD, *Heredity in Relation to Eugenics*, 102, 259. See also Garland Allen, "The Eugenics Record Office at Cold Spring Harbor, 1910–1940," *Osiris*, 2nd ser. (1986), 225–64; Alan R. Rushton, *Genetics and Medicine in the United States, 1800–1922* (Baltimore: Johns Hopkins University Press, 1994), 118. Rafter argues that eugenic researchers "began by assuming that which they then set out to prove"; *White Trash*, 22.
16. For information on Elizabeth B. Muncey and Daniel T. Muncey, I have used the U.S. censuses of Bucks County, Pennsylvania, for 1860 to 1880 and of Washington, D.C., from 1890 to 1920; the *Bucks County Gazette* (April 5, 1883); *Directories* of the American Medical Association; *Howard University Medical Department: A Historical Biographical and Statistical Souvenir* (1900; rpt.

Freeport, N.Y.: Books for Libraries Press, 1971), 201–2; Gloria Moldow, *Women Doctors in Gilded-Age Washington: Race, Gender, and Professionalization* (Urbana: University of Illinois Press, 1987); Amy Sue Bix, "Experiences and Voices of Eugenics Field Workers: 'Women's Work' in Biology," *Social Studies of Science* 27 (1997), 625–68.

17. See Moldow, *Women Doctors*, 37–47; *Howard University*, 201–2.
18. Moldow, *Women Doctors*. On hopes unfulfilled for women doctors see Regina Markell Morantz-Sanchez, *Sympathy and Science: Women Physicians in American Medicine* (Oxford: Oxford University Press, 1985), 232–65.
19. See AMA *Directory* for 1909 and after; *Howard University*, 201–2; EBM to CBD, September 28, 1920, July 10, 1911, Davenport papers, series IIb.
20. Moldow, *Women Doctors*, 12.
21. See EBM to CBD, July 10, 1911, Davenport papers, series IIb; Moldow, *Women Doctors*, 2–4, 12, 166–68. Davenport hired Muncey at a monthly salary of seventy-five dollars a month, with thirty dollars for "maintenance," one dollar per diem while in the field, and two weeks' paid vacation, with two additional weeks at half-pay, an extremely modest income at the time for someone of her qualifications; Davenport papers, series IIb.
22. On making pedigrees see Bateson, *Mendel's Principles*, 15, 205–34; CBD, *Heredity in Relation to Eugenics*, 9, 16; Mayr, *Growth of Biological Thought*, 782–83; also Yoshio Nukaga and Alberto Cambrosio, "Medical Pedigrees and the Visual Production of Family Disease in Canadian and Japanese Genetic Counselling Practice," in M. A. Elston, ed., *The Sociology of Medical Science and Technology* (Oxford: Blackwell, 1997).
23. On the methodology of the ERO pedigree studies see Bix, "Eugenics Field Workers," 637–45; also Allen, "Eugenics Record Office," 242–45. I am grateful to Jacqueline M. Jackson, Shelley D. Burnham, and Emily M. Perkins of the Hereditary Genomics Division, Department of Medical and Molecular Genetics, Indiana University School of Medicine, for their recalculation of Muncey's figures. Muncey attributed chorea to the husband of Phebe Hedges rather than to Phebe herself, although she had Henry P. Hedges's 1908 letter indicating the reverse; this error also led her to make erroneous diagnoses in earlier generations. See CHD, B-3.
24. On the development of the neurological examination see Fielding H. Garrison, *History of Neurology*, rev. and enl. by Lawrence C. McHenry (Springfield, Ill.: Charles C. Thomas, 1969).
25. Early death records indicating magrums or St. Vitus's dance as the cause of death show that this diagnosis was familiar in certain communities. See, for instance, Stamford Deaths, 1847–1890 (family history film 1434311): Zuba Weed died February 7, 1864, from "St. Vitus Dance"; Richard Crabb, fifty-eight, died July 22, 1867, of "St. Vitus dance." Stamford Births, Marriages, and Deaths, 1872–1897 (FHF 1434312), lists Silas Weed, age thirty-five, who died March 28, 1876, Ellen Selleck, forty-seven, who died October 19, 1882, and Anne Amelia Stevens, thirty-eight, who died September 28, 1882, all of "magrums." Some persons from families associated later with Huntington's chorea died with distinct but related diagnoses, like "insanity" and "palsy." Occasional records listed "chorea" as cause of death: Miles Stevens, for example, died October 15, 1873, at age thirty-five, of "chorea." See Stamford Death Records vol. 3. Other diagnoses of persons in affected families indicated "Paralysis Agitans and Chorea General Debility" for a fifty-five-year-old woman ill for three years whose father had confirmed Huntington's chorea and "Locomotor Ataxia" for a thirty-seven-year-old man whose mother had Huntington's. See Stamford Deaths 1897–1906

(FHF 1434313). On the willingness of physicians and superintendents to accept familial diagnoses see Ellen Dwyer, *Homes for the Mad: Life inside Two Nineteenth-Century Asylums* (New Brunswick: Rutgers University Press, 1987).

26. On physicians' broad use of the category *chorea* see Howard J. Kushner, *A Cursing Brain? The Histories of Tourette Syndrome* (Cambridge: Harvard University Press, 1999), 32–39. Muncey explained that "if the term [palsy] was used as the cause of death for several generations of a family, and if there were descendants with Huntington's chorea," she interpreted the term as a reference to chorea, although palsy often referred to stroke and other conditions involving loss of movement. Muncey did not always describe the behavior associated with these names, so it is difficult to know when her informants used the names broadly and when they used it more narrowly in relation to symptoms that knowledgeable clinicians at that time would have interpreted as evidence of Huntington's chorea. Note that the family names I have used in the text to exemplify localized terms for the condition are invented.
27. "She does not remember," CHD, B-81; "his mind remained good," CHD, A-3.
28. "Said she told me all there was to tell," CHD, A-57; ERO, series 7: fieldworker files, 1911–26, box 1, E. B. Muncey 15: 15-357 (EBM, April 13, 1912); see also series 1, box 39, A:31812, 1–5, and A:31812S, 1–3, and box 40, A:31812S nos. 4–5. Two daughters of an affected mother in Connecticut "refuse to discuss their mother's condition," an expression, Muncey believed, of their being "neurotic"; CHD, A-64. Others simply ignored her. "Both she and her brother acted as if I were not present," she wrote of one pair of siblings near Greenwich. "He laughed and acted silly and refused to let me wait on his porch for a car although it was raining very hard. She ignored my request entirely; said she had important business to attend to, went in and shut the door." Muncey concluded, "they are both degenerates," CHD, A-54; "when not drinking," CHD, A-73.
29. CHD, 2.
30. Diagnosis was such a fraught aspect of all the eugenic family studies that by 1915 Davenport was advising fieldworkers, "*Do not diagnose*," urging them rather to make the case histories so complete that the person analyzing the data would be able to make the diagnosis, as if that would somehow be more accurate. See "Cold Spring Harbor: Meeting of Field Workers," June 23, 1915, image 143, MSC77, box 1, www.eugenicsarchive.org/eugenics/list2.pl. See also Allen, "Eugenics Record Office," 243.
31. CHD, B-105, A-9, B-117, A-62, A-5. For other examples of family memory tracing the disease back many generations see Clarence King, "A Third Case of Hereditary Chorea," *Medical News* 55 (July 13, 1889), 40. King reported a patient born around 1851 whose grandmother, probably born around 1800, was also said to have had the disease. Eugene Riggs in 1901 reported a forty-two-year-old patient, born about 1859, whose great-grandfather was said to have been affected; C. Eugene Riggs, "Three Cases of Huntington's Chorea," *JNMD* 38 (1901), 519. On disputing the origin of Huntington's in Connecticut see ERO, fieldworker files 15, EBM, April 13, 1912, 15-357. On the legend of Ann Millington see ERO, fieldworker files 15, EBM, June 5, 1912, 15-402.
32. "The family is said to have been choreic," CHD, A-25; "his son reports," CHD, A25; "the neighbors, knowing the heredity," CHD, B-61; "a pretty young girl," CHD, A-6.
33. "His family says," CHD, B-8; "they are taken," CHD, B-111.
34. "Both children are nervous over the heredity," CHD, A-24; "they are both very anxious about the heredity of chorea," CHD, B-75; "fears the onset of chorea and has made his best friend promise

to tell him when he sees any signs of the trouble," CHD, B-5; "is quite nervous over the possibility of heredity," CHD, B-5; "was beginning to shake," CHD, B-105; "he committed suicide because," CHD, A-61; "when he realized," CHD, A-70.

35. "Wounds received in the army," CHD, C-8; "the result of a fall," CHD, C-6; "fell from a wagon," CHD, B-99; "a complete nervous breakdown," CHD, B-35; "after a slight paralytic attack," CHD, B-13. Clinicians too sometime pointed to precipitating events, as when Eugene Riggs in 1901 noted that "mental stress or shock preceded the onset of the disease" in two different families he observed. See Riggs, "Three Cases," 521; also Nicholas J. Dynan, "The Physical and Mental States in Chronic Chorea," *AJI* 7 (1914), 589–636, especially 591–92. Dynan laid out a range of explanations which "the patients' friends and relatives use to excuse the presence of the disease." One cited alcoholism, another referred to head trauma, a third thought domestic trouble had caused the problem. In other cases, a patient blamed his symptoms on alcoholism, his own as well as his father's, and on "sexual excesses" and a case of typhoid fever eight years earlier. A woman believed the loss of her mother when she was thirty-three had aggravated her "nervous" condition. Another patient was said to have suffered heat exhaustion and also alcoholism. Chicken pox, diphtheria, malaria, sunstroke, and other disorders were all cited as precipitating causes. On the lay belief in a district of Nova Scotia that the disease is a result of alcoholism, see W. H. Hattie, "Huntington's Chorea," *AJI* 66 (July 1909), 125.

36. "No one would allow," CHD, A-55; "they were shunned," A-70; "there was much opposition," B-118; "children in the villages," B-105; "the combination was appalling," B-73.

37. "Great business sagacity," CHD, A-62; "fine character," CHD, A-46; "extensive medical practice," A-58; "a man of wealth," A-57.

38. "Original proprietor," CHD, A-30; "a lawyer," CHD, B-25; "a prominent man," CHD, B-80.

39. For Muncey's notes on Ann Millington, see CH, B-97; also Chapter 2, n. 63; on Elinor Knapp see CHD, B-98; on Elizabeth Knapp see CHD, B-121.

40. On numbers of patients in U.S. state mental hospitals see Abraham Myerson et al., *Eugenical Sterilization: A Reorientation of the Problem* (New York: Macmillan, 1936), 24. Robley Dunglison, *The Practice of Medicine* (Philadelphia: Lea and Blanchard, 1848), 312–13; C. M. Hay, "Hereditary Chorea, with a Contribution of Eight Additional Cases of the Disease," *University Medical Magazine* 2 (June 1890), 464; C. R. McKinniss, "The Value of Eugenics in Huntington's Chorea," *Medical Record* 86 (1914), 105. Nicholas J. Dynan, an assistant physician at the U.S. Government Hospital for the Insane in Washington, D.C., noted the high number of former soldiers among his nineteen patients; other occupations included seamstress and dressmaker, farmers, a printer, a laborer, a painter, and a musician. See Dynan, "The Physical and Mental States in Chronic Chorea: Summary of Nineteen Cases," *AJI* 7 (January 1914), 592. Patients with Huntington's chorea remained a tiny percentage of all patients in mental hospitals.

41. Poor and marginal, CHD, B-104; "fisherman and tramp," CHD, B-109, "peddlers," CHD, B-73; "small businessmen," CHD, B-61, B-77, B-82; "school principal," CHD, B-2; "professor of surgery," CHD, A-58; physician's wife, CHD, A-56; shipping line president, CHD, B-36; family of teachers and successful businessmen, CHD, B-20; New York state legislator, CHD, B-11; town supervisor, CHD, B-5; judges and justices of the peace, CHD, A-38, A-50, B-64; a physician, CHD, B-5; clergymen and deacons, CHD, A-77, A-39, A-44; wealthy farmer, CHD, A-7; magazine editor CHD, A-20.

42. CBD and EBM, "Huntington's Chorea in Relation to Heredity and Eugenics," *AJI* 73 (October

1916), 211; Estella Hughes, "Social Significance of Huntington's Chorea," *American Journal of Psychiatry* 4 (1925), 566; Paul Popenoe and Kate Brousseau, "Huntington's Chorea," *Journal of Heredity* 22 (March 1930), 117. I am grateful to Lynn Sacco for calling my attention to this article.

43. "Vassar graduates," CHD, A-43; "ignorant laborer," CHD, B-107.
44. CHD, "Submerged class," B-71; "ignorant laborer," B-107; "fine personality," A-72; "writes poetry," B-85.
45. E. J. Melville, "Some Remarks on Huntington's Chorea; with Genealogical and Case Histories of a Family of Choreics," *Annals of Medicine* (N.Y.) 9 (1914), 418–24.
46. CBD and EBM, "Huntington's Chorea," 211; Hughes, "Social Significance," 538–39, 566; Popenoe and Brousseau, "Huntington's Chorea," 117. See also T. Edward Reed, Joseph H. Chandler, Estella M. Hughes, and Ruth T. Davidson, "Huntington's Chorea in Michigan: Demography and Genetics," *American Journal of Human Genetics* 10 (1958), 215.
47. George W. Bruyn, "Huntington's Chorea: Historical, Clinical, and Laboratory Synopsis," in P. J. Vinken and G. W. Bruyn, eds., *Handbook of Clinical Neurology*, vol. 6 (Amsterdam: North Holland Publishing, 1968), 304; Mary B. Hans and Thomas H. Gilmore, "Social Aspects of Huntington's Chorea," *American Journal of Psychiatry* 114 (1968), 97. See also Peter Harper and Michael Morris, "Introduction: A Historical Background," in Peter S. Harper, ed., *Huntington's Disease* (London: W. B. Saunders, 1991), 182; Rafter, *White Trash*, 12–17.
48. Cited in Popenoe and Brousseau, "Huntington's Chorea," 114. See Hughes, "Social Significance," 538. For numbers of patients in mental hospitals see Abraham Myerson et al., *Eugenical Sterilization: A Reorientation of the Problem* (New York: Macmillan, 1936), 24; Theodore Diller, "Chorea in the Adult as Seen among the Insane," *American Journal of the Medical Sciences* 99 (April 1890), 348. A 1919 survey suggested 1.1 cases per thousand first hospital admissions, while other estimates indicate 2.3 per thousand. The state hospital at Kalamazoo, Michigan, took in 46 patients with a diagnosis of Huntington's chorea out of a total of nearly 20,000 patients admitted from the time it opened, in 1859, to 1925; a second state hospital in Michigan admitted 5 Huntington's cases out of a total 4,310 between 1895 and 1923, while a third admitted 16 Huntington's cases out of 7,113 between 1903 and 1923. See Hughes, "Social Significance," 538–39. Reed and Chandler reported that 23.5 percent of persons with Huntington's in Michigan (47 out of 200) were in mental institutions on April 1, 1940. See Reed et al., "Huntington's Chorea in Michigan," 204. These figures probably represent a small proportion of the total number of those affected: the 46 patients of the Kalamazoo hospital had some 209 relatives with Huntington's (or probable Huntington's).
49. CHD, "none of the Crabbes," A-61; "the most intelligent member," A-18. In response to a 1911 query from ERO superintendent Harry Laughlin regarding patients with Huntington's chorea in sanitariums, the director of a private sanitarium in Stamford, Connecticut—home to many affected families—replied that "we have no cases of Huntington's Chorea in our institution." It was his experience that "most of these cases are treated at home and seldom sent to private sanitariums." F. H. Barnes to H. H. Laughlin, April 22, 1911, ERO, series 1, box 39, A:3181.
50. CHD, B-24; "Sagg Cemetery," typescript 131, PLIC-EHL. The Sagaponack cemetery has the gravestones of this family.
51. CHD, B-77.
52. Emily Abel, *Hearts of Wisdom: American Women Caring for Kin, 1850–1940* (Cambridge: Harvard University Press, 2000), 37, 60, 263.

53. See Harry Laughlin, "Eugenics Record Office Report #1," Cold Spring Harbor, June, 1913, 30; for Elinor Knapp and Ann Millington see CHD, B-98, B-97.
54. See, for instance, *Sag Harbor Express*, December 22, 1910; January 18, April 25, September 19, 1912; March 27, May 1, June 27, 1913; *East Hampton Star*, June 27, 1913.
55. See Abel, *Hearts of Wisdom*, passim; also Linda Gordon, *Heroes of Their Own Lives: The Politics and History of Family Violence* (New York: Penguin, 1988), 59–81. In her excellent study of eugenics in Vermont, Nancy L. Gallagher argues that "the simple fact that Harriet Abbott or other social workers appeared in town asking questions about the character, problems, and reputation of the family would have fueled prejudice, validated suspicions, and amplified neighbors' 'selective noticing' of the problems of the broken family." See Gallagher, *Breeding Better Vermonters: The Eugenics Project in the Green Mountain State* (Hanover, N.H.: University Press of New England, 1999), 126.
56. Bix, "Eugenics Field Workers," 651; CBD to "Gentlemen," February 16, 1918; CBD to Muncey, September 14, 1920, Davenport papers, series IIb, no. 2. Despite her dissatisfactions, Muncey remained on the payroll of the Eugenics Record Office for more than a decade, carrying out several different studies and ultimately acting as curator of the ERO archives. See *Eugenical News*, 1916–20, passim.
57. EBM to CBD, September 28, 1920, Davenport papers; Harry H. Laughlin, *Report* no. 1 (Cold Spring Harbor, N.Y.; ERO, 1913), 29–31.
58. Peter S. Harper, "Huntington's Disease: A Historical Background," in Gillian Bates, Peter S. Harper, and Lesley Jones, eds., *Huntington's Disease*, 3rd ed. (Oxford: Oxford University Press, 2002), 17; Ntinos C. Myrianthopoulos, "Huntington's Chorea," *Journal of Medical Genetics* 3 (1966), 306, 298. Garland Allen has noted that "most of the data collected [at the ERO] were of a subjective impressionistic nature," and thus impossible to verify. Allen cites Sheldon Reed's estimate that "most of the data collected by the ERO are worthless from a genetic point of view"; Allen, "Eugenics Record Office," 243.
59. Elizabeth B. Muncey, *Classical Huntington's Disease (Huntington's Chorea) Families*, ed. Sheldon C. Reed (1913; Minneapolis: Dight Institute for Human Genetics, University of Minnesota, 1964), inside cover. The Muncey manuscript was ultimately transferred to the library of the American Philosophical Society in Philadelphia. The Papers of Smith Ely Jelliffe at the Manuscript Division, Library of Congress, in Washington, D.C., contain an additional copy.

6. MYTHS OF ORIGINS AND ENDINGS

1. CBD and EBM, "Huntington's Chorea in Relation to Heredity and Eugenics," *AJI* 73 (October 1916), 195–222. On the use of this study to legitimize Mendelian studies of behavior, see Philip R. Reilly, *The Surgical Solution: A History of Involuntary Sterilization in the United States* (Baltimore: Johns Hopkins University Press, 1991), 111. CHD, A-72. On references to the number 962, see Abraham Myerson et al., *Eugenical Sterilization: A Reorientation of the Problem* (New York: Macmillan, 1936), 145; Charles S. Stone, "Huntington's Chorea: A Sociological and Genealogical Study," *Mental Hygiene* 15 (1931), 352; Theodore T. Stone and Eugene I. Falstein, "Genealogical Studies in Huntington's Chorea," *JNMD* 89 (June 1939), 797–98; Simon Stone, "Chronic Progressive Chorea," *New England Journal of Medicine* 207 (December 1, 1932), 975; Eugene I. Falstein and Theodore T. Stone, "Huntington's Chorea as a Psychiatric and Social Problem in

Illinois," *Illinois Medical Journal* 75 (February 1939), 164; J. V. Neel, "The Detection of the Genetic Carriers of Hereditary Disease," *American Journal of Human Genetics* 1 (1948), 26; Ntinos Myrianthopoulos, "Huntington's Chorea," *Journal of Medical Genetics* 3 (1966), 298. As late as 1972 John S. Pearson, a Kansas clinician, praised Davenport and Muncey's eugenic approach, noting that they had "proposed eloquently that somebody ought to do something." Twenty years later, Peter Harper cited the tensions inherent in Davenport's argument between public health aims of preventing disease and genetic counseling that respects individual autonomy, noting that Davenport's advocacy of sterilization "foreshadows later developments in Germany." See John S. Pearson, "Behavioral Aspects of Huntington's Chorea," in Andre Barbeau, Thomas N. Chase, and George W. Paulson, eds., *Advances in Neurology*, vol. 1, *Huntington's Chorea, 1872–1972* (New York: Raven, 1973), 701; also Peter Harper, "Huntington Disease and the Abuse of Genetics," *American Journal of Human Genetics* 50 (1992), 460–64. Kenneth Ludmerer cites the 1916 paper in *Genetics and American Society: A Historical Appraisal* (Baltimore: Johns Hopkins University Press, 1972), 62. See also Jon Beckwith, "On the Social Responsibility of Scientists," *Annali dell'Istituto Superiore di Sanita* 37 (2000), 189–94.

2. See preliminary versions of this paper: CBD, "Some Practical Lessons for Neurologists Drawn from Recent Eugenic Studies," *JNMD* 39 (1912), 402–5; SEJ, EBM, and CBD, "Huntington's Chorea: A Study in Heredity," *JNMD* 40 (1913): 796–99; CBD, "Huntington's Chorea in Relation to Heredity and Eugenics," *Proceedings of the National Academy of Sciences of the United States of America* 1 (May 15, 1915), 283–85; CBD, "Inheritance of Huntington's Chorea," *Science* 41 (1915), 570–71. See also CBD, "Huntington's Chorea in Relation to Heredity and Eugenics," *Bulletin* 17 (Cold Spring Harbor, N.Y.: Eugenics Record Office, 1916).
3. CBD and EBM, "Huntington's Chorea," 202–4; see also Myrianthopoulos, "Huntington's Chorea," 302–4.
4. CBD and EBM, "Huntington's Chorea," 202–4. That the phenomenon of anticipation in transmission of Huntington's from fathers to sons did exist was demonstrated in the late 1980s. See Gillian Bates, Peter S. Harper, and Lesley Jones, eds., *Huntington's Disease*, 3rd ed. (Oxford: Oxford University Press, 2002), 130.
5. CBD and EBM, "Huntington's Chorea," 200; Florence Danielson and CBD, "The Hill Folk: Report on a Rural Community of Hereditary Defectives," in Nicole Hahn Rafter, ed., *White Trash: The Eugenic Family Studies, 1877–1919* (Boston: Northeastern University Press, 1988), 82, 92, 128. Davenport wrote of the Hill folk that "the method of inheritance of feeblemindedness shows that it cannot be considered a unit character. It is evidently a complex of quantitatively and qualitatively varying factors." "Large number of early deaths," B-76; "limited extent," B-82; "lack of mental balance," B-85.
6. CBD and EBM, "Huntington's Chorea," 198–210, 219; CBD, "Inheritance," 284.
7. On biotypes see William Johannsen, "Does Hybridisation Increase Fluctuating Variability?" in *Report of the Third International Conference on Genetics 1906* (London: Spottiswoode, 1906), 98, 111. In stressing "to a certain degree, [the] accidental association of the diagnostic traits" in Huntington's chorea, Davenport also applied to Huntington's chorea Jelliffe's reasoning regarding insanity, namely, "that a great error is made in speaking of insanity as an entity, and I feel when you do it it is 'spiritual wickedness in high places.'" Jelliffe argued, "Hereditary studies will be of immense service in hunting out the defective parts of the mechanisms, but I fear it will only be so when it searches for these in the detail of the conglomerate—rather than in the comparisons

of the conglomerates themselves." See SEJ to CBD, December 26, December 28, 1910, Davenport papers, CBD and EBM, "Huntington's Chorea," *AJI* (1916), 196–97, 200. Myrianthopoulos, "Huntington's Chorea," 302–4, rejected Davenport's biotype theory.

8. CBD and EBM, "Huntington's Chorea," *AJI*, 202–4; see also Myrianthopoulos, "Huntington's Chorea," 302–4.
9. See EBM, "Complete Summary," ERO, series 7, fieldworker files, box 1, 15-731; CBD and EBM, "Huntington's Chorea," 210.
10. CBD and EBM, "Huntington's Chorea," 210.
11. CBD, "Huntington's Chorea" (1915), 284; GH, "On Chorea," *Medical and Surgical Reporter* (1872), 320–21; Clarence King had emphasized the "close relationship between hereditary chorea and other diseases of the nervous centres, notably epilepsy and insanity" (an observation he attributed to his East Hampton–born father). See Clarence King, "A Third Case of Hereditary Chorea," *Medical News* 55 (July 13, 1889), 41; Wharton Sinkler, "Two Additional Cases of Hereditary Chorea," *JNMD* 14 (February 1889), 285; see also C. M. Hay, "Hereditary Chorea, with a Contribution of Eight Additional Cases of the Disease," *University Medical Magazine* 2 (June 1890), 464. Hay wrote, "When actual insanity is absent from the family history, 'eccentricity' and 'nervousness' are commonly ascertained to exist." Even Joseph H. Chandler, T. Edward Reed, and Russell N. DeJong, in one of the most careful studies in 1960, repeated the claim that "it has long been apparent to clinicians and investigators of Huntington's chorea that mental deficiency, convulsive disorders, alcoholism, abnormalities of behavior, suicide, criminal tendencies, and 'insanity' occur commonly in families of patients with this disease." These authors cite Estella Hughes's study of 1925, which in fact claimed precisely the opposite. See Joseph H. Chandler, T. Edward Reed, and Russell N. DeJong, "Huntington's Chorea in Michigan: III. Clinical Observations," *Neurology* 10 (1960), 151; Hughes, "Social Significance of Huntington's Chorea," *American Journal of Psychiatry* 4 (1925), 562–63.
12. Arthur Hamilton, "A Report of Twenty-Seven Cases of Chronic Progressive Chorea," *AHI* 64 (January 1908), 459; Nicholas Dynan, "The Physical and Mental States in Chronic Chorea," *AJI* (January 1914), 632–34.
13. See Julia Bell, "Huntington's Chorea," in *The Treasury of Human Inheritance*, vol. 4, *Nervous Diseases and Muscular Dystrophies*, ed. R. A. Fisher and L. S. Penrose (1934; Cambridge: Cambridge University Press, 1948), 18; Myerson et al., *Eugenical Sterilization*, 145: "To us, however, this represents a not unusual or significant distribution of those diseases in a population." See also Pearson, "Behavioral Aspects," 707: "I have repeatedly been impressed by the low incidence of the major psychoses (schizophrenia and manic-depressive psychoses) among the non-choreic individuals."
14. Gail Bederman, *Manliness and Civilization: A Cultural History of Gender and Race in the United States, 1880–1917* (Chicago: University of Chicago Press, 1995), 11–13, 25, 285. As the cultural critic Sander Gilman has argued, negative portrayals of the ill project deep cultural anxieties onto the Other, turning fears of loss of control and personal disintegration into stereotype and stigma. "The construction of the image of the patient," he writes, "is thus always a playing out of this desire for a demarcation between ourselves and the chaos represented in culture by disease." See Sander Gilman, *Disease and Representation: Images of Illness from Madness to AIDS* (Ithaca: Cornell University Press, 1988), 2–4; also Rosemarie Garland Thomson, *Extraordinary Bodies: Figuring Physical Disability in American Culture and Literature* (New York: Columbia University Press, 1997).

15. Diane B. Paul, *Controlling Human Heredity, 1865 to the Present* (Amherst, N.Y.: Humanity Books, 1998), 44, 62.
16. See CHD, 1–3; CBD, *Heredity in Relation to Eugenics* (New York: Henry Holt, 1911), 181–82. See Rafter, *White Trash*, 2. Muncey named specific families that were dying out, in some cases describing the reasons for their demise. In one family that was "practically extinct," she wrote in her field notes, "chorea seemed to be of such a severe form that it developed rapidly and wore out the patient, or it affected the brain centers so that there were many deaths from convulsions or hydrocephalus in infancy" (CHD, A-10). Although she did no statistical calculations—she left that to Davenport—Muncey's field notes showed a number of families on the brink of extinction: "By the death of Lemuel, the descendants in the male line . . . became extinct" (CHD, A-48); "his choreic children are all dead. The family is dying out" (CHD, B-72); "they all died unmarried" (CHD, B-24).
17. For Davenport's calculations of the percentages of unmarried individuals in each of the three main families included in the Muncey pedigree, see CBD and EBM, "Huntington's Chorea," 213.
18. See Hughes, "Social Significance," 544. For comparisons between the Michigan population in 1940 and members of affected families, with and without Huntington's disease, see T. Edward Reed and Joseph H. Chandler, "Huntington's Chorea in Michigan: I. Demography and Genetics," *American Journal of Human Genetics* 10 (June 1958), 201–24. On marriage rates of white women generally in the nineteenth century see Linda Gordon, *Woman's Body, Woman's Right: A Social History of Birth Control* (New York: Penguin, 1976), 48–49. On the absence of marriage discrimination see Susan E. Folstein, *Huntington's Disease: A Disorder of Families* (Baltimore: Johns Hopkins University Press, 1989), 117: "In general experience suggests that social stigma does not have much impact on reproduction in HD families." Audrey Tyler writes from the U.K. in 1991, "There has never been any evidence presented to the authors that at-risk persons were, or are, discriminated against in their choice of marriage partners." See Tyler, "Social and Psychological Aspects of Huntington's Disease," in Peter Harper, ed., *Huntington's Disease* (London: W. B. Saunders, 1991), 186.
19. Wharton Sinkler, "Two Additional Cases of Hereditary Chorea," *JNMD* 14 (February 1889), 89; Clarence A. Good, "A Review of Chronic Progressive Chorea (Huntington's), with Report of a Case," *AJI* 57 (July 1900), 28, reports that "many of the women are especially prolific," though he offers no evidence for this claim. See also Rafter, *White Trash*, 2; Margaret Marsh and Wanda Ronner, *The Empty Cradle: Infertility in America from Colonial Times to the Present* (Baltimore: Johns Hopkins University Press, 1996), 122; Gordon, *Woman's Body, Woman's Right*, 48–49. Hughes, "Social Significance," 543–44.
20. See also CHD, 1–3; CBD and EBM, "Huntington's Chorea," 220–21.
21. See Stone, "Chronic Progressive Chorea," 981; Bell, "Huntington's Chorea," 4: 17: "Individuals of both sexes have been noted to have very large families."
22. S. C. Reed and J. D. Palm, "Social Fitness versus Reproductive Fitness," *Science* 113 (March 16, 1951), 294–96.
23. T. Edward Reed and James V. Neel, "Huntington's Chorea in Michigan II: Selection and Mutation," *American Journal of Human Genetics* 11 (June 1959), 124, 134.
24. John Terry Maltsberger, "Even unto the Twelfth Generation: Huntington's Chorea," *Journal of the History of Medicine and Allied Sciences* 16 (1961), 13; MacDonald Critchley, "Hunting-

ton's Chorea: Historical and Geographical Considerations," in *The Black Hole and Other Essays* (London: Pitman Medical, 1964), 219; Pearson, "Behavioral Aspects," 711; Myrianthopoulos, "Huntington's Chorea," 306; see also Hughes, "Social Significance," 544–45. See Reed and Neel, "Huntington's Chorea in Michigan," 107–36. Reed and Neel noted that if the fertility of those with Huntington's were higher than that of persons without it, "it would be a rare—not to say unique—situation in human genetics: individuals affected with a severely debilitating disease whose onset is often during the reproductive period nevertheless actually achieving a greater-than-normal fertility." If this were the case, the authors add, "it then becomes necessary to explain why Huntington's chorea is a rare disease today" (107). Although some credible studies in the 1970s and 1980s argued that women with Huntington's did have slightly more children than white women from unaffected families, by the 1990s geneticists generally concluded that reproductive rates within families with Huntington's were close to those of the general population, with little robust evidence for any meaningful difference. See Harper, *Huntington's Disease*, 295; Bates, Harper, and Jones, *Huntington's Disease*, 183–86.

25. CBD and EBM, "Huntington's Chorea," 215.
26. Ibid.
27. SEJ, EBM, and CBD, "Huntington's Chorea," 798; CBD and EBM, "Huntington's Chorea," 211.
28. Referring to the "admixture of good and primarily bad work in the field" of eugenics, Kenneth Ludmerer cites Davenport's study of Huntington's chorea as an example of a paper "still quoted today" that stood apart from other papers "which are now in disrepute." See Ludmerer, *Genetics and American Society*, 62. See also Charles E. Rosenberg, "Charles Benedict Davenport and the Beginning of American Genetics," *Bulletin of the History of Medicine* 35 (1961), 270; Daniel J. Kevles, *In the Name of Eugenics: Genetics and the Uses of Human Heredity* (Berkeley: University of California Press, 1985), 48, 67; Reilly, *Surgical Solution*, 111.
29. See, for example, Stone, "Chronic Progressive Chorea," 975; Falstein and Stone, "Huntington's Chorea," 164; James V. Neel, "The Detection of Genetic Carriers of Hereditary Disease," *American Journal of Human Genetics* 1 (September 1949), 26; John S. Pearson, et al., "An Educational Approach to the Social Problem of Huntington's Chorea," *Proceedings of the Staff Meetings of the Mayo Clinic* 30 (August 10, 1955), 349; Myrianthopoulos, "Huntington's Chorea" (1966), 298; Russell N. DeJong, "The History of Huntington's Chorea in the United States of America," in Barbeau, Chase, and Paulson, *Advances in Neurology*, 1: 25. As we have seen, hospital statistics did not appear to support Davenport's claim of a mounting Huntington's chorea crisis.
30. See Janet Farrell Brodie, *Contraception and Abortion in Nineteenth-Century America* (Ithaca: Cornell University Press, 1994), 2, 255. While the average number of children born to white women in 1800 was around 7.04, that number had dropped a century later to 3.56, a 49 percent decline. On sterilization see Reilly, *Surgical Solution*, 87, 98; Gordon, *Woman's Body, Woman's Right*, 259–60.
31. Hughes, "Social Significance," 573. See also C. R. McKinniss, "The Value of Eugenics in Huntington's Chorea," *Medical Record* 86 (July 18, 1914), 106: "We can not emphasize the danger too much, and should advise always against marriage of these individuals"; Stone, "Huntington's Chorea," 363: "There is no doubt that the facts here presented would be considered by many as positive evidence in favor of legalization of birth control and sterilization of mental defectives"; Stone, "Chronic Progressive Chorea," 983: "Suggestions of birth control or restraint from having children, whenever possible, should be made to the unaffected members of families who wish to

marry and are in danger of developing the disease in later life." Simon Stone also recommended that patients in state hospitals for the insane be sterilized as a condition of their release. Stone and Falstein, "Genealogical Studies in Huntington's Chorea," 809: "Prospects of its eradication appear to be remote without adequate legislative measures of the type exemplified by legalized sterilization."

32. See G. W. Bruyn, F. Baro, and N. C. Myrianthopoulos, *A Centennial Bibliography of Huntington's Chorea, 1872–1972* (Louvain: Leuven University Press, 1973).

33. See Ludmerer, *Genetics and American Society*, 66. In Germany in the 1920s, as the "race hygiene" movement grew, interest in Huntington's chorea increased, possibly due to the influence of such longtime researchers as J. L. Entres and especially Friedrich Panse, a psychiatrist who testified as an "expert" identifying mental patients to be murdered under the Third Reich. See Benno Muller-Hill, *Murderous Science: Elimination by Scientific Selection of Jews, Gypsies, and Others in Germany, 1933–1945* (Cold Spring Harbor, N.Y.: Cold Spring Harbor Laboratory Press, 1988), 44, 47, 90.

34. Although Vessie later said he had graduated from the Cleveland-Pulte Medical College, that college did not come into existence until 1910, when Cleveland Homeopathic merged with the Pulte Medical College in Cincinnati. On homeopathy see Paul Starr, *The Social Transformation of American Medicine* (New York: Basic, 1982), 96–108. Vessie appears in directories of the American Medical Association starting in 1914.

35. Vessie became a member of the American Psychiatric Association in 1925, but he evidently never joined the American Neurological Association, although he was listed in the AMA Directory as a specialist in neurology and psychiatry. See Nils Kerschus, "Blythewood," ms., GHS; see also Vessie to SEJ, April 21, August 22, 1933, Jelliffe papers, LC; on Vessie's efforts to write a novel about Huntington's in colonial New England see SEJ to Vessie, December 5, 1935, January 21, January 23, 1936; Vessie to SEJ, December 7, 1935, January 22, 1936, Jelliffe papers, Manuscript Division, LC.

36. Davenport had had a slightly different interpretation; it was understandable, he wrote, that at a time when many nervous disorders were attributed to witchcraft, ordinary people might think "that the choreic was bewitched or even capable of bewitching others, especially her own children!" CBD and EBM, "Huntington's Chorea," 202. See Percy R. Vessie, "On the Transmission of Huntington's Chorea for Three Hundred Years: The Bures Family Group," *JNMD* 76 (December 1932), 553–73; Mary B. Hans and Thomas H. Gilmore, "Huntington's Chorea and Genealogical Credibility," *JNMD* 148 (1969), 5–6. Vessie rehearsed his 1932 paper in a second article, "Hereditary Chorea: St. Anthony's Dance and Witchcraft in Colonial Connecticut," *Journal of the Connecticut State Medical Society* 3 (1939), 596–600. The English medical authors Adrian Caro and Sheila Haines called Vessie's 1932 paper one of "the two most quoted classics" in the literature on Huntington's (the other being MacDonald Critchley's 1934 paper, as we shall see). See Caro and Haines, "Medical History: The History of Huntington's Chorea," *Update* (1975), 91–95.

37. Vessie to SEJ, November 2, 1931, April 25, 1932; SEJ to Vessie, November 4, 1931, April 25, 1932, Jelliffe papers, LC. Vessie, "On the Transmission of Huntington's Chorea," 562–63, 557, 573. Although Muncey incorrectly makes Elizabeth Knapp the granddaughter of Elinor and Nicholas, Vessie accurately describes her as the granddaughter of William Knapp, who was probably unrelated to Nicholas.

38. Vessie, "On the Transmission of Huntington's Chorea," 556–59; see *The Public Records of the*

Colony of Connecticut, May 1665 (Hartford: Brown and Parsons, 1850), 44–45; also *Records of the Court of Assistants of the Colony of Massachusetts Bay, 1630–1692* (Boston: Suffolk County, 1904), 9–13, 26, 50–52, 68, 99, 107, 108, 136–37.

39. Vessie, "Hereditary Chorea," 596, 598; Vessie, "On the Transmission of Huntington's Chorea," 556, 573.
40. Vessie, "Hereditary Chorea," 596–600; Vessie, "On the Transmission of Huntington's Chorea" (1932), 556, 573. "Sorrowful march of victims" comes straight out of John M. Taylor, *The Witchcraft Delusion in Colonial Connecticut, 1647–1697* (New York: Grafton, 1908), 37.
41. Vessie, "On the Transmission of Huntington's Chorea," 556; "Hereditary Chorea," 600.
42. "Huntington's Chorea," *Lancet* 221 (April 22, 1933), 869; "The Witchcraft Disease," *Literary Digest*, May 27, 1933, 27–28.
43. MacDonald Critchley, "Huntington's Chorea and East Anglia," *Journal of State Medicine* 42 (October 1934), 587; Critchley, "Huntington's Chorea: Historical and Geographical Considerations," 210–19; also MacDonald Critchley, "The History of Huntington's Chorea," *Psychological Medicine* 14 (1984), 725–27; and MacDonald Critchley, "Great Britain and the Early History of Huntington's Chorea," in Barbeau, Chase, and Paulson, *Advances in Neurology*, 1: 13–17; also Maltsberger, "Even unto the Twelfth Generation," 1–17; Myrianthopoulos, "Huntington's Chorea," 299; Eric R. Kandel and James H. Schwartz, *Principles of Neural Science*, 2nd ed. (New York: Elsevier, 1985), 532.
44. See Bell, "Huntington's Chorea," 17–18; James V. Neel, "Detection of Genetic Carriers," *American Journal of Human Genetics* 1 (September 1949), 26. Although his version was the one most often cited, Vessie was not the first writer to portray families with Huntington's in a highly negative way. A 1927 Vermont eugenics study focused on the "Pirate" family, the "Gypsy" family, and the "Chorea" family as exemplars of "undesirable citizens" and "degeneracy." See Nancy Gallagher, *Breeding Better Vermonters: The Eugenics Project in the Green Mountain State* (Hanover, N.H.: University Press of New England, 1999), 82–83. See also Henry F. Perkins, *The First Annual Report of a Eugenics Survey of Vermont* (Burlington: University of Vermont, 1927), 9. Like Muncey, Perkins thought the disease was dying out and the family becoming smaller, "partly due to the debilitating factor that goes along with the disease."
45. Steven Selden, *Inheriting Shame: The Story of Eugenics and Racism in America* (New York: Teachers College Press, Columbia University, 1999), 69; Alan R. Rushton, *Genetics and Medicine in the United States, 1800–1922* (Baltimore: Johns Hopkins University Press, 1994), 125; Alexandra Minna Stern, *Eugenic Nation: Faults and Frontiers of Better Breeding in Modern America* (Berkeley: University of California Press, 2005), 149.
46. Hans and Gilmore, "Huntington's Chorea and Genealogical Credibility," 5–13; on Goodwife Knapp see Taylor, *Witchcraft Delusion*, 122–41; Elizabeth Schenck, *The History of Fairfield County, Connecticut* (New York: self-published, 1889), 324–93; Charles J. Hoadley, *New Haven Records of the Colony or Jurisdiction of New Haven Colony* (Hartford: Case, Lockwood, 1858), 2: 77–89. Contrary to Vessie's claims, there is no extant transcript of the trial of Goodwife Knapp; all information comes from a subsequent trial in which both plaintiffs and defendants recalled Goodwife Knapp. Although Vessie cited primary sources, he did not reconcile his account of Goodwife Knapp's execution in 1653 with the *Records of the Colony or Jurisdiction of New Haven*, 2: 80–84, nor did he check the account of Elinor Knapp's death in 1658 in Stamford, recorded in James

Savage, *A Genealogical Dictionary of the First Settlers of New England* (1860–62; rpt. Baltimore: Genealogical Publishing, 1969), 2: 34. Vessie also omits mention of a classic 1911 history of Greenwich, which included genealogies of Jeffrey Ferris and of Elinor and Nicholas Knapp that make clear Muncey's error about Elinor. See Spencer P. Mead, *Ye Historie of Ye Town of Greenwich* (New York: Knickerbocker, 1911), 536–45, 595–607.

47. In late 1671 the sixteen-year-old Elizabeth, a servant in the house of a prominent minister, suddenly began to suffer a series of strange symptoms diagnosed at the time as possession. What impressed Vessie as evidence of Huntington's chorea were her intermittent "fits" in which she was "violent in bodily motions, leapings, strainings and strange agitations . . . violent also in roarings and screamings, representing a dark resemblance of hellish torments." At times also "her tongue was for many hours together drawn into a semicircle up to the roof of her mouth and not to be removed." Elizabeth Knapp also had periods of "intermission," however, during which she was quiet, self-accusatory, and responsive. This episode was well documented by the minister in whose house she resided, Samuel Willard, and also by the historian of witchcraft John Demos. Her symptoms do not sound like Huntington's chorea, nor was there any indication, either at the time of her possession or later, that townspeople equated her behavior with St. Vitus's dance. Although Muncey described Elizabeth Knapp as the granddaughter of Elinor, in fact she was the granddaughter of William Knapp or Knopp, as Vessie had indicated. See Samuel Willard, "A briefe account of a strange & unusuall Providence of God befallen to Elizabeth Knap of Groton," http://history.hanover.edu/texts/groton/grointro.html; Carol F. Carlson, *The Devil in the Shape of a Woman: Witchcraft in Colonial New England* (New York: Norton, 1987), 236–41; John F. Demos, *Entertaining Satan: Witchcraft and the Culture of Early New England* (New York: Oxford University Press, 1982), 97–131; Hans and Gilmore, "Huntington's Chorea and Genealogical Credibility," 12.

48. Adrian Caro, "A Genetic Problem in East Anglia," Ph.D. diss., University of East Anglia, Norwich, 1977; Caro and Haines, "History of Huntington's Chorea," 91–95.

49. According to Demos, "Numerous and varied forms of evidence suggest that insanity was recognized, understood, accepted—without reference to supernatural cause—whenever and wherever it might appear." Demos also notes that "there are no signs whatsoever" of mental illness among those accused of witchcraft, "no incoherence of speech, no extreme irregularities of behavior, no very substantial disorder of thought or feeling." See *Entertaining Satan*, 90–91. For an example of the earlier view see Albert Deutsch, *The Mentally Ill in America* (New York: Columbia University Press, 1946).

50. Michael MacDonald, *Mystical Bedlam: Madness, Anxiety, and Healing in Seventeenth-Century England* (Cambridge: Cambridge University Press, 1981), 209; William Buchan, *Domestic Medicine*, 2nd ed. (London: W. Strahan, 1772), 551–52.

51. Vessie, "On the Transmission of Huntington's Chorea," 553–71; Vessie, "Hereditary Chorea," 596–600.

52. It is unclear how much Vessie as well as Hans and Gilmore may have relied on Muncey and merely copied her genealogy although they all claimed to have secured information from their patients. In any case, Vessie's three couples and their immediate descendants appear to have been typical, and in one case prominent, early New England settlers. William Knapp or Knopp (1580/81–1658), a carpenter, was the eldest among Vessie's three male emigrants, about fifty-one when he arrived

in America in 1630. Although Vessie portrays Knopp as the most disreputable of the three men ("from the beginning he and his sons were notorious principals in unsavory colonial history"), his legal infractions (swearing, making speeches against the governor, and selling beer without a license) could be considered social or political rebellion, and in any event they were minor. His wife's license to operate a "house of entertainment" (tavern) was entirely legitimate and certainly not "public prostitution" as Vessie claimed. According to later sources, Knopp died with a modest estate of £129, including a house and lands. Although he may have been non compos mentis at the end of his life, at his death he was old, "about eighty." One son was evidently involved in several thefts. But another son, James Knapp (the father of Elizabeth Knapp), after going through a period of drinking and an episode of adultery, became prominent in public affairs in Groton. There were no close descendants with Huntington's chorea that we know of. On William Knopp see Robert Charles Anderson, *The Great Migration Begins: Immigrants to New England, 1620–1633* (Boston: New England Historic Genealogical Society, 1995), 2: 1143–45. See also Demos, *Entertaining Satan*, 111–12. For historical records see *Records of the Court of Assistants of the Colony of Massachusetts Bay, 1630–1692* (Boston: Suffolk County, 1904), 9–13, 26, 50–52, 68, 99, 107, 108, 136–37. William Knopp remained in Massachusetts and evidently had no genealogical relationship to the other two families in Vessie's Connecticut pedigree.

Vessie described Nicholas Knapp (ca. 1606–70) as William's younger brother, but this relationship is unconfirmed. While William remained in Boston, Nicholas, a weaver, moved to Stamford, where he became the owner of extensive lands, although he was not a church member and therefore could not hold local office. For Vessie, Nicholas's main offense was selling medicine for scurvy "of no worth nor value," for which he was fined, although part of the payment was remitted in a general amnesty. After Elinor died in 1658, Nicholas married again. At his death in 1670, when he was about sixty-four, he left a modest estate of £166. On Nicholas Knapp, see Anderson, *The Great Migration Begins*, 2: 1135–37; also *Public Records of the Colony of Connecticut*, 44–45.

Jeffrey Ferris (ca. 1610–60), evidently the wealthiest of the three men, emigrated from England (from Leicestershire, according to family tradition, not Bures, as Vessie claimed) to Watertown, in the Massachusetts Bay colony, sometime around 1634. Later he and his wife were among the founders of Stamford and Greenwich, Connecticut, where Jeffrey was a proprietor and a significant landowner, and was active in town affairs. Jeffrey's wrongdoings in Vessie's eyes consisted mainly of various actions as a jury member, where he rendered "harsh verdicts on his fellows," such as ordering a young man guilty of impregnating a young woman to be publicly whipped, have the letter R burned on his cheek, and then marry the woman. Jeffrey Ferris was also fined for questioning the impartiality of a jury that had fined him for failing to maintain his fences. Vessie claimed that Jeffrey's first wife was a woman "to whom his family objected," although he did not explain why. After this wife died, Jeffrey married twice more, assuming financial responsibility for the children of his second wife, who had also died before him. At his death in 1666, he left a significant estate, about £493. One of Jeffrey's sons ran into serious trouble as a youth. In 1657 John Ferris was prosecuted for "bestialitie," as Vessie claimed. Although not uncommon, this was considered a major offense, punishable by execution in colonial New England. However, after being publicly whipped, fined, imprisoned, and forced to wear a halter around his neck for two years, John Ferris went on to live a long life in Westchester County, where he became a Quaker. At his death in 1715, at the age of seventy-five, he was a relatively wealthy man. Many descendants of Jeffrey Ferris in particular became prominent and highly respected; they were known as "one of the old historic families" in Connecticut and across the border in Westchester. For the most reliable information on Jeffrey Ferris see Anderson, *The Great Migration Begins*, 2: 517–21. On the "bestialitie" of John Ferris see Hoadley, *Records of the Colony or Jurisdiction of New Haven*, 2: 223–24, 293.

53. Vessie, "On the Transmission of Huntington's Chorea," 554, 573, 565. See CHD, B-98; Hans and Gilmore, "Huntington's Chorea and Genealogical Credibility" (1969), 12.
54. Critchley, "Great Britain and the Early History," 15; Critchley, "Huntington's Chorea: Historical and Geographical Considerations," 214; Ian McEwan, *Saturday* (New York: Doubleday, 2005); Nancy S. Wexler and Michael D. Rawlins, "Prejudice in a Portrayal of Huntington's Disease," *Lancet* 366 (September 24, 2005).
55. For the expansion of Vessie's original thesis see Kandel and Schwartz, *Principles of Neural Science*, 532; Stanley M. Aronson, "Witchcraft Was Not Sorcery but a Too Human Disease," *Providence Journal*, July 22, 2002. *Report: Commission for the Control of Huntington's Disease and Its Consequences* (Washington, D.C.: National Institutes of Health; Department of Health, Education, and Welfare; and Public Health Service, 1977), DHEW pub. no. (NIH) 78-1051; vol. 5, "Public Testimony" (New York), 336. (Hereafter cited as Commission *Report*.)
56. Quotation from Nancy Leys Stepan, *"The Hour of Eugenics": Race, Gender, and Nation in Latin America* (Ithaca: Cornell University Press, 1991), 5; Paul, *Controlling Human Heredity*, 72–91.
57. Robert Proctor, *Racial Hygiene: Medicine under the Nazis* (Cambridge: Harvard University Press, 1988), 94–111; Benno Müller-Hill, *Murderous Science: Elimination by Scientific Selection of Jews, Gypsies, and Others in Germany, 1933–1945* (Cold Spring Harbor, N.Y.: Cold Spring Harbor Laboratory Press, 1998), 35; Peter Harper, "Huntington Disease and the Abuse of Genetics," *American Journal of Human Genetics* 50 (1992), 460–64.
58. See Paul, *Controlling Human Heredity*, 128; Stern, *Eugenic Nation;* Reilly, *Surgical Solution*, 94; Selden, *Inheriting Shame*, 69. See also John Whittier, "Clinical Aspects of Huntington's Disease," in Andrew Barbeau and Jean-Real Brunette, eds., *Progress in Neuro-Genetics* (Amsterdam: Excerpta Medica Foundation, 1969), 640. Whittier notes that "from a questionnaire sent to several hundred gynecologists and urologists our unit [Creedmoor Institute, Queens, New York] learned that sterilizations have been performed for H.d. in the United States." He does not indicate the numbers. Marjorie Guthrie also testified that she had heard of children at risk for Huntington's in the United States who were sterilized. See Commission *Report*, vol. 4, part 3, 121. See also Myerson et al., *Eugenical Sterilization*, 40, 57, 179–83.
59. Myerson et al., *Eugenical Sterilization*, 40, 57, 179–83.
60. Ibid., 179–83. Other disorders for which the report recommended sterilization included Friedreich's ataxia, "feeblemindedness of familial type," schizophrenia, "manic-depressive psychosis," and epilepsy. See also Reilly, *Surgical Solution*, 123.
61. Pearson, "Behavioral Aspects," 711.
62. Stepan, *"Hour of Eugenics,"* 134. See Thomson, *Extraordinary Bodies*, 10: "From folktales and classical myths to modern and postmodern 'grotesques,' the disabled body is almost always a freakish spectacle, presented by the mediating narrative voice." See also Gilman, *Disease and Representation*, 4. See also Ernest G. Lion and Eugen Kahn, "Experiential Aspects of Huntington's Chorea," *American Journal of Psychiatry* 95 (November 1938), 724–25: "Our choreatics and their

parents tried to keep the hereditary taint in the family tree a secret. They all denied their illnesses were in any way alike or transmissible. They were selfish in their desire to marry and rather unconcerned as to the possibility of transmitting the hereditary taint."

63. For an overview see Commission *Report*, vol. 1. Unless otherwise specified, all subsequent references to the *Report* refer to vol. 4. I also cite unedited transcripts of Commission hearings and unedited testimony submitted to the Commission for the record.
64. Ibid., part 5 (New York), 325; part 3 (Chicago), 139; "Unedited Transcript" (Los Angeles), 37; part 5 (New York), 250.
65. Ibid., part 5 (New York), 251, 540; "Unedited Transcript" (Los Angeles), 35.
66. Ibid., part 5 (New York), 71; (New Orleans), 162–63, 398, 490.
67. Ibid., part 5 (New Orleans), 171, 63, 81; "Unedited Transcript" (Los Angeles), 5, 39.
68. John R. Whittier, "Management of Huntington's Chorea: The Disease, Those Affected, and Those Otherwise Involved," in Barbeau, Chase, and Paulson, *Advances in Neurology*, 1: 740; Paul, *Controlling Human Heredity*, 146–47; Myrianthopoulos, "Huntington's Chorea," 312.
69. *Report*, "Testimony Submitted for the Record" (Ann Arbor), 55, 91, 570; (Los Angeles), 108. See also Nancy S. Wexler, "Genetic 'Russian Roulette': The Experience of Being 'At-Risk' for Huntington's Disease," in Seymour Kessler, ed., *Genetic Counseling: Psychological Dimensions* (New York: Academic Press, 1979), 213. In this study, "approximately two-thirds of the subjects said, with varying degrees of conviction, that they would take a predictive test."
70. See David L. Stevens, "Test for Huntington's Chorea," *New England Journal of Medicine* 285 (August 12, 1971,) 413–14; also Steven Cedarbaum, "Test for Huntington's Chorea," *New England Journal of Medicine* 284 (May 6, 1971), 1045; *Report*, vol. 1, "Overview," 24–25.
71. *Report*, part 5 (Seattle), 592.
72. *Report*, part 5 (New York), 400; also "Unedited Transcript" (Boston), 141; part 5 (New York), 592; "Unedited Transcript" (Ann Arbor), 47, 49; "Unedited Transcript" (New York), 5–400.
73. "Unedited Transcript" (Ann Arbor), 158; part 5 (New York), 423, 248; (Seattle), 495, 519. See also Stern, *Eugenic Nation*, 3; Paul, *Controlling Human Heredity*, 125–29; Wendy Kline, *Building a Better Race: Gender, Sexuality, and the Turn of the Century to the Baby Boom* (Berkeley: University of California, 2001), 6. See also Mary B. Hans and Thomas H. Gilmore, "Social Aspects of Huntington's Chorea," *American Journal of Psychiatry* 114 (1968), 93–98.
74. *Report*, part 5 (Seattle), 457.
75. "Unedited Transcript" (Ann Arbor), 97; Paul Rabinow, "Artificiality and Enlightenment: From Sociobiology to Biosociality," in Jonathan Crary and Sanford Kwinter, eds., *Incorporations* (New York: Zone, 1992), 234–52; "Unedited Transcript" (Boston), 28.
76. See Jesse F. Ballenger, *Self, Senility, and Alzheimer's Disease in Modern America: A History* (Baltimore: Johns Hopkins University Press, 2006), 183–85; "Unedited Transcript" (Boston), 66; *Report*, part 5 (New York), 344; "Unedited Transcript" (Boston), 36; "Unedited Transcript" (Los Angeles), 34–36.
77. "Unedited Transcript" (Seattle), 458; *Report*, part 3 (Chicago), 49.
78. See James W. Trent Jr., *Inventing the Feeble Mind: A History of Mental Retardation in the United States* (Berkeley: University of California Press, 1994), 164; Paul, *Controlling Human Heredity*, 62; Charles E. Rosenberg, "The Bitter Fruit: Heredity, Disease, and Social Thought in Nineteenth-Century America," in Donald Fleming and Bernard Bailyn, eds., *Perspectives in American History*,

vol. 8 (Cambridge: Cambridge University Press, 1974), 217–23; Thomson, *Extraordinary Bodies*, 36–46.

79. Davenport published in *Science*, the *Proceedings of the National Academy of Science*, the *Journal of Nervous and Mental Disease*, and the *American Journal of Insanity*. Vessie published his first paper in the *Journal of Nervous and Mental Disease* and the second in the *Journal of the Connecticut Medical Society*. Critchley's papers appeared in the *British Journal of State Medicine* and in the 1973 *Advances in Neurology* dedicated to Huntington's, as well as in his own collection of essays, *The Black Hole and Other Essays*.

80. *Report*, part 5, 200; quotation from Stepan, "*The Hour of Eugenics*," 201.

81. On the persistence of eugenics see Paul, *Controlling Human Heredity*, Kline, *Building a Better Race*, and Stern, *Eugenic Nation*. The periodization proposed by these authors partly parallels that described by George Chauncey Jr. for the gay subculture of New York City. Chauncey argues that this world that flourished in the 1910s and 1920s was "forced into hiding in the 1930s, '40s, and '50s," and that "gay life was *less* tolerated, *less* visible to outsiders, and *more* rigidly segregated in the second third of the century than the first." See *Gay New York: Gender, Urban Culture, and the Making of the Gay Male World, 1890–1940* (New York: Basic, 1994). On family members redefining a predictive test see *Report*, vol. 1, "Overview," 24–25.

INDEX

Page numbers in **boldface** refer to illustrations.